Breast Cancer

Editor

HAROLD J. BURSTEIN

HEMATOLOGY/ONCOLOGY CLINICS OF NORTH AMERICA

www.hemonc.theclinics.com

Consulting Editors
GEORGE P. CANELLOS
H. FRANKLIN BUNN

August 2013 • Volume 27 • Number 4

ELSEVIER

1600 John F. Kennedy Boulevard • Suite 1800 • Philadelphia, Pennsylvania, 19103-2899

http://www.theclinics.com

HEMATOLOGY/ONCOLOGY CLINICS OF NORTH AMERICA Volume 27, Number 4
August, 2013 ISSN 0889-8588, ISBN 13: 978-0-323-18606-3

Editor: Patrick Manley
Developmental Editor: Donald Mumford

Hematology/Oncology Clinics (ISSN 0889-8588) is published bimonthly by Elsevier Inc., 360 Park Avenue South, New York, NY 10010-1710. Months of issue are February, April, June, August, October, and December. Business and Editorial Offices: 1600 John F. Kennedy Blvd., Ste. 1800, Philadelphia, PA 19103–2899. Customer Service Office: 3251 Riverport Lane, Maryland Heights, MO 63043. Periodicals postage paid at New York, NY and at additional mailing offices. Subscription prices are $367.00 per year (domestic individuals), $599.00 per year (domestic institutions), $179.00 per year (domestic students/residents), $417.00 per year (Canadian individuals), $732.00 per year (Canadian institutions) $496.00 per year (international individuals), $732.00 per year (international institutions), and $241.00 per year (international and Canadian students/residents). International air speed delivery is included in all *Clinics* subscription prices. All prices are subject to change without notice. **POSTMASTER:** Send address changes to *Hematology/Oncology Clinics of North America*, Elsevier Health Sciences Division, Subscription Customer Service, 3251 Riverport Lane, Maryland Heights, MO 63043. Customer Service (orders, claims, online, change of address): Elsevier Health Sciences Division, Subscription Customer Service, 3251 Riverport Lane, Maryland Heights, MO 63043. Tel: 1-800-654-2452 (U.S. and Canada); 314-447-8871 (outside U.S. and Canada). Fax: 314-447-8029. E-mail: journalscustomerservice-usa@elsevier.com (for print support); journalsonlinesupport-usa@elsevier.com (for online support).

Reprints. For copies of 100 or more, of articles in this publication, please contact the Commercial Reprints Department, Elsevier Inc., 360 Park Avenue South, New York, New York 10010-1710; Tel.: 212-633-3813, Fax: 212-462-1935, E-mail: reprints@elsevier.com.

Hematology/Oncology Clinics of North America is covered in *MEDLINE/PubMed (Index Medicus), EMBASE/ Excerpta Medica, and BIOSIS.*

Printed and bound by CPI Group (UK) Ltd, Croydon, CR0 4YY

Transferred to digital print 2012

Contributors

CONSULTING EDITORS

GEORGE P. CANELLOS, MD
William Rosenberg Professor of Medicine, Department of Medical Oncology, Dana-Farber Cancer Institute, Boston, Massachusetts

H. FRANKLIN BUNN, MD
Professor of Medicine, Division of Hematology, Brigham and Women's Hospital, Boston, Harvard Medical School, Massachusetts

EDITOR

HAROLD J. BURSTEIN, MD, PhD
Dana-Farber Cancer Institute, Brigham and Women's Hospital, Harvard Medical School, Boston, Massachusetts

AUTHORS

FARIN AMERSI, MD, FACS
Assistant Professor of Surgery, Associate Program Director General Surgery Residency, Division of Surgical Oncology, Department of Surgery, Cedars-Sinai Medical Center, Samuel Oschin Comprehensive Cancer Institute, Saul and Joyce Brandman Breast Center, Los Angeles, California

CAREY K. ANDERS, MD
Assistant Professor of Medicine, Division of Hematology-Oncology, Department of Medicine, Lineberger Comprehensive Cancer Center, University of North Carolina at Chapel Hill, Chapel Hill, North Carolina

ADAM BRUFSKY, MD, PhD
Professor of Medicine, University of Pittsburgh, Magee-Women's Hospital, Pittsburgh, Pennsylvania

LISA A. CAREY, MD
Division of Hematology-Oncology, Department of Medicine, Lineberger Comprehensive Cancer Center, University of North Carolina at Chapel Hill, Chapel Hill, North Carolina

MARCO COLLEONI, MD
Division of Medical Senology, European Institute of Oncology, Milan, Italy

GIUSEPPE CURIGLIANO, MD, PhD
Division of Early Drug Development, European Institute of Oncology, Milan, Italy

ANDREA DECENSI, MD
Division of Cancer Prevention and Genetics, European Institute of Oncology, Milan; Division of Medical Oncology, E.O. Ospedali Galliera, Genoa, Italy

ELENA B. ELKIN, PhD
Associate Attending Outcomes Research Scientist, Department of Epidemiology and Biostatistics, Memorial Sloan-Kettering Cancer Center, New York, New York

ARMANDO E. GIULIANO, MD, FACS
Division of Surgical Oncology, Department of Surgery, Cedars-Sinai Medical Center, Professor of Surgery, Executive Vice-Chair of Surgery, Surgical Oncology, Associate Director of Surgical Oncology, Samuel Oschin Comprehensive Cancer Institute, Co-Director, Saul and Joyce Brandman Breast Center, Los Angeles, California

MICHAEL J. HASSETT, MD, MPH
Assistant Professor of Medicine, Department of Medicine, Harvard Medical School; Medical Director of Clinical Information Systems, Department of Medical Oncology, Dana-Farber Cancer Institute, Boston, Massachusetts

NITIN JAIN, MD
Assistant Professor of Medicine, Department of Leukemia, MD Anderson Cancer Center, Houston, Texas

ELLEN JONES, MD, PhD
Professor and Vice Chair Radiation Oncology, Clinical and Residency Director, University of North Carolina, Chapel Hill, North Carolina

MATTEO LAZZERONI, MD
Division of Cancer Prevention and Genetics, European Institute of Oncology, Milan, Italy

KATHLEEN LOKAY, BBA
President and CEO, D3 Oncology Solutions, University of Pittsburgh Medical Center, Pittsburgh, Pennsylvania

CHARLES L. LOPRINZI, MD
Regis Professor of Breast Cancer Research, Medical Oncology, Mayo Clinic, Rochester, Minnesota

BERYL MCCORMICK, MD, FACR
Clinical Director, Radiation Oncology, Memorial Sloan Kettering Cancer Center, New York, New York

ELISABETTA MUNZONE, MD
Division of Medical Senology, European Institute of Oncology, Milan, Italy

HYMAN B. MUSS, MD
Director of Geriatric Oncology, Lineberger Comprehensive Cancer Center; Professor of Medicine, University of North Carolina, Chapel Hill, North Carolina

SUSAN O'BRIEN, MD
Professor of Medicine, Department of Leukemia, MD Anderson Cancer Center, Houston, Texas

MARK D. PEGRAM, MD
Susy Yuan-Huey Hung Professor of Medical Oncology; Director, Stanford Breast Oncology Program; Co-director, Molecular Therapeutics Program, Stanford Cancer Institute, Stanford University School of Medicine, Stanford, California

KATHRYN J. RUDDY, MD, MPH
Instructor in Medicine, Medical Oncology, Dana-Farber Cancer Institute, Harvard Medical School, Boston, Massachusetts

GAIA SCHIAVON, MD, PhD
Clinical Fellow in Medical Oncology, Breast Unit, The Royal Marsden NHS Foundation Trust; The Institute of Cancer Research, London, United Kingdom

IAN E. SMITH, MD, FRCP, FRCPE
Head of Breast Unit, Consultant Medical Oncologist, Professor of Cancer Medicine, The Royal Marsden NHS Foundation Trust; The Institute of Cancer Research, London, United Kingdom

DANIELA STAN, MD
Assistant Professor of Medicine, Division of General Internal Medicine, Mayo Clinic, Rochester, Minnesota

GUNTER VON MINCKWITZ, MD
Associate Professor, German Breast Group, Neu-Isenburg; Department of Obstetrics and Gynecology, University Women's Hospital, Frankfurt, Germany

GRANT R. WILLIAMS, MD
Geriatric Oncology Fellow, University of North Carolina, Chapel Hill, North Carolina

TIMOTHY M. ZAGAR, MD
Department of Radiation Oncology, Lineberger Comprehensive Cancer Center, University of North Carolina at Chapel Hill, Chapel Hill, North Carolina

Contents

Breast cancer is the most common cancer in women worldwide. The selective estrogen-receptor (ER) modulators tamoxifen and raloxifene are approved by the Food and Drug Administration for the preventive therapy of breast cancer. Other drugs have shown promise but need further assessment. In the present review, we present an update of the chemoprevention of ER-positive breast cancer and discuss the potential role of metformin and aspirin, 2 drugs other than the specific "antihormones."

Duct carcinoma in situ (DCIS) is a common but non–life-threatening breast cancer. Four large prospective randomized trials comparing radiation therapy (RT) with none after breast-conservation surgery have all concluded that the use of RT reduces the risk of a local recurrence (LR) in the ipsilateral breast by at least 50%. More information is needed to assess the role of antiestrogen therapy when RT is not given. When markers are validated to predict which patients will have an invasive LR versus another DCIS or no LR, it is hoped that the discussion with the patient will clarify the situation further.

The development and wide acceptance of sentinel lymph node biopsy (SLNB) has profoundly affected the management of breast cancer. SLNB has spared the additional morbidity of axillary lymph node dissection (ALND) without compromising diagnostic accuracy and prognostic information in patients with clinically node-negative early-stage breast cancer. It has become an invaluable tool to clinicians to guide decisions regarding adjuvant treatment. The management of breast cancer continues to advance to more minimally invasive approaches, and the role of ALND is likely to become less important in the future.

Estrogen Receptor–positive/HER-2 negative breast cancers represent a heterogeneous group of tumors. Luminal A and B tumor subtypes can be identified through immunohistochemical assessment of estrogen and progesterone receptor, Ki-67 and HER-2 status. Patients with high levels of expression of steroid hormone receptors and low proliferation (Luminal A) are commonly cured with endocrine therapy alone. Patients with doubtful endocrine responsiveness or with high proliferation index (Luminal B/Her-negative) require the addition of chemotherapy to the best endocrine therapy. Controversies still exist on the identification of those patients who do not benefit from chemotherapy. Tailored adjuvant treatments should be considered in the therapeutic algorithm of patients with luminal tumors.

First-line endocrine therapy by estrogen antagonism or suppression of estrogen achieves objective responses (ORs) and clinical benefit (CB) in around 30% and 50% of estrogen receptor-positive metastatic breast cancer patients, respectively. Aromatase inhibitors (AIs) are the most effective treatment in previously untreated postmenopausal women. Tamoxifen is an effective alternative. The optimal endocrine therapy on relapse remains uncertain. Tamoxifen and fulvestrant achieve CB in around 50% of patients and ORs of 10%. CB of exemestane after nonsteroidal AIs is 30% to 50% but ORs are rare. Targeted agents (eg, everolimus) plus endocrine therapy are likely to become increasingly important in overcoming endocrine resistance.

Triple-negative breast cancer (TNBC), defined as lacking expression of the estrogen receptor, progesterone receptor, and HER2, comprises approximately 15% of incident breast cancers and is over-represented among those with metastatic disease. There are several biologically distinct subtypes within TNBC. Although the incidence of BRCA mutations across all subsets of breast cancer is low, BRCA mutations are more common among those with TNBC and may have therapeutic implications. The general principles guiding the use of chemotherapy and radiation therapy do not differ dramatically between early-stage TNBC and non-TNBC.

ERBB2 gene amplification occurs in ~20% of human breast cancers (BC) and is associated with an adverse clinical prognosis, indicating that it may be playing a critical role in disease pathogenesis. Therapeutic strategies targeting pathologic ERBB2 overexpression have revolutionized the diagnosis and treatment of BC. Indeed, humanized anti-ERBB2 antibodies, small molecule ERBB2 kinase inhibitors and ERBB2-targeting antibody-drug conjugates have proven safety and efficacy based upon evidence from randomized phase III clinical trials. Recent progress in targeting ERBB2 alteration will be reviewed, with focus on data that has informed changes in clinical practice for the treatment of BC.

Lessons have recently been learned in the use of neoadjuvant chemo-therapy. This article explains how diagnosis of a pathologic complete response (pCR) can avoid an unfavorable prognosis in patients with high-risk breast cancer; how the surrogacy of pCR for long-term survival remains questionable; how translational biomarker studies have not been helpful in identifying patients with a high chance of treatment benefit; assessment of the prognosis of patients without a pCR for identifying patients at high risk and which clinical trials will be available for these patients in the near future; and which patients might require less locore-gional treatment.

As the population ages, oncologists will be faced with managing an exploding number of older patients with breast cancer. The primary chal-lenge of caring for older cancer patients is providing treatment options that maximize long-term survival while accounting for comorbidities, life expectancy, and effects of treatment. There is a paucity of data from trials on the risks and benefits of effective treatments in elderly breast cancer patients. This article discusses how to evaluate older breast cancer patients and provides guidelines for optimal therapies in the adjuvant and metastatic treatment settings.

Survivors of breast cancer are confronted with a plethora of cancer treatment-related long-term symptoms, the most common being fatigue, hot flashes, sexual dysfunction, arthralgias, neuropathy, and cognitive dysfunction. Survivors of breast cancer also face cancer treatment-related disease states, such as osteoporosis, cardiac dysfunction, obesity, infer-tility, and secondary cancers. Evidence-based recommendations for screening, prevention, and early intervention should be implemented to improve quality of life and decrease comorbidities in this population.

The costs of breast cancer care are substantial and growing, and they extend across the spectrum of care. Medical therapies and hospitalizations account for a significant proportion of these costs. Cost-effectiveness analysis (CEA) is the preferred method for assessing the health benefits of medical interventions relative to their costs. Although many CEAs have been conducted for a wide range of breast cancer treatments, these anal-yses are not used routinely to guide coverage or utilization decisions in the United States. Currently, patients and providers may not consider costs when making most treatment decisions; this is likely to change as payment reform spreads.

The results from the UPMC Cancer Center's experience with Via Pathways and those reported by other pathways programs suggest that these are effective models for improving quality, reducing unwarranted variability in care, and reducing the rate of growth in the cost of cancer care. A robust pathways program that reduces unwarranted variability can serve as the vehicle to improve the value of cancer care to patients, payers, and providers through increasing quality and decreasing costs. Oncologists must take an active role in defining and implementing cost-effective care for patients, payers, and referring physicians.

B-cell receptor (BCR) signaling is essential for chronic lymphocytic leukemia (CLL) cell survival. Many kinases in the BCR signaling pathway are being studied as potential therapeutic targets. Ibrutinib (PCI-32765) is a novel first-in-class selective inhibitor of Bruton tyrosine kinase. Preclinical evidence suggests that ibrutinib inhibits CLL cell survival and proliferation and affects CLL cell migration and homing. Early clinical data in patients with CLL and non-Hodgkin lymphoma is encouraging. It is likely that ibrutinib and other drugs targeting the BCR pathway will become an integral component of CLL therapy.

HEMATOLOGY/ONCOLOGY CLINICS OF NORTH AMERICA

Preface

Breast Cancer Treatment in the Era of Individualized Care

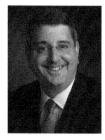

Harold J. Burstein, MD, PhD
Editor

Breast cancer management has entered the era of personalized medicine. It is widely appreciated that breast cancers differ in their biology and treatment needs. It is also understood that there are "subsets of subsets": divisions within the broad separations of tumor type that are increasingly appreciated as clinically relevant. Indeed, the realization that breast cancer is not a single disease is so broadly recognized that phrases like "one size doesn't fit all" or "tailored therapy" have rapidly transitioned from powerful insight to tired cliche.

But individualized care for breast cancer patients is not just a slogan; it is the current reality and represents the alignment of scientific discoveries with clinical practice. As we are in the age of tailored approaches to care, we have a whole new set of questions. Who is the tailor, and how good are they? Who picked out the cloth, and where was it made? When does the client show up to be measured? Who handles the alterations? Does the garment really fit better than one off the rack? And can we afford bespoke care?

For breast cancer patients expecting tailored treatment, those questions hold powerful resonance. The articles in this issue of *Hematology/Oncology Clinics of North America* seek to address these many questions.

Classifying the breast cancer is the first step in individualized care. As more of our treatment decisions hinge on the fundamental biology of the cancer, and not on the surgical or anatomical stage, the correct classification of the tumor is a sine qua non for appropriate therapy. This realization moves the pathologist to the center of the treatment team in breast cancer medicine. High-quality pathology and diagnostic testing are critical for correctly assigning tumors into the various treatment subsets. Rigorous pathology can still make for fraught clinical decisions; tumors are rarely homogeneous, and natural variations in "simple" things like histological grade,

Hematol Oncol Clin N Am 27 (2013) xiii–xv
http://dx.doi.org/10.1016/j.hoc.2013.05.013
0889-8588/13/$ – see front matter © 2013 Elsevier Inc. All rights reserved.

estrogen receptor status, and HER2 status still post vexing clinical challenges. But superb pathology, fully integrated into the multidisciplinary treatment team, is now essential for the best breast cancer care. As clinicians increasingly lean on molecular diagnostics to make treatment choices, the importance of quality control and careful attention to tumor biology will grow greater, and not diminish, in the pathology laboratory.

Our systemic treatment approaches are all driven by the underlying classification of the breast cancer. For estrogen-receptor-positive breast cancers, endocrine therapy remains the mainstay of treatment. For HER2-driven breast cancers, it is anti-HER2 therapy. Having a powerful target fuels successful drug discovery. New innovations in targeting ER and HER2 pathways have led to dramatic transformations in management of these tumor subsets in recent years and hold promise of more to come. Chemotherapy plays a role in many breast cancer types including triple-negative, HER2, and HER2 positive tumors. A particular challenge has been to ascertain reliably which ER-positive cancers can safely be treated without chemotherapy. Here again, the decisive piece of information lies within the tumor pathology, and the debate centers on how to most accurately classify tumors for treatment.

The reliance on tumor biology for choosing systemic therapies has altered the ways we think about integrating local and adjuvant therapy for breast cancer. One immediate consequence has been the opportunity to lessen the extent of surgery for breast cancer, and in particular, to avoid axillary dissection. Because the "die is cast" for treatment based on basic staging and tumor pathology, we no longer have to remove the full axillary node basin to justify the likely adjuvant therapies. The result is less morbidity for the patient, without any negative impact on treatment outcomes. Similarly, we can often employ neoadjuvant therapy based purely on tumor pathology—and not stage—as our initial treatment for breast cancer. But the use of neoadjuvant therapy poses new dilemmas, such as what to do when our initial therapy seems more—or less—successful than we had anticipated and hoped for. Can we respond to these dynamic interactions between tumor and treatment to individualize the care of the patient based on the actual treatment response, and if so, how?

But tailoring treatment based on tumor biology is not the full measure of individualized care for the breast cancer patient. Indeed, more than ever, it seems important to "put the person" back in personalized medicine. Not all breast cancer patients are the same people, even if they have the same kind of breast cancer. Individuals struggle with the physical, social, and psychological consequences of diagnosis and treatment and need support as cancer survivors. Older patients with breast cancer—the vast majority of all breast cancer patients—warrant special consideration because of real-world consequences of aging and comorbid conditions. Even when treatments work, there are tradeoffs between benefit and side effects. The fields of prevention and DCIS management are checkered by such tradeoffs and being able to frame the likely gains versus real pains are a critical part of caring for patients who are at risk for but have not yet developed breast cancer. Because of the generally good outcomes for such women, the calculation of treat versus not treat is especially difficult to add up, and personal preferences will matter a great deal when actually choosing treatments.

In an age of tailored approaches to breast cancer, it is tempting to think that the treatment plan for each individual will be different. But, of course, those plans are not. In fact, within the confines of breast cancer subtypes, rather clear treatment approaches are well-documented, and increasingly there is pressure to standardize our approaches. This of course is a paradox of the modern era in medicine—the pursuit of pathways-based treatments build on strong evidence, to achieve higher quality and efficiency while simultaneously appreciating the uniqueness of each patient and tumor. Not everyone needs a tailored suit; off the rack works pretty well for many, especially with a few alterations. Implementing guidelines that include both tailored and premeasured approaches is a key task for academic and community oncologists.

While everyone wants progress in breast cancer, there is growing concern that we cannot afford the progress we are making. Not everyone can afford a couture garment. What are the real costs of cancer care, and what is worth paying for? Defining those criteria is proving every bit as essential as defining breast cancer sub- sets. This issue, with its theme of individualized care for breast cancer, seeks to frame and discuss these many and varied meanings of personalized, tailored, and targeted treatment.

Harold J. Burstein, MD, PhD
Dana-Farber Cancer Institute
450 Brookline Avenue
Brigham and Women's Hospital
Harvard Medical School
Boston, MA 02215, USA

E-mail address:
hburstein@partners.org

Breast Cancer Prevention by Antihormones and Other Drugs

Where Do We Stand?

Matteo Lazzeroni, MD[a], Andrea DeCensi, MD[a,b],*

KEYWORDS

- Breast cancer chemoprevention • Aromatase Inhibitors • Metformin
- Selective estrogen receptor modulators • Aspirin

KEY POINTS

- Tamoxifen and raloxifene have been shown in randomized clinical trials to reduce the risk of developing primary invasive breast cancer in high-risk women.
- The aromatase inhibitor exemestane is a viable option but further follow-up is needed, as well as on other aromatase inhibitors in the prevention setting.
- Metformin and aspirin also show promise. However, preventive therapy needs to be integrated into wider strategies of risk reduction, weight control, and increase in physical activity.

INTRODUCTION

Excluding cancers of the skin, breast cancer remains the most frequently diagnosed cancer in women. Although the incidence rate began to decline in 2000 because of reductions in the use of menopausal hormone therapy, an estimated 226,870 new cases of invasive breast cancer were expected to occur among women in the United States in 2012.[1] The idea of preventing breast cancer dates back at least a century, when the first positive associations between environmental or individual factors and increased risk of breast cancer development were asserted. Although the precise mechanisms that promote a breast cancer are not completely established, the success of several recent clinical trials in preventive settings in selected high-risk populations suggests that chemoprevention is a rational and appealing strategy. The term "chemoprevention" was coined by Michael B. Sporn in a 1976 article to define "the use of

Competing Interests: The authors declare that they have no financial or nonfinancial competing interests.
[a] Division of Cancer Prevention and Genetics, European Institute of Oncology, Via Ripamonti 435, 20141, Milan, Italy; [b] Division of Medical Oncology, E.O. Ospedali Galliera, Mura delle Cappuccine 14, Genoa 16128, Italy
* Corresponding author. Medical Oncology Unit, E.O. Ospedali Galliera, Mura delle Cappuccine 14, Genoa 16128, Italy.
E-mail address: andrea.decensi@galliera.it

pharmacologic or natural agents that inhibit the development of invasive breast cancer either by blocking the DNA damage that initiates carcinogenesis, or by arresting or reversing the progression of premalignant cells in which such damage has already occurred."[2] Progress has been made since then, and now 2 medications are currently approved by the Food and Drug Administration (FDA) to reduce the risk of primary breast cancer. In this review, we present an update of the chemoprevention of estrogen receptor (ER)-positive breast cancer and discuss the potential role of metformin and aspirin, 2 drugs other than the specific "antihormones."

SELECTIVE ER MODULATORS: RANDOMIZED CLINICAL TRIALS AND META-ANALYSIS

Selective ER modulators (SERMs) are synthetic ER ligands. They are characterized by different chemical structures, which may influence their specific activities, but they all work by binding to the ER and preventing the cell division stimulus induced by estrogen. Nine randomized clinical trials have analyzed the effect of a SERM in preventing breast cancer (**Table 1**).

Tamoxifen

The International Breast Cancer Intervention Study (IBIS-I)[3] is a double-blind placebo-controlled randomized trial of tamoxifen, 20 mg per day for 5 years, in 7152 women, aged 35 to 70 years, at increased risk of breast cancer. The primary outcome measure was the frequency of invasive and in situ breast cancer. After a median follow-up of 96 months, 142 breast cancers were diagnosed in the 3579 women in the tamoxifen group and 195 in the 3575 women in the placebo group (4.97 vs 6.82 per 1000 woman-years, respectively; risk ratio [RR] 0.73, 95% confidence interval [CI] 0.58–0.91, $P = .004$). The prophylactic effect of tamoxifen was constant for the entire follow-up period, and no diminution of benefit was observed for up to 10 years after randomization. On the contrary, side effects in the tamoxifen group were much lower after completion of the active treatment period than during active treatment. Deep vein thrombosis and pulmonary embolism were statistically significantly higher in the tamoxifen arm than in the placebo arm during active treatment (52 vs 23 cases, RR 2.26, 95% CI 1.36–3.87) but not after tamoxifen was stopped (16 vs 14 cases, RR 1.14, 95% CI 0.52–2.53). The 2 arms did not differ in the risk of ER-negative invasive tumors (35 in each arm, RR 1.00, 95% CI 0.61–1.65) across the entire follow-up period, but the risk of ER-positive invasive breast cancer was 34% lower in the tamoxifen arm (87 vs 132 cases, RR 0.66, 95% CI 0.50–0.87). In conclusion, the risk-reducing effect of tamoxifen appears to persist for at least 10 years, but most side effects of tamoxifen do not continue after the 5-year treatment period.[4]

The Italian Tamoxifen Prevention Study[5] included 5408 healthy hysterectomized women aged 35 to 70 years who were randomized to 20 mg per day of tamoxifen or placebo for 5 years. After 11 years of follow-up,[6] 136 women (74 placebo, 62 tamoxifen) developed breast cancer (RR 0.84, 95% CI 0.60–1.17; annual rates were 2.48 and 2.07 per 1000 women-years, respectively). The rates of breast cancer in the 2 groups were similar among women who had had bilateral oophorectomy and among women at low risk for ER-positive disease but were much lower in the tamoxifen group among women at high risk (placebo, 6.26 per 1000 women-years, tamoxifen, 1.50 per 1000 women-years; RR 0.24, 95% CI 0.10–0.59). During the treatment period, women in the tamoxifen group reported more hot flashes (RR 1.78, 95% CI 1.57–2.00), vaginal discharge (RR 3.44, 95% CI 2.90–4.09), and urinary disturbances (RR 1.52, 95% CI 1.23–1.89), but fewer headaches (RR 0.68, 95% CI 0.50–0.94), than women in the placebo group. Hypertriglyceridemia (RR 4.33, 95% CI 1.96–9.53), thromboembolic events (RR 1.63, 95% CI 1.02–2.62), and cardiac arrhythmia or atrial fibrillation (RR 1.73, 95% CI 1.01–2.98) were also more frequent in the tamoxifen group than in the placebo group.[6] Withdrawal rate was mainly because of menopausal symptoms and differed according to estrogen replacement therapy (ERT) use, with compliance being 78% and 75% at 3 and 5 years, respectively, for women who never took ERT, and 92% and 88% at 3 and 5 years, respectively, for women not on ERT at baseline, but who took ERT at some time during the trial.[7]

The Royal Marsden Hospital tamoxifen randomized chemoprevention trial[8] accrued 2494 healthy women between 30 and 70 years with a family history of breast cancer. They were randomized to receive tamoxifen 20 mg per day orally or placebo for up to 8 years. The 20-year follow-up (median follow-up = 13 years) analysis[9] reported 186 invasive breast cancers (82 on tamoxifen and 104 on placebo; hazard ratio [HR] 0.78, 95% CI 0.58–1.04; P = .1). Of these 186 cancers, 139 were ER positive (53 on tamoxifen and 86 on placebo; HR 0.61, 95% CI 0.43–0.86; P = .005). The risk of ER-positive breast cancer was not statistically significantly lower in the tamoxifen arm than in the placebo arm during the 8-year treatment period (30 cancers in the tamoxifen arm and 39 in the placebo arm; HR 0.77, 95% CI 0.48–1.23; P = .3) but was statistically significantly lower in the posttreatment period (23 in the tamoxifen arm and 47 in the placebo arm; HR 0.48, 95% CI 0.29–0.79; P = .004). Fifty-four participants in each arm have died from any cause (HR 0.99, 95% CI 0.68–1.44; P = .95). The clinically significant adverse events, including other cancers, thromboembolisms, and non–breast cancer deaths were low, occurred predominantly during the treatment period, and were similar to those reported in the interim analysis.[8]

In the National Surgical Adjuvant Breast and Bowel Project P-1 study,[10] women (n = 13,388) at increased risk for breast cancer (60 years of age or older; 35–59 years of age with a 5-year predicted risk for breast cancer of at least 1.66% [chances in 100 of invasive breast cancer developing within 5 years]; women with a history of lobular carcinoma in situ) were randomly assigned to receive placebo (n = 6707) or 20 mg per day tamoxifen (n = 6681) for 5 years. Tamoxifen reduced the risk of invasive breast cancer by 49% (2-sided P<.00001), with cumulative incidence through 69 months of follow-up of 43.4 versus 22.0 per 1000 women in the placebo and tamoxifen groups, respectively. The decreased risk occurred in women aged 49 years or younger (44%), 50 to 59 years (51%), and 60 years or older (55%); risk was also reduced in women with a history of lobular carcinoma in situ (56%) or atypical hyperplasia (86%) and in those with any category of predicted 5-year risk. Tamoxifen reduced the risk of non-invasive breast cancer by 50% (2-sided P<.002) and the occurrence of ER-positive tumors by 69%, but no difference in the occurrence of ER-negative tumors was seen. After 7 years of follow-up,[11] the effects were similar to those seen in the initial report.[10] The cumulative rate of invasive breast cancer was reduced from 42.5 per 1000 women in the placebo group to 24.8 per 1000 women in the tamoxifen group (RR 0.57, 95% CI 0.46–0.70) and the cumulative rate of noninvasive breast cancer was reduced from 15.8 per 1000 women in the placebo group to 10.2 per 1000 women in the tamoxifen group (RR 0.63, 95% CI 0.45–0.89).[10] Tamoxifen administration did not alter the average annual rate of ischemic heart disease; however, a reduction in hip, radius, and spine fractures was observed. The rate of endometrial cancer was increased in the tamoxifen group (RR 2.53, 95% CI 1.35–4.97) and this increased risk occurred predominantly in women aged 50 years or older. All endometrial cancers in the tamoxifen group were stage I (localized disease) and no endometrial cancer deaths have occurred in this group. No increase in other tumors was observed in the tamoxifen group. The rates of stroke, pulmonary embolism, and deep vein thrombosis were elevated in the tamoxifen group; these events occurred more frequently in

Table 1
Study results for selective estrogen receptor modulators, aromatase inhibitors, metformin, and aspirin as potential preventive agents for breast cancer

	No. of Patients	Population	Median Duration of Follow-up, mo	RR	Comment
Tamoxifen					
IBIS-I[3,4]	7139	High risk	96	0.66 (0.50–0.87)	
Italian Study[5–7]	5408	Normal risk; hysterectomy	132	0.77 (0.51–1.16)	
Royal Marsden Trial[8,9]	2471	High risk	158	0.61 (0.43–0.86)	
NSABP[10,11]					
Raloxifene					
MORE[13]	7705	Osteoporosis; postmenopausal	48	0.28 (0.17–0.46)	3 arms: 60 mg, 20 mg, placebo in 1:1:1 ratio; BC as secondary end point
CORE[14]	4011	Osteoporosis; postmenopausal	96	0.24 (0.22–0.40)	BC as secondary end point
RUTH[15]	10,101	Postmenopausal and CHD	67	0.45 (0.28–0.72)	
STAR[16,17]	19,747	High risk and postmenopausal	81	1.24 (1.05–1.47) vs tamoxifen	Estimated RR 0.77 vs placebo
Lasofoxifene					
PEARL[18,19]	8556	Osteoporosis; age 59–80 y	60	0.19 (0.07–0.56)	Two doses of lasofoxifene (0.25 and 0.5 mg) or placebo for 5 y in a 1:1:1 ratio; RR reduction only for 0.5-mg daily group
Arzoxifene					
Generations[20,21]	9354	Osteoporosis; age ≥ years	48	0.30 (0.14–0.63)	

Study	No.	Population	Follow-up	RR (95% CI)	Comments
Anastrozole					
IBIS-II[25]	Total of 6844 women enrolled (3864 to Prevention and 2980 to DCIS)	High risk and postmenopausal	//	//	IBIS-II Prevention (anastrozole 1 mg vs placebo); IBIS-II DCIS (anastrozole 1 mg vs tamoxifen 20 mg)
Exemestane					
MAP.3[27]	4560	High risk and postmenopausal	35	0.35 (0.18–0.70)	
Metformin					
Chlebowski et al,[41] 2012	68,019, 3401 with diabetes at study entry, 3273 invasive breast cancers diagnosed	Postmenopausal women participating in Women's Health Initiative clinical trials	11.8	0.75 (0.57–0.99)	
MA 32[47]	Planned 3582, randomized to 850 mg (or placebo) twice daily for 5 y	Patients with early-stage and resected breast cancer	Ongoing	N.A.	
Aspirin					
Holmes et al,[69] 2010	4164	Nurses' Health Study, stage I, II, III breast cancer	Maximum 30	//	Breast cancer mortality 0.51 (0.41–0.65)
Li et al,[71] 2012	1024	Cases from a population-based case-control study followed as a cohort	7.3	//	Breast cancer mortality 0.89 (0.52–1.52)

Abbreviations: BC, breast cancer; CHD, coronary heart disease; CORE, Continuing Outcomes of Relevant to Evista; DCIS, ductal carcinoma in situ; IBIS, International Breast Cancer Intervention Study; MAP.3, Mammary Prevention 3; MORE, Multiple Outcomes of Raloxifene Evaluation; N.A., not applicable; NSABP, National Surgical Adjuvant Breast and Bowel Project; PEARL, Postmenopausal Evaluation and Risk-Reduction with Lasofoxifene; RR, risk ratio; RUTH, Raloxifene Use for The Heart; STAR, National Surgical Adjuvant Breast and Bowel Project Study of Tamoxifen and Raloxifene.

women aged 50 years or older. Tamoxifen led to a 32% reduction in osteoporotic fractures (RR 0.68, 95% CI 0.51–0.92). Relative risks of stroke, deep vein thrombosis, and cataracts (which increased with tamoxifen) and of ischemic heart disease and death (which were not changed with tamoxifen) were also similar to those initially reported.[10] Risks of pulmonary embolism were approximately 11% lower than in the original report, and risks of endometrial cancer were about 29% higher, but these differences were not statistically significant. The net benefit achieved with tamoxifen varied according to age, race, and level of breast cancer risk.

In 2003, Cuzick and colleagues[12] performed a meta-analysis including the 4 previously mentioned clinical trials and showed that ER-positive cancers were decreased by 48% (36–58; P<.0001) by tamoxifen treatment. Rates of endometrial cancer and venous thromboembolic events were increased in all tamoxifen prevention trials (consensus relative risk 2.4 [1.5–4.0]; P = .0005, and 1.9 [1.4–2.6] ; P<.0001, respectively). Overall, there was no effect on non–breast cancer mortality; the only cause showing a mortality increase was pulmonary embolism (6 vs 2).[12]

Raloxifene

Two trials investigated the role of raloxifene in postmenopausal women with osteoporosis. The Multiple Outcomes of Raloxifene Evaluation (MORE) trial randomized 7705 women to either placebo or raloxifene at 60 mg or 120 mg daily for 4 years in a 1:1:1 ratio.[13] Women were a mean of 66.5 years old at trial entry, 19 years postmenopause, and osteoporotic (low bone mineral density and/or prevalent vertebral fractures). In the completed 4-year trial, raloxifene decreased the incidence of all breast cancers by 62% and invasive breast cancers by 72% compared with placebo (RR 0.28, 95%; CI 0.17–0.46). This reduction was largely attributable to the 84% reduction in invasive ER-positive breast cancers in the raloxifene group. Raloxifene had no effect on ER-negative breast cancers (RR 0.16, 95% CI 0.09–0.30). These data indicate that 93 osteoporotic women would need to be treated with raloxifene for 4 years to prevent 1 case of invasive breast cancer. Raloxifene was generally safe and well tolerated; however, thromboembolic disease occurred more frequently with raloxifene compared with placebo (P = .003).[13]

The Continuing Outcomes of Relevant to Evista (CORE) trial examined the effect of continuing raloxifene for additional 4 years on the incidence of invasive breast cancer in women in MORE who agreed to continue in CORE (n = 6511).[14] The study compared only the 60-mg dose with placebo so that these women who were initially randomized to 120 mg daily had their dose reduced to 60 mg. During the CORE trial, the 4-year incidences of invasive breast cancer and ER-positive invasive breast cancer were reduced by 59% (HR 0.41, 95% CI 0.24–0.71) and 66% (HR 0.34, 95% CI 0.18–0.66), respectively, in the raloxifene group compared with the placebo group. There was no difference between the 2 groups in incidence of ER-negative invasive breast cancer. Over the 8 years of both trials, the incidences of invasive breast cancer and ER-positive invasive breast cancer were reduced by 66% (HR 0.34, 95% CI 0.22–0.50) and 76% (HR 0.24, 95% CI 0.15–0.40), respectively, in the raloxifene group compared with the placebo group. During the CORE trial, the relative risk of thromboembolism in the raloxifene group compared with that in the placebo group was 2.17 (95% CI 0.83–5.70). This increased risk, also observed in the MORE trial, persisted over the 8 years of both trials.[14]

The Raloxifene Use for The Heart (RUTH) trial randomly assigned 10,101 postmenopausal women (mean age, 67.5 years) with established cardiovascular disease, coronary heart disease (CHD), or risk factor for heart disease to either 60 mg per day of raloxifene or matching placebo and followed them for a median of 5.6 years.[15] The

2 primary outcomes were coronary events and invasive breast cancer. As compared with placebo, raloxifene did not significantly affect the risk of CHD but it reduced the risk of invasive breast cancer (40 vs 70 events; HR 0.56, 95% CI 0.38–0.83; absolute risk reduction, 1.2 invasive breast cancers per 1000 women treated for 1 year); the benefit was primarily attributable to a reduced risk of ER-positive invasive breast cancers. There was no significant difference in the rates of death from any cause or total stroke according to group assignment, but raloxifene was associated with an increased risk of fatal stroke (59 vs 39 events; HR 1.49, 95% CI 1.00–2.24; absolute risk increase, 0.7 per 1000 woman-years) and venous thromboembolism (103 vs 71 events; HR 1.44, 95% CI 1.06–1.95; absolute risk increase, 1.2 per 1000 woman-years).[15]

The National Surgical Adjuvant Breast and Bowel Project Study of Tamoxifen and Raloxifene (STAR) compared raloxifene with tamoxifen among women at increased risk of developing breast cancer.[16] The trial randomized a total of 19,747 postmeno-pausal women (mean age 58.5 years) to either tamoxifen 20 mg per day or raloxifene 60 mg per day for 5 years in a double dummy blind fashion. From 1999 to 2005, there were 163 cases of invasive breast cancer in women assigned to tamoxifen and 168 in those assigned to raloxifene (incidence, 4.30 per 1000 vs 4.41 per 1000; RR 1.02, 95% CI 0.82–1.28). There were fewer cases of noninvasive breast cancer in the tamoxifen group (57 cases) than in the raloxifene group (80 cases) (incidence, 1.51 vs 2.11 per 1000; RR 1.40, 95% CI 0.98–2.00). There were 36 cases of endometrial cancer with tamoxifen and 23 with raloxifene (RR 0.62, 95% CI 0.35–1.08). No differences were found for other invasive cancer sites, for ischemic heart disease events, or for stroke. Thromboembolic events occurred less often in the raloxifene group (RR 0.70, 95% CI 0.54–0.91). The number of osteoporotic fractures in the groups was similar. There were fewer cataracts (RR 0.79, 95% CI 0.68–0.92) and cataract surgeries (RR 0.82, 95% CI 0.68–0.99) in the women taking raloxifene. There was no difference in the total number of deaths (101 vs 96 for tamoxifen vs raloxifene) or in causes of death. An updated anal-ysis with an 81-month median follow-up[17] showed that the RR of raloxifene:tamoxifen for invasive breast cancer was 1.24 (95% CI 1.05–1.47) and for noninvasive disease, 1.22 (95% CI 0.95–1.59). Compared with initial results, the RRs increased for invasive and decreased in width for noninvasive breast cancer. Toxicity RRs were 0.55 (95% CI 0.36–0.83; $P = .003$) for endometrial cancer (this difference was not significant in the initial results), 0.19 (95% CI 0.12–0.29) for uterine hyperplasia, and 0.75 (95% CI 0.60–0.93) for thromboembolic events. There were no significant mortality differences. In conclusion, long-term raloxifene retained 76% of the effectiveness of tamoxifen in preventing invasive disease and grew closer over time to tamoxifen in preventing noninvasive disease, with significantly less endometrial cancer.[17]

Lasofoxifene

The Postmenopausal Evaluation and Risk-Reduction with Lasofoxifene (PEARL) trial recruited 8556 postmenopausal healthy women aged 59 to 80 years with low bone density and normal mammograms. Subjects were randomly assigned to 2 doses of lasofoxifene (0.25 and 0.50 mg) or placebo for 5 years in a 1:1:1 ratio.[18] The primary end points were incidence of ER-positive breast cancer and nonvertebral fractures at 5 years. Lasofoxifene at a dosage of 0.5 mg per day, as compared with placebo, was associated with reduced risks of ER-positive breast cancer (0.3 vs 1.7 cases per 1000 person-years; HR 0.19, 95% CI 0.07–0.56). A nested case-control study of 49 case patients with incident breast cancer and 156 unaffected control subjects from the PEARL trial was performed to evaluate treatment effects on risk of total and ER-positive invasive breast cancer by baseline serum estradiol and sex hormone–binding globulin levels.[19] Compared with placebo, 0.5 mg of lasofoxifene statistically significantly reduced the risk of total breast cancer by 79% (HR 0.21, 95% CI 0.08–0.55) and ER-positive invasive breast cancer by 83% (HR 0.17, 95% CI 0.05–0.57). The effects of 0.5 mg of lasofoxifene on total breast cancer were similar regardless of Gail score, whereas the effects were markedly stronger for women with baseline estradiol levels greater than the median (odds ratio [OR] 0.11, 95% CI 0.02–0.51) versus those with levels less than the median (OR 0.78, 95% CI 0.16 to 3.79; P for interaction = .04).[19] Both the lower and higher doses, as compared with placebo, were associated with an increase in venous thromboembolic events (3.8 and 2.9 cases vs 1.4 cases per 1000 person-years; HR 2.67, 95% CI 1.55–4.58, and HR 2.06, 95% CI 1.17–3.60, respectively). Endometrial cancer occurred in 3 women in the placebo group, 2 women in the lower-dose lasofoxifene group, and 2 women in the higher-dose lasofoxifene group.

Arzoxifene

The Generations trial, a multicenter, placebo-controlled, double-blind trial, compared arzoxifene 20 mg per day and placebo in 9354 postmenopausal women with osteoporosis (n = 5252) or low bone mass (n = 4102). Primary outcomes were vertebral fracture in the osteoporotic population and invasive breast cancer in all study participants.[20] The detailed breast cancer findings from the trial were reported recently by Powles and colleagues.[21] After 48 months of follow-up there were a total of 75 breast cancers, 53 in the placebo group and 22 in the arzoxifene group (HR 0.41, 95% CI 0.25–0.68, P<.001), with a 59% reduction in overall breast cancer incidence with arzoxifene compared with placebo. Although generally well tolerated, there was a significant increase in venous thromboembolism, vasomotor symptoms, muscle cramps, and some gynecologic events with arzoxifene.[21]

THE AROMATASE INHIBITORS

Aromatase inhibitors (AIs) work by inhibiting the action of the enzyme aromatase, which converts androgens into estrogens by a process called "aromatization." Evidence for a preventive effect of aromatase inhibitors against breast cancer derives from an assessment of new contralateral breast cancers in adjuvant trials involving women with early disease. This risk has been lower in women receiving an aromatase inhibitor than in those receiving tamoxifen in virtually all adjuvant trials, leading to an overall reduction in risk of about 50% below that achieved with tamoxifen.[22] Because tamoxifen is associated with a reduced risk of new ER-positive tumors of about 50%, a 75% reduction in risk of ER-positive breast cancer risk is projected for aromatase inhibitors.[23]

Anastrozole

The Arimidex, Tamoxifen, Alone or in Combination (ATAC) trial was undertaken to compare the efficacy and safety data of the third-generation, oral, nonsteroidal aromatase inhibitor anastrozole (Arimidex) against tamoxifen. Participants were postmenopausal patients with invasive operable breast cancer who had completed primary therapy and were eligible to receive adjuvant hormonal therapy. The primary end points were disease-free survival and occurrence of adverse events. Analysis for efficacy was by intention to treat. The trial recruited 9366 patients, of whom 3125 were randomly assigned anastrozole, 3116 tamoxifen, and 3125 combination. After a median follow-up of 100 months, a significant 40% reduction (HR 0.60, 95% CI 0.42–0.85) in contralateral breast cancers with anastrozole compared with tamoxifen was reported.[24] Side effects appear to be fewer with the aromatase inhibitors, with no excess of gynecologic (including endometrial cancer) or thromboembolic events, but an increase in fracture risk and joint symptoms does occur. Fracture rates were higher in patients receiving anastrozole than in those receiving tamoxifen during active treatment (annual rate 2.93% vs 1.90%; incidence rate ratio [IRR] 1.55, 95% CI 1.31–1.83, P<.0001), but were not different after treatment was completed (off treatment: 1.56% vs 1.51%; IRR 1.03, 95% CI 0.81–1.31, P = .79).[24]

Anastrozole is currently being tested in the International Breast Cancer Intervention Study-II[25] (IBIS-II) for its ability to reduce the risk of invasive breast cancer in postmenopausal women at increased risk of disease. The overall IBIS-II design comprises 2 independent strata, one testing anastrozole in comparison with tamoxifen in women with ductal carcinoma in situ (DCIS) and the other testing this AI versus placebo in postmenopausal women at increased risk of breast cancer. The eligibility criteria for this "high-risk" portion of IBIS-II were similar to those used in IBIS-I, including risk based on family history, history of benign breast biopsies, lobular carcinoma in situ (LCIS) and/or atypical hyperplasia, and nulliparity. All women (aged 35–70 years) were postmenopausal. Exclusion criteria included a dual-energy x-ray absorptiometry (DXA) T score of 4 or lower or more than 2 fragility fractures. The IBIS-II trial stopped the accrual in December 2012, with a total of 6844 women enrolled (3864 to Prevention and 2980 to DCIS). Results are expected shortly.

Exemestane

Exemestane is 1 of the 2 types of aromatase inhibitors approved to treat breast cancer. It is an irreversible steroidal inhibitor (better defined inactivator) able to form a permanent and deactivating bond with the aromatase enzyme. Because its steroidal nature suggested that it might behave like a weak androgen in bone, the possible counteraction of the resorptive effect of estrogen depletion[26] by exemestane might be responsible for less bone toxicity than seen with other AIs.

The National Cancer Institute of Cancer (NCIC) Mammary Prevention 3 (MAP.3) Trial[27] was a randomized, placebo-controlled, double-blind trial of exemestane administered to postmenopausal women 35 years or older with at least one of the following risk factors: 60 years or older; Gail 5-year risk score greater than 1.66%; prior atypical ductal or lobular hyperplasia or LCIS; or DCIS with mastectomy. A total of 4560 women (median age 62.5 years, median Gail risk score 2.3%) were randomly assigned to either exemestane or placebo. At a median follow-up of 35 months, 11 invasive breast cancers were detected in those given exemestane and in 32 of those given placebo, with a 65% relative reduction in the annual incidence of invasive breast cancer (0.19% vs 0.55%; HR 0.35, 95% CI 0.18–0.70; P = .002). The annual incidence of invasive plus noninvasive (DCIS) breast cancers was 0.35% on exemestane and 0.77% on placebo (HR 0.47, 95% CI 0.27–0.79; P = .004). Adverse events occurred in 88% of the exemestane group and 85% of the placebo group (P = .003), with no significant differences between the 2 groups in terms of skeletal fractures, cardiovascular events, other cancers, or treatment-related deaths. Minimal quality-of-life differences were observed. However, subsequent results in a selected subgroup showed that the loss of cortical thickness induced by 2 years of exemestane over placebo assessed by high-resolution peripheral quantitative computed tomography (CT) was substantial and underestimated by DEXA compared with CT.[28]

OTHER DRUGS
Metformin

Metformin represents the first-line medication for type 2 diabetes management and acts by increasing insulin sensitivity and improving glycemic control.[29] Data from literature show that hyperinsulinemia and insulin resistance worsen breast cancer prognosis and increase breast cancer risk.[30,31] Interestingly, preclinical studies have identified some properties suggestive of anticancer activity that may be independent of insulin effects.[32] The mechanism by which metformin may influence mammary cancer is not established. Preclinical studies suggest that metformin may have different mechanisms of tumor inhibition, including activation of adenosine monophosphate kinase (AMPk) and inhibition of the mammalian target of rapamycin (mTOR) pathway, as well as indirect, insulin-mediated effects.[32–35] Consequently, observational studies have examined associations between metformin use and cancer incidence. In 2010, Decensi and colleagues[36] performed a comprehensive literature search and meta-analysis of epidemiologic studies to assess the effect of metformin on cancer incidence and mortality in diabetic patients until May 2009, with no language or time restrictions. Eleven studies were selected for relevance in terms of intervention, population studied, independence, and reporting of cancer incidence or mortality data, reporting 4042 cancer events and 529 cancer deaths. A 31% reduction in overall summary relative risk (0.69, 95% CI 0.61–0.79) was found in subjects taking metformin compared with other antidiabetic drugs. The inverse association was significant for pancreatic and hepatocellular cancer, and nonsignificant for colon, breast, and prostate cancer. A trend to a dose-response relationship was noted.[36]

Another recent meta-analysis supported a protective effect of metformin on breast cancer risk among postmenopausal women with diabetes,[37] but all 7 studies included in the analyses were observational and thus precluded any causal interpretation (combined OR of all 7 studies for metformin use and breast cancer incidence was 0.83, 95% CI 0.71–0.97). Furthermore, emerging clinical proof-of-principle studies support a potential role of metformin in the control of breast cancer cell proliferation.[38–40]

Chlebowski and colleagues[41] recently assessed associations among diabetes, metformin use, and breast cancer in postmenopausal women participating in Women's Health Initiative clinical trials. All the postmenopausal women (68,019), including 3401 with diabetes at study entry, were observed over a mean of 11.8 years with 3273 invasive breast cancers diagnosed. Women with diabetes who were given metformin had lower breast cancer incidence (HR 0.75, 95% CI 0.57–0.99). An important issue is if clinical activity against breast cancer might be limited to women with impaired glucose homeostasis or high body mass index (BMI), as suggested by Bonanni and colleagues.[40] Notably, Bonanni and colleagues[40] conducted a randomized, phase II, double-blind, placebo-controlled trial in nondiabetic women with early breast cancer who were candidates for elective surgery and who received either metformin 850 mg twice per day (n = 100) or placebo (n = 100) for 4 weeks. The primary outcome measure was the difference between arms in Ki-67 after 4 weeks adjusted for baseline values, as the change in Ki-67 between pretreatment biopsy and posttreatment surgical specimen has prognostic value and may predict antitumor activity in breast cancer.[42–44] Given the different effect of metformin on diabetes incidence depending on BMI or glucose intolerance,[45] the investigators also assessed whether metformin had a greater effect in women with insulin resistance, as assessed by the homeostasis model assessment (HOMA) index (fasting blood glucose [mmol/L] × insulin [mU/L]/22.5).[46] Overall, the metformin effect on Ki-67 change relative to placebo was not statistically significant, with a mean proportional increase of 4.0% (95% CI −5.6%–14.4%) 4 weeks apart. However, there was a different drug effect depending on insulin resistance (HOMA index >2.8; P(interaction) = .045), with a nonsignificant mean proportional decrease in Ki-67 of 10.5% (95% CI −26.1%–8.4%) in women with HOMA more than 2.8 and a nonsignificant increase of 11.1% (95% CI −0.6%–24.2%) with HOMA less than or equal to 2.8. A different effect of metformin according to HOMA index was noted also in luminal B tumors (P for interaction = .05). Similar trends to drug effect modifications were observed according to BMI (P = .143), waist/hip girth-ratio (P = .058), moderate alcohol consumption (P = .005), and C-reactive protein (P = .080).

Several other clinical studies are proceeding to address metformin and cancer issues (http://www.clinicaltrials.gov/ct2/results?term=Metformin+and+breast+cancer& recr=Open) and in particular the NCIC MA 32 is an ongoing, full-scale clinical trial that will enroll 3582 patients with early-stage and resected breast cancer receiving standard breast cancer therapy. Subjects will be randomized to receive metformin 850 mg (or placebo) twice daily for 5 years.[47]

Aspirin

In 1997, the world celebrated the centenary of the discovery of aspirin by Felix Hoffmann, and this 100-year-old drug can be now considered one of the most successful agents ever produced. Commonly known as a pain reliever, aspirin may also influence breast cancerogenesis through a number of mechanisms, including the decreased production of prostaglandins, which can stimulate angiogenesis and inhibit apoptosis, and the inhibition of the cyclo-oxygenase (COX) enzymatic pathways.[48–51] Furthermore, prostaglandin E2 (PGE2) has shown to increase aromatase gene expression and thereby estrogen production in cultured cells[52] and, consistent with this, a positive correlation has been observed between the level of COX and expression of CYP19 in human breast cancer.[53] Progesterone synthesis can also be stimulated by PGE2.[54] Thus, the use of aspirin to inhibit prostaglandin-driven production of estrogen or progesterone may be a means to prevent breast cancer.

Large prospective observational studies have shown a potential mortality reduction among women with breast cancer who use aspirin.[55–67] In 2004, Terry and colleagues[68] reported an inverse association between aspirin use and breast cancer incidence in a population-based case-control study of women with breast cancer (1442 cases and 1420 controls). Ever use of aspirin or other nonsteroidal anti-inflammatory drugs (NSAIDs) at least once per week for 6 months or longer was reported in 301 cases (20.9%) and 345 controls (24.3%) (OR 0.80, 95% CI 0.66–0.97 for ever vs nonusers). The inverse association was most pronounced among frequent users (≥7 tablets per week) and among current and recent users (OR 0.72, 95% CI 0.58–0.90). The reduction in risk with aspirin use was seen among those with hormone receptor–positive tumors (OR 0.74, 95% CI 0.60–0.93) but not for women with hormone receptor–negative tumors (OR 0.97, 95% CI 0.67–1.40).[68]

In the Nurses' Health Study, breast cancer mortality risk according to number of days per week of aspirin use (0, 1, 2–5, or 6–7 days) was analyzed in 4164 female nurses with early breast cancer.[69] The RR of dichotomous aspirin use (yes or no) in relation to breast cancer mortality was 0.51 (95% CI 0.41–0.65). Adjusted RRs for 1, 2 to 5, and 6 to 7 days of aspirin use per week compared with no use were 1.07 (95% CI 0.70–1.63), 0.29 (95% CI 0.16–0.52), and 0.36 (95% CI 0.24–0.54), respectively (test for linear trend, $P<.001$). This association did not differ appreciably by stage, menopausal status, BMI, or ER status. Results were similar for distant recurrence.[69] Among a subset of 2001 subjects for whom we had tumor samples to perform COX-2 immunohistochemistry, a similar association for aspirin use was seen among those with COX-2–positive tumors (RR 0.64, 95% CI 0.43–0.96) and COX-2–negative tumors (RR 0.57, 95% CI 0.44–0.74), suggesting that the aspirin mechanism for breast cancer may be independent of COX-2.[70]

Recently, Li and colleagues[71] reported that lifetime use of aspirin up to diagnosis was not significantly associated with either all-cause mortality (RR 0.82, 95% CI 0.54–1.24) or breast cancer–specific mortality (RR 0.89, 95% CI 0.53–1.52) among 1024 breast cancer cases from a population-based case-control study followed as a cohort for an average of 7 years.

In addition to the prospective studies, randomized trial data have demonstrated an effect of aspirin on cancer recurrence. Rothwell and colleagues[72] included in their analysis all 5 large randomized trials of daily aspirin ($\geq$75 mg daily) versus control for the prevention of vascular events in the United Kingdom. The investigators showed that aspirin was able to reduce risk of cancer with distant metastasis (RR 0.52, 95% CI 0.35–0.75). Notably, patients with no metastasis from adenocarcinoma from any site at initial diagnosis and who remained on aspirin up to or after diagnosis had a markedly reduced risk of metastasis during follow-up (RR 0.31, 95% CI 0.15–0.76). Reliable estimation of effects of aspirin on case-fatality in individual primary cancers was limited by small numbers, but there was also some evidence of reduced case fatality for breast cancer (RR 0.16, 95% CI 0.02–1.19).[72]

Finally, a recent meta-analysis compared data from observational studies with those from randomized trials. Regular use of aspirin or NSAIDs was associated with a trend to a reduced proportion of breast cancers with distant metastasis, consistent with the effect in the randomized trials (OR 0.58, 95% CI 0.20–1.71).

Altogether, the effect of aspirin on breast cancer incidence is probably too small to justify its use as a single preventive agent. However, phase 2 biomarker trials may better elucidate its breast cancer preventive potential (http://www.clinicaltrials.gov/ct2/results?term=Aspirin+and+breast+cancer&Search=Search).

Moreover, taking into account the risk reduction seen with other cancers (eg, gastrointestinal cancers), as well as the beneficial cardiovascular effects, this drug may be part of a broad pharamacological intervention approach, such as the polypill.[73]

SUMMARY

So far, 2 SERMs, tamoxifen and raloxifene, are licensed for use in the United States, although neither is being widely used. Possible explanations are a perceived concern about side effects and poor ability to identify women at high risk. Two newer SERMs, lasofoxifene and arzoxifene, seem to have good risk-benefit profiles and trials in women at high risk of breast cancer are needed to confirm initial findings. Aromatase inhibitors also show promise and are being studied in large trials. Newer agents, notably metformin and aspirin, also show promise, but less costly and time-consuming approaches need to be established to assess these and other new agents. Large-scale phase III chemoprevention trials with cancer incidence as the end point require large populations, long time for accrual and follow-up, and are extremely expensive. It is therefore crucial to proceed with short-term clinical phase II chemoprevention trials testing the efficacy of potential agents by evaluating the modulation of intermediate surrogate end points in an appropriate cohort of individuals. Finally, to reduce the impact of breast cancer to a minimum, preventive therapy needs to be integrated into wider strategies of risk reduction, weight control, and increase in physical activity.

REFERENCES

1. American Cancer Society. Cancer Facts & Figures 2012. Atlanta: American Cancer Society; 2012.

2. Sporn MB. Approaches to prevention of epithelial cancer during the preneoplastic period. Cancer Res 1976;36:2699–702.

3. Cuzick J, Forbes J, Edwards R, et al. First results from the International Breast Cancer Intervention Study (IBIS-I): a randomised prevention trial. Lancet 2002; 360:817–24.

4. Cuzick J, Forbes JF, Sestak I, et al. Long-term results of tamoxifen prophylaxis for breast cancer—96-month follow-up of the randomized IBIS-I Trial. J Natl Cancer Inst 2007;99:272–82.

5. Veronesi U, Maisonneuve P, Costa A, et al. Prevention of breast cancer with tamoxifen: preliminary findings from the Italian randomised trial among hysterectomised women. Italian Tamoxifen Prevention Study. Lancet 1998;352:93–7.

6. Veronesi U, Maisonneuve P, Rotmensz N, et al. Tamoxifen for the prevention of breast cancer: late results of the Italian Randomized Tamoxifen Prevention Trial among women with hysterectomy. J Natl Cancer Inst 2007;99:727–37.

7. Guerrieri-Gonzaga A, Galli A, Rotmensz N, et al. The Italian breast cancer prevention trial with tamoxifen: findings and new perspectives. Ann N Y Acad Sci 2001;949:113–22.

8. Powles T, Eeles R, Ashley S, et al. Interim analysis of the incidence of breast cancer in the Royal Marsden Hospital tamoxifen randomised chemoprevention trial. Lancet 1998;352:98–101.

9. Powles TJ, Ashley S, Tidy A, et al. Twenty-year follow-up of the Royal Marsden randomized, double-blinded tamoxifen breast cancer prevention trial. J Natl Cancer Inst 2007;99:283–90.

10. Fisher B, Costantino JP, Wickerham DL, et al. Tamoxifen for prevention of breast cancer: report of the National Surgical Adjuvant Breast and Bowel Project P-1 Study. J Natl Cancer Inst 1998;90:1371–88.

11. Fisher B, Costantino JP, Wickerham DL, et al. Tamoxifen for the prevention of breast cancer: current status of the National Surgical Adjuvant Breast and Bowel Project P-1 study. J Natl Cancer Inst 2005;97:1652–62.

12. Cuzick J, Powles T, Veronesi U, et al. Overview of the main outcomes in breast-cancer prevention trials. Lancet 2003;361:296–300.

13. Cauley JA, Norton L, Lippman ME, et al. Continued breast cancer risk reduction in postmenopausal women treated with raloxifene: 4-year results from the MORE trial. Multiple outcomes of raloxifene evaluation. Breast Cancer Res Treat 2001; 65:125–34.

14. Martino S, Cauley JA, Barrett-Connor E, et al. Continuing outcomes relevant to Evista: breast cancer incidence in postmenopausal osteoporotic women in a randomized trial of raloxifene. J Natl Cancer Inst 2004;96:1751–61.

15. Barrett-Connor E, Mosca L, Collins P, et al. Effects of raloxifene on cardiovascular events and breast cancer in postmenopausal women. N Engl J Med 2006; 355:125–37.

16. Vogel VG, Costantino JP, Wickerham DL, et al. Effects of tamoxifen vs raloxifene on the risk of developing invasive breast cancer and other disease outcomes: the NSABP study of tamoxifen and raloxifene (STAR) P-2 trial. JAMA 2006; 295:2727–41.

17. Vogel VG, Costantino JP, Wickerham DL, et al. Update of the National Surgical Adjuvant Breast and Bowel Project Study of Tamoxifen and Raloxifene (STAR) P-2 Trial: preventing breast cancer. Cancer Prev Res (Phila) 2010;3: 696–706.

18. Cummings SR, Ensrud K, Delmas PD, et al. Lasofoxifene in postmenopausal women with osteoporosis. N Engl J Med 2010;362:686–96.

19. LaCroix AZ, Powles T, Osborne CK, et al. Breast cancer incidence in the randomized PEARL trial of lasofoxifene in postmenopausal osteoporotic women. J Natl Cancer Inst 2010;102:1706–15.
20. Cummings SR, McClung M, Reginster JY, et al. Arzoxifene for prevention of fractures and invasive breast cancer in postmenopausal women. J Bone Miner Res 2011;26:397–404.
21. Powles TJ, Diem SJ, Fabian CJ, et al. Breast cancer incidence in postmenopausal women with osteoporosis or low bone mass using arzoxifene. Breast Cancer Res Treat 2012;134:299–306.
22. Cuzick J. Aromatase inhibitors for breast cancer prevention. J Clin Oncol 2005; 23:1636–43.
23. Cuzick J, Decensi A, Arun B, et al. Preventive therapy for breast cancer: a consensus statement. Lancet Oncol 2011;12:496–503.
24. Forbes JF, Cuzick J, Buzdar A, et al. Effect of anastrozole and tamoxifen as adjuvant treatment for early-stage breast cancer: 100-month analysis of the ATAC trial. Lancet Oncol 2008;9:45–53.
25. Cuzick J. IBIS II: a breast cancer prevention trial in postmenopausal women using the aromatase inhibitor anastrozole. Expert Rev Anticancer Ther 2008;8: 1377–85.
26. Goss PE, Qi S, Josse RG, et al. The steroidal aromatase inhibitor exemestane prevents bone loss in ovariectomized rats. Bone 2004;34:384–92.
27. Goss PE, Ingle JN, Alés-Martínez JE, et al. Exemestane for breast-cancer prevention in postmenopausal women. N Engl J Med 2011;364(25):2381–91.
28. Cheung AM, Tile L, Cardew S, et al. Bone density and structure in healthy postmenopausal women treated with exemestane for the primary prevention of breast cancer: a nested substudy of the MAP.3 randomised controlled trial. Lancet Oncol 2012;13:275–84.
29. Nathan DM, Buse JB, Davidson MB, et al. Medical management of hyperglycaemia in type 2 diabetes mellitus: a consensus algorithm for the initiation and adjustment of therapy: a consensus statement from the American Diabetes Association and the European Association for the Study of Diabetes. Diabetologia 2009;52:17–30.
30. Decensi A, Gennari A. Insulin breast cancer connection: confirmatory data set the stage for better care. J Clin Oncol 2011;29:7–10.
31. Gunter MJ, Hoover DR, Yu H, et al. Insulin, insulin-like growth factor-I, and risk of breast cancer in postmenopausal women. J Natl Cancer Inst 2009;101:48–60.
32. Gonzalez-Angulo AM, Meric-Bernstam F. Metformin: a therapeutic opportunity in breast cancer. Clin Cancer Res 2010;16:1695–700.
33. Alimova IN, Liu B, Fan Z, et al. Metformin inhibits breast cancer cell growth, colony formation and induces cell cycle arrest in vitro. Cell Cycle 2009;8:909–15.
34. Ben Sahra I, Regazzetti C, Robert G, et al. Metformin, independent of AMPK, induces mTOR inhibition and cell-cycle arrest through REDD1. Cancer Res 2011;71:4366–72.
35. Martin M, Marais R. Metformin: a diabetes drug for cancer, or a cancer drug for diabetics? J Clin Oncol 2012;30:2698–700.
36. Decensi A, Puntoni M, Goodwin P, et al. Metformin and cancer risk in diabetic patients: a systematic review and meta-analysis. Cancer Prev Res (Phila) 2010;3:1451–61.
37. Col NF, Ochs L, Springmann V, et al. Metformin and breast cancer risk: a meta-analysis and critical literature review. Breast Cancer Res Treat 2012;135(3): 639–46.

38. Hadad S, Iwamoto T, Jordan L, et al. Evidence for biological effects of metformin in operable breast cancer: a pre-operative, window-of-opportunity, randomized trial. Breast Cancer Res Treat 2011;128:783–94.

39. Jiralerspong S, Palla SL, Giordano SH, et al. Metformin and pathologic complete responses to neoadjuvant chemotherapy in diabetic patients with breast cancer. J Clin Oncol 2009;27:3297–302.

40. Bonanni B, Puntoni M, Cazzaniga M, et al. Dual effect of metformin on breast cancer proliferation in a randomized presurgical trial. J Clin Oncol 2012;30: 2593–600.

41. Chlebowski RT, McTiernan A, Wactawski-Wende J, et al. Diabetes, metformin, and breast cancer in postmenopausal women. J Clin Oncol 2012;30: 2844–52.

42. Dowsett M, Smith IE, Ebbs SR, et al. Prognostic value of Ki67 expression after short-term presurgical endocrine therapy for primary breast cancer. J Natl Cancer Inst 2007;99:167–70.

43. Ellis MJ, Tao Y, Luo J, et al. Outcome prediction for estrogen receptor-positive breast cancer based on postneoadjuvant endocrine therapy tumor characteristics. J Natl Cancer Inst 2008;100:1380–8.

44. Decensi A, Guerrieri-Gonzaga A, Gandini S, et al. Prognostic significance of Ki-67 labeling index after short-term presurgical tamoxifen in women with ER-positive breast cancer. Ann Oncol 2010;22:582–7.

45. Knowler WC, Barrett-Connor E, Fowler SE, et al. Reduction in the incidence of type 2 diabetes with lifestyle intervention or metformin. N Engl J Med 2002; 346:393–403.

46. Bonora E, Kiechl S, Willeit J, et al. Prevalence of insulin resistance in metabolic disorders: the Bruneck Study. Diabetes 1998;47:1643–9.

47. Goodwin PJ, Stambolic V, Lemieux J, et al. Evaluation of metformin in early breast cancer: a modification of the traditional paradigm for clinical testing of anti-cancer agents. Breast Cancer Res Treat 2011;126:215–20.

48. Sharma S, Sharma SC. An update on eicosanoids and inhibitors of cyclooxygenase enzyme systems. Indian J Exp Biol 1997;35:1025–31.

49. Leahy KM, Ornberg RL, Wang Y, et al. Cyclooxygenase-2 inhibition by celecoxib reduces proliferation and induces apoptosis in angiogenic endothelial cells in vivo. Cancer Res 2002;62:625–31.

50. Tsujii M, DuBois RN. Alterations in cellular adhesion and apoptosis in epithelial cells overexpressing prostaglandin endoperoxide synthase 2. Cell 1995;83: 493–501.

51. Kaiser J. Wondering how the wonder drug works. Science 2012;337:1472.

52. Zhao Y, Agarwal VR, Mendelson CR, et al. Estrogen biosynthesis proximal to a breast tumor is stimulated by PGE2 via cyclic AMP, leading to activation of promoter II of the CYP19 (aromatase) gene. Endocrinology 1996;137:5739–42.

53. Brueggemeier RW, Quinn AL, Parrett ML, et al. Correlation of aromatase and cyclooxygenase gene expression in human breast cancer specimens. Cancer Lett 1999;140:27–35.

54. Elvin JA, Yan C, Matzuk MM. Growth differentiation factor-9 stimulates progesterone synthesis in granulosa cells via a prostaglandin E2/EP2 receptor pathway. Proc Natl Acad Sci U S A 2000;97:10288–93.

55. Schreinemachers DM, Everson RB. Aspirin use and lung, colon, and breast cancer incidence in a prospective study. Epidemiology 1994;5:138–46.

56. Harris RE, Namboodiri K, Stellman SD, et al. Breast cancer and NSAID use: heterogeneity of effect in a case-control study. Prev Med 1995;24:119–20.

57. Rosenberg L. Nonsteroidal anti-inflammatory drugs and cancer. Prev Med 1995; 24:107–9.
58. Harris RE, Kasbari S, Farrar WB. Prospective study of nonsteroidal anti-inflammatory drugs and breast cancer. Oncol Rep 1999;6:71–3.
59. Harris RE, Namboodiri KK, Farrar WB. Nonsteroidal antiinflammatory drugs and breast cancer. Epidemiology 1996;7:203–5.
60. Coogan PF, Rao SR, Rosenberg L, et al. The relationship of nonsteroidal anti-inflammatory drug use to the risk of breast cancer. Prev Med 1999;29:72–6.
61. Sharpe CR, Collet JP, McNutt M, et al. Nested case-control study of the effects of non-steroidal anti-inflammatory drugs on breast cancer risk and stage. Br J Cancer 2000;83:112–20.
62. Johnson TW, Anderson KE, Lazovich D, et al. Association of aspirin and nonsteroidal anti-inflammatory drug use with breast cancer. Cancer Epidemiol Biomarkers Prev 2002;11:1586–91.
63. Paganini-Hill A, Chao A, Ross RK, et al. Aspirin use and chronic diseases: a cohort study of the elderly. BMJ 1989;299:1247–50.
64. Egan KM, Stampfer MJ, Giovannucci E, et al. Prospective study of regular aspirin use and the risk of breast cancer. J Natl Cancer Inst 1996;88:988–93.
65. Langman MJ, Cheng KK, Gilman EA, et al. Effect of anti-inflammatory drugs on overall risk of common cancer: case-control study in general practice research database. BMJ 2000;320:1642–6.
66. Harris RE, Chlebowski RT, Jackson RD, et al. Breast cancer and nonsteroidal anti-inflammatory drugs: prospective results from the Women's Health Initiative. Cancer Res 2003;63:6096–101.
67. Cotterchio M, Kreiger N, Sloan M, et al. Nonsteroidal anti-inflammatory drug use and breast cancer risk. Cancer Epidemiol Biomarkers Prev 2001;10:1213–7.
68. Terry MB, Gammon MD, Zhang FF, et al. Association of frequency and duration of aspirin use and hormone receptor status with breast cancer risk. JAMA 2004; 291:2433–40.
69. Holmes MD, Chen WY, Li L, et al. Aspirin intake and survival after breast cancer. J Clin Oncol 2010;28:1467–72.
70. Holmes MD, Chen WY, Schnitt SJ, et al. COX-2 expression predicts worse breast cancer prognosis and does not modify the association with aspirin. Breast Cancer Res Treat 2011;130:657–62.
71. Li Y, Brasky TM, Nie J, et al. Use of nonsteroidal anti-inflammatory drugs and survival following breast cancer diagnosis. Cancer Epidemiol Biomarkers Prev 2012;21:239–42.
72. Rothwell PM, Wilson M, Price JF, et al. Effect of daily aspirin on risk of cancer metastasis: a study of incident cancers during randomised controlled trials. Lancet 2012;379:1591–601.
73. Wald NJ, Morris JK, Law MR. Aspirin in the prevention of cancer. Lancet 2011; 377:1649 [author reply: 1651–2].

Radiation Therapy for Duct Carcinoma in Situ
Who Needs Radiation Therapy, Who Doesn't?

Beryl McCormick, MD

KEYWORDS

- DCIS • Radiation therapy • Breast cancer • Duct carcinoma in situ

KEY POINTS

- Assessing the pathology details.
- Age and presentation of the patient.
- Assessing the patient's expectations from possible radiation therapy.

INTRODUCTION

Duct carcinoma in situ (DCIS) is an early form of breast cancer, which is commonly diagnosed in Western countries with robust screening mammography programs. Of new breast cancers detected through screening, DCIS diagnoses make up 20% to 25% of the total cases.

Women with DCIS have 2 surgical options, simple mastectomy or breast-conservation surgery (BCS). This article focuses on the issue of who benefits from radiation therapy (RT) after BCS. Four large prospective trials have been completed, comparing RT with observation after BCS. The results of the trials are consistent: RT after BCS reduces the risk of an ipsilateral breast cancer recurrence by 50% or more.

So why does the controversy continue about the role of RT in DCIS management? First, the randomized trials also show excellent survival rates, with no differences noted with or without the RT. A University of Michigan study of patients and close family members reported that the benefit of RT in these circumstances is perceived as less important than for invasive carcinomas, which carries both a local control and breast cancer survival benefit from RT.[1]

Second, many physicians also favor the use of no RT in certain subsets of women with DCIS; the several versions of the Van Nuys Prognostic Indices published by Silverstein and colleagues[2–4] received widespread acclaim. Several studies, both of

Radiation Oncology, Memorial Sloan-Kettering Cancer Center, 1275 York Avenue, New York, NY 10065, USA
E-mail address: mccormib@mskcc.org

Hematol Oncol Clin N Am 27 (2013) 673–686
http://dx.doi.org/10.1016/j.hoc.2013.05.001
hemonc.theclinics.com

the registry and the prospective randomized trial design, have opened over the last decade, focused on identifying women who may not benefit from the addition of RT for their DCIS, because their risk of local recurrence (LR) is so low.

Of LR in DCIS studies, about one-half are recurrence of DCIS and one-half are invasive ductal carcinoma. Predictors of which patients are destined to develop the invasive recurrences would enhance decision making regarding the role of RT, but thus far remain the subject of ongoing research.[5–7]

THE ASYMPTOMATIC PATIENT

Most women with DCIS present without any symptoms. The disease is identified either through a screening study such as a mammogram, or as an incidental finding for a biopsy performed for another indication. Some of these women may be at a relatively low risk for LR. Although the addition of radiation lowers the risk of local failure in all subsets of DCIS, some patient subsets, identified by disease characteristics, age at presentation, and other factors, may start out with a relatively low risk for local failure, and may be considered for no RT, because the absolute benefit is so small.

Grade, Size, and Other Disease Factors

Two groups of pathologists were the first to suggest that low-grade DCIS could be treated by excision alone. Both Betsill and Rosen at Memorial Sloan-Kettering Cancer Center (MSKCC) and Page at Vanderbilt retrospectively identified pathology specimens from women that had been signed out as benign but on re-review showed low-grade DCIS. The women had no planned treatment, just the biopsy, and both studies were designed to track down the patients and study the natural history of low-grade DCIS.[5,6] Page updated the results of the 28 women in his study, with a median interval of 24 years in those who did not develop breast cancer. **Fig. 1** shows those results; the risk of developing invasive breast cancer in those women was 9.10 times greater than women in the general population. Page and colleagues[6] discuss offering these women treatment with a wide excision only, processed with the careful attention to details that modern pathology laboratories use. The results of both studies were similar, and contributed to the controversy concerning which patients need RT.

Silverstein and colleagues[2] published their first version of the Van Nuys Prognostic Index in 1996; this scoring system incorporated grade, presence of necrosis, tumor size, and margin width to calculate a score predicting which patients with a diagnosis of DCIS would be at highest risk for recurrence and thus should benefit from whole-breast RT after BCS (**Fig. 2**). The score was developed from and then

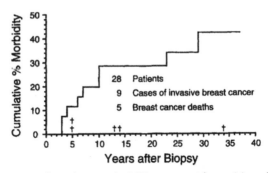

Fig. 1. Results of Page study on low-grade DCIS treatment by excision alone.

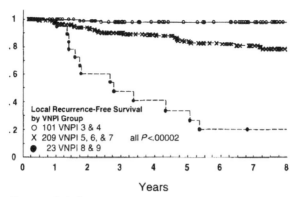

Fig. 2. Van Nuys Prognostic Index.

tested in the same group of patients, those operated on by Dr Silverstein's group in Van Nuys, California. RT was used in some but not all cases. In our own pathology material at MSKCC, we attempted to apply the Van Nuys score to recent cases, but had issues primarily because size is not easily calculated in many DCIS cases. But Silverstein's work was useful as a starting place to define which subsets of DCIS can be identified that may be at very low risk for LR.

Although none of the 4 large prospective trials comparing RT with no RT specifically was designed around the details of pathology subtypes, several of the trials retrospectively looked at pathology and LR. Pathology review of 623 of 814 patients in the NSABP (National Surgical Adjuvant Breast and Bowel Project) B-17 trial[7] was completed for the characteristics shown in **Table 1**. The investigators concluded that many of the factors were related, and further multivariant analysis showed that comedo necrosis was the "significant predictor for ipsilateral breast" LR. But the investigators observed a benefit for RT in each risk group, including the lowest-risk groups.

The similar European Organisation for Research and Treatment of Cancer (EORTC) DCIS trial also performed a central pathology review of most of the women enrolled in the trial. **Table 2** shows the hazard ratios in the various pathology subsets, with well-differentiated histology, clinging or micropapillary architecture, and free margins all associated with the lowest risk of local failure. The randomized treatment arm (ie, RT versus no RT) also was highly significantly associated with risk of LR. The investigators stated that although RT benefited all subsets, in the well-differentiated DCIS with clinging or micropapillary growth, the LR at 10 years was less than 10%, and thus the absolute benefit for the RT was small.[8]

Another trial, the UKCCCR (UK Coordinating Committee on Cancer Research)/ANZ study from the United Kingdom, Australia and New Zealand, randomized 1701 women

Table 1 Study information			
Variable	Lumpectomy	Lumpectomy and Radiotherapy	All Patients
Randomized	405	413	818
Ineligible	6	12	18
No follow-up	2	2	4
Patients included in analysis	403	411	814

Table 2
Multivariate analysis of risk factors related to LR

Variable	Hazard Ratio	95% Confidence Interval	P Value
Age (y)			
>40	1		
≤40	1.89	1.12–3.19	.026
Method of detection			
Radiograph finding only	1		
Clinical symptoms	1.55	1.11–2.16	.012
Histologic type			
Well	1		
Intermediate	1.85	1.18–2.90	.024
Poor	1.61	0.93–2.79	
Architecture			
Clinging/micropapillary	1		
Cribriform	2.39	1.41–4.03	.002
Solid/comedo	2.25	1.21–4.18	
Margins			
Free	1		
Not free	1.84	1.32–2.56	.0005
Treatment			
Local excision + radiotherapy	1		
Local excision	1.82	1.33–2.49	.0002

to receive RT and tamoxifen, RT only, tamoxifen only, or no treatment. **Fig. 3** is a Forest plot for new breast events, with RT and without RT, stratified by tamoxifen use. The study later performed a pathology review on most of the patients, and also concluded that "high grade, large size and young age were significant predictors" for a high LR (see later discussion). This cooperative group proposed a new pathology system for DCIS based on their pathology findings. The subsets at lowest risk for LR were the women with the low-grade and intermediate-grade lesions. In addition to classic high-grade lesions associated with a higher risk of LR, the group proposed a new definition of "very high grade" lesions to include DCIS with greater than 50% solid architecture, and with comedo-type necrosis involving more than 50% of the ducts.[9,10]

The SweDCIS trial[11] is the fourth prospective randomized trial comparing RT with no RT; because of the health care system in Sweden providing mammograms, almost all of the women enrolled had only mammographic findings. With a shorter median follow-up time than the other studies, of just more than 5 years, those enrolled in the RT arm had a hazard ratio of 0.33 for LR compared with those in the observation arm. There was also central pathology review, but primarily to confirm the diagnosis of DCIS.

Margin Issues

The width of the surgical margin is another pathology feature associated with the LR rate. Silverstein and colleagues[3] were the first to suggest this factor, in their 1999 version of the Van Nuys Prognostic Index. They categorized margin width as follows: less than

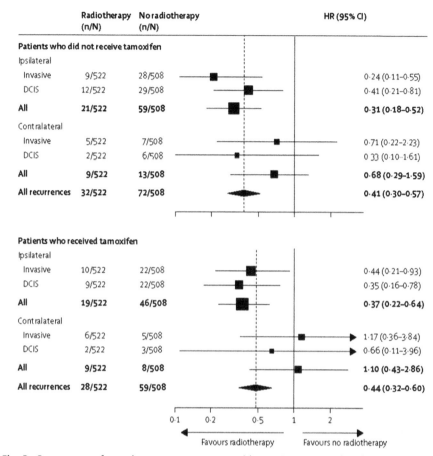

	Radiotherapy (n/N)	No radiotherapy (n/N)		HR (95% CI)
Patients who did not receive tamoxifen				
Ipsilateral				
Invasive	9/522	28/508		0·24 (0·11–0·55)
DCIS	12/522	29/508		0·41 (0·21–0·81)
All	21/522	59/508		0·31 (0·18–0·52)
Contralateral				
Invasive	5/522	7/508		0·71 (0·22–2·23)
DCIS	2/522	6/508		0·33 (0·10–1·61)
All	9/522	13/508		0·68 (0·29–1·59)
All recurrences	32/522	72/508		0·41 (0·30–0·57)
Patients who received tamoxifen				
Ipsilateral				
Invasive	10/522	22/508		0·44 (0·21–0·93)
DCIS	9/522	22/508		0·35 (0·16–0·78)
All	19/522	46/508		0·37 (0·22–0·64)
Contralateral				
Invasive	6/522	5/508		1·17 (0·36–3·84)
DCIS	2/522	3/508		0·66 (0·11–3·96)
All	9/522	8/508		1·10 (0·43–2·86)
All recurrences	28/522	59/508		0·44 (0·32–0·60)

Favours radiotherapy   Favours no radiotherapy

Fig. 3. Occurrence of new breast events measured by patients treated with tamoxifen.

1 mm, 1 mm to 10 mm, and 10 mm or greater. In **Figs. 4–6**, the LR rate is shown within these margin categories with and without RT. The investigators concluded that RT did not benefit any of the patients, except those with margin widths of less than 1 mm.

Based in part on the results of the Van Nuys group, a prospective trial for observation only after BCS for women with low-grade or intermediate-grade DCIS, not exceeding 2.5 cm in size, and excised with margins of 1 cm or larger, or with a reexcision showing no residual DCIS, was opened at the Dana Farber Cancer Center and Harvard Hospitals. The accrual goal was 200 women, but the study was closed after just 158 patients were enrolled, because the LR rate passed the stopping rules of the study. With a median follow-up time of 40 months, the projected LR rate at 5 years was 12%.[12] It is hypothesized that the different results without RT, between the Van Nuys and Harvard studies, may reflect more aggressive surgery in Van Nuys.

Two other studies were also opened, from the Eastern Cooperative Oncology Group (ECOG) and Radiation Therapy Oncology Group (RTOG) cooperative trials. Both studies were designed around defining a low-risk group of women with DCIS diagnoses, who may not need RT. The ECOG study was observational; in the low-grade stratum, patients were eligible if they had low-grade or intermediate-grade DCIS, no larger than 2.5 cm, excised with a minimum margin width of 3 mm. In the high-grade stratum,

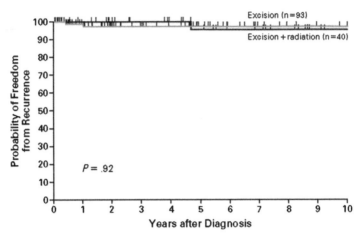

Fig. 4. Van Nuys Prognostic Index with <1 mm, 1 mm to 10 mm, and >10 mm LR rate.

patients were eligible if they had high-grade DCIS measuring 1 cm or less, and excised with the same minimum margin width of 3 mm. **Fig. 7** shows the LR rate in the low-grade group, compared with the rate of a contralateral breast event in the same patient. At 7 years, 10.5% of women had an ipsilateral LR. The addition of RT would be expected to decrease that LR rate by half, so for some women and physicians, this may not be a large enough benefit to justify the treatment with RT. In the high-grade group, as noted in **Fig. 8**, the LR rate was 18% in the ipsilateral breast; the investigators concluded that "excision alone is inadequate treatment" for this high-grade group.[13] Approximately 30% of all women in these studies also took tamoxifen.

The RTOG study had similar entry criteria as the low-grade stratum of the ECOG study, namely, no symptoms, low or intermediate grade, size 2.5 cm or less, and a minimal margin width of 3 mm. Patients were stratified by tamoxifen use (62%) and age (<50 or >50 years), and then randomized to whole-breast RT or observation. The study did not meet accrual goals and was closed with 636 patients, followed for a median of 7 years. The LR rate in the RT arm was 0.9%, and in the observation arm, 6.4%. This difference in LR between the 2 studies (ECOG with a 10.5% LR rate

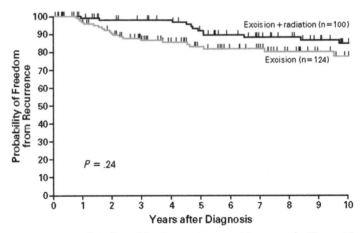

Fig. 5. Van Nuys Prognostic Index with <1 mm, 1 mm to 10 mm, and >10 mm LR rate.

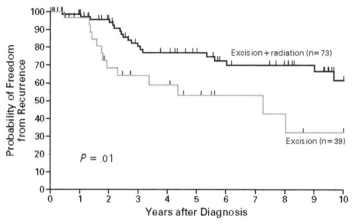

Fig. 6. Van Nuys Prognostic Index with <1 mm, 1 mm to 10 mm, and >10 mm LR rate.

and RTOG with 6.4%) may in part be related to tamoxifen use, which is discussed later.[14]

Age

The relationship of young age to LR for women with DCIS has been observed in numerous retrospective trials. The EBCTCG (Early Breast Cancer Trialists'

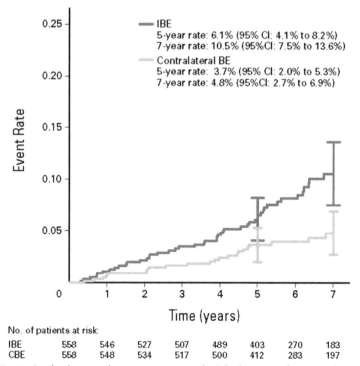

Fig. 7. LR rate in the low-grade group, compared with the rate of a contralateral breast event in the same patient.

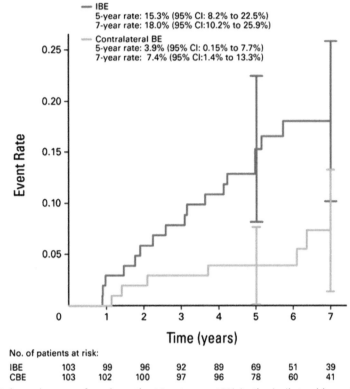

Fig. 8. High-grade group for whom the LR rate was 18% in the ipsilateral breast.

Collaborative Group) published an overview of the 4 prospective randomized DCIS trials discussed earlier[15] and, in addition to confirming that the addition of RT reduced the risk of LR in all subsets of DCIS, found a significant relationship between age at diagnosis and LR. This trial defined age as less than or greater than 50 years. **Fig. 9**

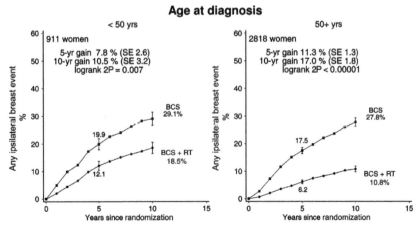

Fig. 9. DCIS relationship between age at diagnosis and LR.

shows those data, with the risk of an LR both with RT or without, higher in those younger than age 50 years.

The French Cancer Centers pooled their retrospective data for women with DCIS, also noting the effect of age on the risk of local failure. They grouped women as younger than 40 years, 40 to 60 years, and older than 60 years. **Table 3** shows their data with a median follow-up time of 7 years, by these age groups and the quality of the excision. The increase in LR is especially noted in those younger than 40 years.[16] Similar results relating young age to LR using this age scheme were also shown by the group at MSKCC, with and without RT.[17]

Markers for Predicting Recurrence

Predicting which patients with a diagnosis of DCIS are at highest risk for an LR, particularly an invasive LR, would be helpful information in making a recommendation for the use of RT after BCS. A research group from the University of California in San Francisco conducted a case-control study of 1162 women diagnosed with DCIS who were treated with BCS but no RT. When follow-up information was obtained, those with an LR were designated the case subjects, and those without as the controls. The investigators were also able to obtain the tumor tissue blocks for 72 women with an invasive LR, 71 with a DCIS LR, and 186 controls who did not recur. These samples were then tested for a panel of biomarkers. **Table 4** shows the final multivariable model, which incorporated both markers and clinical information, as well as grade and margin width. For those women with an invasive LR, detection by palpation was associated with the highest hazard ratio. For those with a DCIS LR, several marker groups appeared strong predictors for this event.[18] To the best of my knowledge, this marker evaluation is not yet in clinical use.

In December 2011, Solin[19] reported on a new real-time polymerase chain reaction assay developed by Genomic Health. The company used tissue from the ECOG observation study mentioned earlier, and reported on patient outcomes from that same study. This new assay used 12 of the 21 genes in the widely used Oncotype Score for invasive cancer. The investigators reported that the gene score, divided into high-risk, intermediate-risk, and low-risk subsets and with a 10-year follow-up, was able to predict both LR and invasive LR in the patients in the study. However, the new assay is not yet validated in another patient group, and Solin's presentation not yet published. The LR rate at 10 years for those with a low score was 12%. For

Table 3			
Local failure rates according to significant Cox factors			
Age (y)	Quality Excision	Conservative Surgery + Radiotherapy Number (%)	Conservative Surgery Number (%)
<40	Complete	6/25 (24)	3/7 (43)
	Incomplete/doubtful	5/9 (56)	0/0
	Not specified	2/6 (33.3)	1/4 (25)
40–59	Complete	24/233 (10)	10/40 (25)
	Incomplete/doubtful	15/63 (24)	10/17 (59)
	Not specified	3/38 (8)	18/65 (28)
>60	Complete	9/102 (9)	5/23 (22)
	Incomplete/doubtful	2/25 (8)	3/6 (50)
	Not specified	0/14 (0)	9/28 (32)
Total		66/515 (13)	59/190 (31)

Table 4
Hazard ratios (HRs) and 95% confidence intervals from final multivariable models of clinical and histopathologic characteristics and molecular markers independently associated with subsequent tumor events

Variable	Hazard Ratio (95% Confidence Interval)
Invasive cancer	
Age at diagnosis (y)	1.0 (0.8–1.3)
Detection by palpation (vs mammography)[a]	2.7 (1.4–5.5)
Nuclear grade	
High vs low	1.0 (0.4–2.3)
Intermediate vs low	1.9 (0.8–4.3)
p16/COX-2/Ki67	
Positive/positive/positive	2.2 (1.1–4.5)
All other groupings	1.0 (referent)
DCIS	
Age at diagnosis (y)	0.9 (0.7–1.1)
Margins ordinal (per category increase)[b]	1.3 (1.1–1.7)
Nuclear grade	
High vs low	1.7 (0.6–4.8)
Intermediate vs low	1.3 (0.4–4.1)
p16/COX-2/Ki67	
Positive/negative/positive	3.7 (1.7–7.9)
All other groupings	1.0 (referent)
ER/ERBB2/Ki67	
Negative/positive/positive	5.8 (2.4–14)
All other groupings	1.0 (referent)

Abbreviations: COX-2, cyclooxygenase 2; ER, estrogen receptor; ERBB2, human epidermal growth factor receptor 2 (HER2/neu-oncoprotein).
[a] Palpable mass found by the woman or by her physician on physical examination.
[b] Margins ordinal defined as margin ≥10 mm disease free = 0; margin ≥2 to <10 mm disease free = 1; margin 1–1.9 mm disease free = 2; margin uncertain = 3; margin positive = 4.

some patients and their physicians, that LR may still be viewed as high enough to consider radiation after BCS.

THE PATIENT WITH DCIS WITH SYMPTOMS

The patient who has her DCIS present with symptoms is not a good candidate for BCS without RT. The NSABP group first reported that method of detection, that is, clinical examination findings versus mammographic finding only, increased the rate of LR for women in both arms of the B-17 study.[7] In the EORTC 10853 trial for DCIS, presentation with clinical symptoms increased the hazard ratio for LR to 1.55.[8] Not surprisingly, this same relationship was observed in the EBCTCG DCIS overview, as seen in **Fig. 10.**[15]

THE ESTROGEN RECEPTOR, TAMOXIFEN, AND RT

The NSABP Cooperative Group was the first to report a benefit of 5 years of tamoxifen with whole-breast radiation, compared with RT treatment alone. Allred and

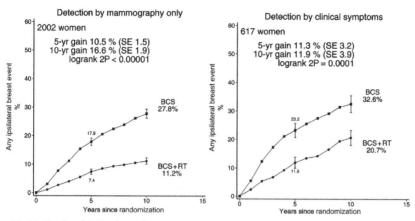

Fig. 10. Methods of DCIS detection.

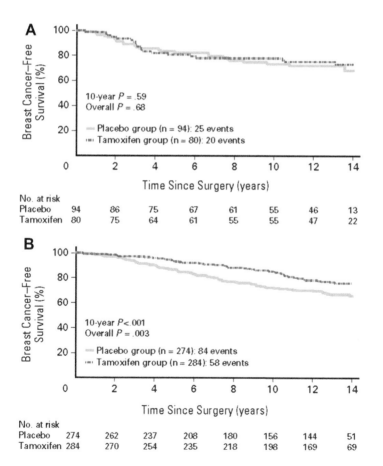

Fig. 11. Tamoxifen was confined to those women whose DCIS was positive for ER. ER-negative patients (*A*) and ER-positive patients (*B*).

colleagues[20] later confirmed this benefit of tamoxifen was confined to those women whose DCIS was positive for the estrogen receptor (ER). These data are shown in **Fig. 11**, with the ER-negative patients in the A graph, and the ER-positive patients in the B graph. Both ipsilateral and contralateral events were included.

For a woman with a low-risk breast cancer considering not having RT after BCS, the possible benefit of tamoxifen is less well defined. In the UKCCCR/ANZ trial, women not assigned to receive RT had a reduction in the risk of ipsilateral LR, when randomized to receive tamoxifen. As discussed earlier, both the RTOG and the ECOG trials also suggest a benefit for tamoxifen alone after BCS.

RT TECHNIQUE

For those women receiving RT, whole-breast RT remains the standard of care. The 4 large prospective trials used a dose of 50 Gy over 5 weeks; none of the trials required the use of an additional boost dose to the lumpectomy site. The RTOG 9804 trial did allow for the shorter-course, hypofractionated RT, to allow participation by Canadian centers. A dose of 42.5 Gy was delivered in 16 fractions, or just more than 3 weeks of treatment time. With 7 years of follow-up, there seems to be no disadvantage to this shorter RT course.[14] Again, no boost was allowed in the RTOG trial.

Formenti and colleagues reported on the use of a similar hypofractionated RT (42 Gy in 15 fractions) for women with DCIS. They concluded that "accelerated hypofractionation regimens of RT is a viable option for DCIS." The use of a boost in some of their patients did not seem to affect the risk of LR.[21]

SUMMARY

DCIS is a common but non–life-threatening breast cancer, usually found through mammographic screening programs. Four large prospective randomized trials comparing RT with no RT after BCS have all concluded that the use of RT reduces the risk of an LR in the ipsilateral breast by at least 50%.

However, the risk of an LR for an individual patient varies by age, presentation of the cancer, grade and other disease characteristics, size, and margin results. As well, the patient's perception of risk needs to be considered in finalizing a decision to recommend RT after BCS or simply observation.

In my practice, I consider the no-RT option for women who present with no symptoms, and who are 50 years of age or older. I also look at the pathology details. There should be no high-grade DCIS anywhere in the specimen, and I use the ECOG and RTOG trial guidelines, specifying a size not exceeding 2.5 cm and a minimum margin width of 3 mm. For any patient not fitting these DCIS characteristics, I firmly recommend a course of whole-breast RT, without a boost.

More information is needed to assess the role of antiestrogen therapy when RT is not given. In the future, when markers are validated to predict which patients will have an invasive LR versus another DCIS or no LR, it is hoped that the discussion with the patient will clarify the situation further.

REFERENCES

1. Hayman JA, Kabeto MU, Schipper MJ, et al. Assessing the benefit of radiation therapy after breast-conserving surgery for ductal carcinoma-in-situ. J Clin Oncol 2005;23:5171–7.
2. Silverstein MJ, Lagios MD, Craig PH, et al. A prognostic index for ductal carcinoma in situ of the breast. Cancer 1996;77:2267–74.

3. Silverstein MJ, Lagios MD, Groshen S, et al. The influence of margin width on local control of ductal carcinoma in situ of the breast. N Engl J Med 1999;340: 1455–61.
4. Silverstein MJ. The University of Southern California/Van Nuys prognostic index for ductal carcinoma in situ of the breast. Am J Surg 2003;186:337–43.
5. Betsill WL Jr, Rosen PP, Lieberman PH, et al. Intraductal carcinoma. Long-term follow-up after treatment by biopsy alone. JAMA 1978;239:1863–7.
6. Page DL, Dupont WD, Rogers LW, et al. Continued local recurrence of carcinoma 15–25 years after a diagnosis of low grade ductal carcinoma in situ of the breast treated only by biopsy. Cancer 1995;76:1197–200.
7. Fisher B, Dignam J, Wolmark N, et al. Lumpectomy and radiation therapy for the treatment of intraductal breast cancer: findings from National Surgical Adjuvant Breast and Bowel Project B-17. J Clin Oncol 1998;16:441–52.
8. Bijker N, Meijnen P, Peterse JL, et al. Breast-conserving treatment with or without radiotherapy in ductal carcinoma-in-situ: ten-year results of European Organisation for Research and Treatment of Cancer randomized phase III trial 10853–a study by the EORTC Breast Cancer Cooperative Group and EORTC Radiotherapy Group. J Clin Oncol 2006;24:3381–7.
9. Cuzick J, Sestak I, Pinder SE, et al. Effect of tamoxifen and radiotherapy in women with locally excised ductal carcinoma in situ: long-term results from the UK/ANZ DCIS trial. Lancet Oncol 2011;12:21–9.
10. Pinder SE, Duggan C, Ellis IO, et al. A new pathological system for grading DCIS with improved prediction of local recurrence: results from the UKCCCR/ANZ DCIS trial. Br J Cancer 2010;103:94–100.
11. Emdin SO, Granstrand B, Ringberg A, et al. SweDCIS: radiotherapy after sector resection for ductal carcinoma in situ of the breast. Results of a randomised trial in a population offered mammography screening. Acta Oncol 2006;45: 536–43.
12. Wong JS, Kaelin CM, Troyan SL, et al. Prospective study of wide excision alone for ductal carcinoma in situ of the breast. J Clin Oncol 2006;24:1031–6.
13. Hughes LL, Wang M, Page DL, et al. Local excision alone without irradiation for ductal carcinoma in situ of the breast: a trial of the Eastern Cooperative Oncology Group. J Clin Oncol 2009;27:5319–24.
14. McCormick B, Moughan J, Hudis C, et al. Low-risk breast ductal carcinoma in situ (DCIS) Results from the Radiation Therapy Oncology Group 9804 phase 3 trial. ASTRO Meeting. Boston, October 28, 2012.
15. Early Breast Cancer Trialists' Collaborative Group (EBCTCG). Overview of the randomized trials of radiotherapy in ductal carcinoma in situ of the breast. J Natl Cancer Inst Monogr 2010;2010:162–77.
16. Cutuli B, Cohen-Solal-le Nir C, de Lafontan B, et al. Breast-conserving therapy for ductal carcinoma in situ of the breast: the French Cancer Centers' experience. Int J Radiat Oncol Biol Phys 2002;53:868–79.
17. Van Zee KJ, Liberman L, Samli B, et al. Long term follow-up of women with ductal carcinoma in situ treated with breast-conserving surgery: the effect of age. Cancer 1999;86:1757–67.
18. Kerlikowske K, Molinaro AM, Gauthier ML, et al. Biomarker expression and risk of subsequent tumors after initial ductal carcinoma in situ diagnosis. J Natl Cancer Inst 2010;102:627–37.
19. Solin L. Evolving strategies in the management of DCIS of the breast. 29th Annual Symposium, New York Metropolitan Breast Cancer Group, New York, February 4, 2012.

20. Allred DC, Anderson SJ, Paik S, et al. Adjuvant tamoxifen reduces subsequent breast cancer in women with estrogen receptor-positive ductal carcinoma in situ: a study based on NSABP protocol B-24. J Clin Oncol 2012;30:1268–73.
21. Ciervide R, Dhage S, Guth A, et al. Five year outcome of 145 patients with ductal carcinoma in situ (DCIS) after accelerated breast radiotherapy. Int J Radiat Oncol Biol Phys 2012;83:e159–64.

Management of the Axilla

Farin Amersi, MD, Armando E. Giuliano, MD*

KEYWORDS

- Axillary node dissection • Sentinel lymph node biopsy • ACOSOG Z0010
- ACOSOG Z0011

KEY POINTS

- The presence of axillary nodal metastasis in breast cancer is the most important predictor of survival and recurrence.
- Sentinel lymph node biopsy (SLNB) allows accurate axillary staging of patients with invasive breast cancer and a clinically negative axilla.
- SLNB has replaced axillary lymph node dissection for staging of the axilla.
- SLNB has less morbidity and fewer complications than standard axillary lymph node dissection.
- Completion axillary lymph node dissection can be avoided in patients with a positive sentinel lymph node who undergo lumpectomy, whole-breast radiation, and systemic therapy.

INTRODUCTION

Over the past 3 decades, there have been significant advances in the surgical and clinical management of patients with breast cancer. Screening mammography, advances in both systemic and radiation therapy, the implementation of breast-conserving surgery, and the use of sentinel lymph node biopsy (SLNB) have substantially affected the care of patients with breast cancer.

The presence or absence of lymph node metastasis and the number of positive lymph nodes with metastasis determines the pathologic stage of the patient. Axillary lymph node metastasis remains the most important predictor of overall recurrence and survival in patients with breast cancer.[1–5] However, the value of axillary lymph node dissection (ALND) has been an area of controversy for more than a decade. The prognostic information gained from an ALND had been deemed so important that removal of clinically uninvolved lymph nodes was widely viewed as a procedure for complete axillary staging and improved local control, with no

Division of Surgical Oncology, Department of Surgery, Cedars-Sinai Medical Center, Samuel Oschin Comprehensive Cancer Institute, Saul and Joyce Brandman Breast Center, 310 North San Vicente Boulevard, 3rd Floor, Los Angeles, CA 90048, USA
* Corresponding author.
E-mail address: armando.giuliano@cshs.org

Hematol Oncol Clin N Am 27 (2013) 687–702
http://dx.doi.org/10.1016/j.hoc.2013.05.002
0889-8588/13/$ – see front matter © 2013 Elsevier Inc. All rights reserved.

measurable survival benefit.[6,7] More recently, decisions by medical oncologists to initiate adjuvant chemotherapy are now individualized and are no longer limited to patients with nodal involvement but include characteristics of the primary tumor including tumor size, grade, histologic subtype, lymphovascular invasion, and receptor status.

ALND has been associated with significant short-term and long-term morbidity including increased risk of infection, pain, cosmetic deformity, and occasionally injury to major vessels or motor nerves. Significant lymphedema may occur early after surgery or years later, with some studies reporting an incidence as high as 30%.[8–10] Because the use of screening mammography has increased over the last few decades, the size of the primary breast lesion has continued to decrease, as did the number of patients who had axillary metastases. For all these reasons, the appeal of a smaller operation as an alternative to ALND for patients with node-negative breast cancer was entertained. This minimally invasive procedure using a vital blue dye to identify the sentinel node, which is the lymph node most likely to harbor metastases, was developed. Patients with early-stage breast cancer could be spared the morbidity and complications without compromising prognostic information.

HISTORY OF BREAST SLNB

The concepts of the spread of metastatic cancer cells in reproducible patterns and the role of lymph nodes as a barrier to distant metastatic spread were established in the 1940s.[11,12] The understanding of a single draining lymph node representing a nodal basin dates back more than half a century. Virchow node for metastatic gastric cancer, Sister Mary Joseph nodule for metastatic intra-abdominal malignancies, and the Delphian node of the thyroid all represent this concept.[13–15] In 1951, Gould and colleagues[16] reported on a frozen section of a single lymph node during a parotidectomy, and on performing a radical neck dissection only if pathology confirmed metastatic disease in this single lymph node. This concept of lymphatic drainage to a single node was subsequently reported in penile cancer and testicular cancer.[17,18] Morton and colleagues[19] developed lymphatic mapping and SLNB as a staging procedure for patients with early-stage melanoma. They defined the sentinel lymph node (SLN) as the first lymph node within the nodal basin to which the primary tumor drains. The SLN was localized by either an intradermal injection with radiolabeled colloid, or vital blue dye, or both together, and strongly predicted the status of the remaining lymph nodes in that basin. This technique was subsequently modified and applied to breast cancer by Giuliano and colleagues[20] in 1991. Their initial experience, which defined the technical aspects, criteria for selecting patients for SLNB, and feasibility, involved 174 patients with T1 to T3 breast cancers, and included patients with or without palpable axillary adenopathy. Using a peritumoral injection of 5 mL of 1% isosulfan blue dye (Lymphazurin), the technique identified SLNs in 114 of the 174 procedures (66%) and accurately predicted the tumor status of the axillary basin in 109 (96%) patients.

The SLNB technique was then prospectively evaluated in 162 clinically node-negative patients with T1 or T2 breast cancers who underwent SLNB followed by ALND compared with 134 patients who only had ALND.[21] The SLNs were analyzed using both hematoxylin and eosin staining (HE) and immunohistochemistry (IHC). A significantly higher rate of detection of metastases was shown in the group that had an SLNB followed by completion ALND than in the group that only had ALND (42% vs 29%), suggesting that a more focused examination of 1 or 2 SLNs was more accurate than the histopathologic evaluation of the lymph node basin by HE alone. Micrometastases were found in 3% of all patients who had ALND and 16% of all patients who had SLNB because of the analysis of a smaller volume of tissue and the addition of IHC analysis. SLNB provides the pathologist with the tissue most likely to contain metastases so that it can be the focus for intense study through multiple sectioning and IHC analyses rather than the large volume of tissue in an ALND that is processed through routine HE staining.

Other investigators subsequently validated the SLNB technique in breast cancer. Albertini and colleagues[22] published the first use of both blue dye and filtered technetium-colloid for identifying the SLN, followed by completion ALND. Of the 62 patients in this study, the SLN was successfully identified in 92% of the patients with 100% specificity. Veronesi and colleagues[23] performed the procedure using a subdermal injection of technetium 99m (^{99m}Tc) –labeled human serum albumin and reported a 98% success rate in 160 of 163 patients, and accurately predicted the axillary status in 97% of the cases. These studies subsequently led to the first multicenter trial of 443 patients who had SLNB followed by ALND using radiotracer alone, which reported identification of the SLN in 93% of the cases, with a false-negative rate of 11.4%.[24] A meta-analysis of 11 published studies was performed with 912 patients and compared injection techniques with lymphoscintigraphy or blue dye, or a combination of both, in patients who had SLNB followed by ALND for in situ and invasive cancer.[25] This study reported a significantly higher rate of identification if both radiocolloid and blue dye were used or radiocolloid alone compared with blue dye alone. Moreover, the SLN reflected the status of the axilla in 97% of the cases with only a 5% false-negative rate reported. These studies show that the status of the SLN accurately predicts the status of the axillary nodal basin.

Veronesi and colleagues[26] then performed the first randomized trial with 516 patients with T1 randomized to either SLNB followed by ALND or SLNB alone. ALND was only performed if the SLN contained metastases. At a median follow-up of 46 months, both groups of patients had the same incidence of SLN metastases. This early trial showed that SLNB alone could predict axillary nodal metastases with a false-negative rate of SLNB of 8.8% in the group that underwent complete ALND. In addition, patients in the SLNB-only group had less pain and better arm mobility. Moreover, these patients developed no axillary recurrences, had the same survival as patients who underwent ALND, and had axillary lymph nodes that were tumor free.

TECHNICAL ASPECTS OF SLNB

The SLN can be localized by either lymphoscintigraphy with injection of ^{99m}Tc-labeled sulfur colloid, or vital blue, or a combination of both. An advantage of lymphoscintigraphy with radiocolloid is that it identifies drainage to areas away from the standard axillary nodal basin, including supraclavicular, infraclavicular, and internal mammary nodes, which could be sampled or treated with postoperative radiation.[27–29]

Before surgery, patients are injected with 0.5 mL of 0.5 mCi of filtered ^{99m}Tc sulfur colloid radiocolloid into the skin, subdermally, or into the peritumoral parenchyma of the breast. Imaging documents the drainage patterns from the tumor through the lymphatics to the regional lymph nodes. During surgery, a gamma probe emits a signal that is used to guide the surgeon in identification of the sentinel node.

Intraoperative injection of isosulfan blue dye (Lymphazurin 1%) or diluted methylene blue injected subcutaneously or into the breast parenchyma surrounding the tumor migrates to the sentinel node with gentle massage. SLNs are located by visual identification of a blue lymphatic tract or blue stained node. During surgery, if the SLN is not identified, regardless of the technique used, a full ALND should be performed. In addition, any additional palpable nodes that look or feel clinically suspicious should be removed at the time of SLNB.

The SLNB technique may be performed with blue dye, radiocolloid, or both. Previous work has shown that the combination of blue dye and radiocolloid has the highest success rate in sentinel node identification and the lowest false-negative rate.[30] In addition, surgeons decrease their false-negative rates and increase their identification rates as their experience increases.[31] A randomized trial by Morrow and colleagues[32] showed no significant difference in identifying the SLN when patients were randomized to either blue due alone or the combination of blue dye and radiocolloid (86% vs 88%, respectively) for surgeons learning the procedure. A significant predictor of SLN identification in this study was surgeon experience.

Several factors determine the success rate of the SLNB technique. These factors include patient selection, injection technique, addition of massage, and time of the incision. Elderly patients and patients with increased body mass index have been shown to have a decreased rate of SLN identification.[33–35] The combination of blue dye and radioisotope enhances the ability to identify the SLN in all patient groups and may be especially helpful for sentinel node identification in obese or elderly patients.

There is no consensus on the optimal injection technique. Although many groups are proponents of peritumoral injections, controversy exists regarding the most appropriate technique for injection of blue dye or radiocolloid, and individual experience and comfort with a particular technique is the most important factor in successful SLNB.[36–38]

SLNB INDICATIONS

As the indications for adjuvant therapy for patients with breast cancer have evolved over the last decade, SLNB has provided a rational basis for identifying high-risk patients who can benefit from the use of systemic chemotherapy or hormonal therapy. SLNB may provide local control if metastases are limited to the SLN. For patients with early-stage breast cancer, the histopathologic status of the lymph nodes has become one of the deciding factors for or against adjuvant chemotherapy.

Although SLNB has become well accepted in the staging and management of patients with early-stage breast cancer, the role of SLNB in the management of patients with ductal carcinoma in situ (DCIS), previous breast and axillary surgery, clinically palpable axillary disease, neoadjuvant treatment, inflammatory breast cancer, and pregnancy-associated breast cancer continues to be debated (**Table 1**).

Prophylactic Mastectomy

Indications for prophylactic mastectomy have become accepted for patients with increased susceptibility to breast cancer including BRCA-1 and BRCA-2 gene mutation carriers, as well as for cosmesis or phobia of developing breast cancer in patients undergoing a contralateral mastectomy for breast cancer. The risk of finding an occult cancer at the time of a prophylactic mastectomy has been reported to be about 5%; in addition, in patients with a history of breast cancer the risk of developing a contralateral breast cancer is about 0.5% to 1% per year.[39,40] Patients who do not undergo an SLNB at the time of prophylactic mastectomy and are found to have invasive cancer in the breast specimen require an ALND to stage the axilla. If SLNB is performed at the time of prophylactic mastectomy, and final pathology shows an invasive cancer with histologically negative SLNs, the morbidity of an ALND can be avoided. King and

Table 1
Indications for SLNB

Approved Indications	Unapproved Indications
Prophylactic mastectomy	Prior axillary surgery
T1–T2 lesions	T3–T4 lesions
Multicentric tumors	Pregnancy
Male breast cancer	Inflammatory breast cancer
Elderly	After neoadjuvant treatment
Obesity	Suspicious palpable axillary nodes
DCIS with mastectomy	—
Before neoadjuvant treatment	—
Prior breast surgery	—

Adapted from Lyman GH, Giuliano AE, Somerfield MR, et al. American Society of Clinical Oncology guideline recommendations for sentinel lymph node biopsy in early- stage breast cancer. J Clin Oncol 2005;23(30):7703–20.

colleagues[41] reported a series of 163 women at high risk for breast cancer or diagnosed with a contralateral breast cancer who underwent prophylactic mastectomy and SLNB. Occult carcinoma was found in 13 (8%) patients. Two patients who had occult carcinoma also had sentinel nodes positive by HE. In a recent meta-analysis performed by Zhou and colleagues[42] the rate of occult invasive cancers among 1343 pooled prophylactic mastectomies was 1.7%, with a rate of positive SLNs of 1.9%. SLNB may be offered to high-risk patients who choose to undergo prophylactic mastectomies.

Previous Breast or Axillary Surgery

There are no large studies reporting success in identifying SLNs in patients who present with either previous breast or axillary surgery. Many of the large clinical trials excluded patients who had previous breast biopsies or previous axillary surgery.[43,44] Limited small studies suggest that identifying the SLN can be achieved after previous breast biopsies, regardless of the size, location, or the length of time between the initial biopsy and the SLNB procedure.[45,46] Based on clinical experience, a prior breast biopsy is not considered a contraindication to SLNB.

Successful identification of the SLN after previous axillary surgery can be limited because of disruption of lymphatic channels during surgery that can lead to aberrant lymphatic drainage patterns. A small series reported 18 patients who underwent a second SLNB after developed recurrent breast cancer after breast conservation and negative SLNB at their initial surgery.[47] All patients had successful identification of the SLN using preoperative lymphoscintigraphy with 2 patients found to have positive SLNs requiring completion ALND and, of the remaining 16 patients with negative SLNs, no recurrences were reported. In patients with prior axillary surgery, SLNB can be performed; however, both preoperative lymphoscintigraphy and blue dye should be used for optimal identification.

DCIS

By definition, DCIS does not have the ability to metastasize to axillary lymph nodes and so, in theory, should not require axillary staging. The decision to perform an SLNB on patients with a core biopsy showing DCIS is based on the possibility that invasive disease may be found on final pathology. Yen and colleagues[48] reviewed 398 patients with DCIS on core biopsy and found that 20% had invasive disease on subsequent examination of the excised specimen. Multivariate analysis showed 4 independent risk factors for invasive disease: age less than 55 years (odds ratio [OR] 2.19, $P = .024$), diagnosis on core biopsy (OR 3.76, $P = .006$), mammographic size of DCIS greater than 4 cm (OR 2.92, $P = .001$), and high-grade DCIS (OR 3.06, $P = .002$).

American Society of Clinical Oncology (ASCO) guidelines during a consensus conference in 2005 recommended that SLNB should not be done routinely for breast conservation for DCIS, and selective use is recommended for patients undergoing mastectomy, palpable lesions, DCIS larger than 40 mm, or high nuclear grade.

Multicentric Lesions

Multicentric cancer, which is defined as distinct cancers found in different quadrants of the same breast or at a distance of 2 to 5 cm from each other, occurs in approximately 10% of patients. Multicentric tumors have been considered a contraindication to SLNB because it is postulated that different drainage patterns may occur with multiple foci of cancer, increasing the false-negative rate of the procedure. However, there is evidence that the breast may drain through the same afferent lymphatic channels to the same axillary sentinel node.[49] Multiple nonrandomized studies have shown success in identifying SLN with false-negative rates similar to those in patients with unifocal lesions.[50–52] In a large single-institution study by Gentilini and colleagues,[53] a mean number of 1.7 SLNs were found in 337 patients, with an identification rate of 100%. At a median follow-up of 5 years, only 3 of 138 patients (2.2%) developed axillary recurrences after a negative SLNB at their initial surgery. SLNB should be offered to clinically node-negative patients with multicentric disease.

Clinically Palpable Axillary Lymph Nodes

Most SLNB studies have excluded patients with clinically positive axillary lymph nodes. Although ALND is the standard of care in patients with clinically palpable suspicious lymph nodes, determination of metastatic axillary disease by clinical examination is often unreliable. The results of several series show that clinical examination of the axilla, even by experienced surgeons, can be inaccurate with false-positive rates as high as 40%.[54–56] For patients with suspicious nodes on clinical examination, axillary ultrasound and ultrasound-guided core biopsy are reliable techniques in the management of these patients. SLNB is not recommended in patients with gross axillary disease. When performing an SLNB, any lymph node that is clinically suspicious for metastatic disease during surgery because of firm texture or enlarged size must be removed. These nodes should be considered and evaluated as sentinel nodes even if they are not radioactive or blue. SLNB can be performed in patients with nodes clinically suspicious for metastatic disease; however, patients with larger primary tumors or lymphovascular invasion are likely to have nodal metastases and subsequently require ALND. ASCO guidelines recommend against performing SLNB in patients with nodes clinically suspicious for metastases.

Neoadjuvant Chemotherapy

Neoadjuvant chemotherapy for patients with locally advanced breast cancer continues to be debated. The rationale for treating patients with large operable tumors is the potential downstaging of tumors, providing the alternative of breast conservation instead of mastectomy. In addition, studies have shown that neoadjuvant chemotherapy can lead to axillary downstaging.[57,58] The use of SLNB continues to be debated in patients who show a significant reduction in the number of nodes with metastatic disease, or who show a complete response. However, there is currently no evidence that ALND can be avoided in patients who had an axillary lymph node core biopsy that had metastatic disease before neoadjuvant chemotherapy, and has a negative SLN after completion of neoadjuvant chemotherapy.

The feasibility and accuracy of SLNB after neoadjuvant treatment in patients who are clinically node negative and who need axillary staging continues to be debated. For patients with large tumors with a clinically negative axilla who are being considered for neoadjuvant chemotherapy, SLNB is important for decisions on nodal radiation and ALND. The feasibility and accuracy remain controversial because difficulties in identification and retrieval of the SLN caused by fat necrosis and fibrosis, which have been reported after neoadjuvant treatment, can be avoided if the procedure is performed before the initiation of therapy.[59–62]

Several studies show an acceptable identification rate and a low false-negative rate after neoadjuvant therapy in clinically node-negative patients (**Table 2**). The largest multicenter trial showing the feasibility and accuracy of SLNB after neoadjuvant chemotherapy was conducted as part of the National Surgical Adjuvant Breast and Bowel Project (NSABP) B-27 study.[63] In this study, 428 patients were randomized to SLNB with either lymphoscintigraphy, isosulfan blue dye, or a combination of both. Accurate identification of the SLN occurred in 85% of patients; however, the rate of identification of the SLN was significantly higher in the group that underwent SLNB with radiocolloid compared with blue dye or both: 90%, 77%, and 88%, respectively. Of the 323 patients who went on to complete ALND, the SLN was the only involved node in 56% of patients. Moreover, no differences were seen in identification of the SLN based on tumor size or clinical status of the axilla.

There are presently no published randomized trials evaluating the efficacy of SLNB in the setting of neoadjuvant chemotherapy. The American College of Surgeons Oncology Group (ACOSOG) Z1071 trial, which is designed to evaluate patients with T1 to T4 N1 to N2, MO breast cancer who underwent preoperative neoadjuvant

Table 2				
Studies of SNB after neoadjuvant chemotherapy				
Study	**Tumor Stage**	**# Patients**	**% SLN Identification Rate**	**% False-negative**
Nason et al,[71] 2000	2–3	15	87	33
Tafra et al,[72] 2000	1–2	29	93	0
Fernandez et al,[73] 2001	1–4	40	90	20
Haid et al,[74] 2001	1–3	33	88	0
Julian et al,[75] 2002	2–3	34	88	6
Miller et al,[76] 2002	1–4	35	91	0
Piato et al,[77] 2003	1–2	42	98	17
Jones et al,[78] 2005	2–3	36	81	11
Mamounas et al,[63] 2005	1–3	428	85	11
Tanaka et al,[79] 2006	1–2	70	90	5
Lee et al,[80] 2007	2–3	219	78	6
Gimbergues et al,[81] 2008	1–3	129	94	15
Hunt et al,[82] 2009	1–3	575	97	6
Classe et al,[83] 2009	1–3	195	90	12

chemotherapy followed by SLNB and ALND, just closed to accrual. The study evaluates the efficacy of SLNB in women with node-positive breast cancer at initial diagnosis who have an SLNB performed after neoadjuvant chemotherapy. However, this study will not address the more important question of whether there is a need to perform a completion ALND for patients with T1 to T4, N1 to N2 disease who have a negative SLN after neoadjuvant chemotherapy.

CONTRAINDICATIONS TO SNB
Pregnancy-associated Breast Cancer

Patients with pregnancy-associated breast cancer may have a delay in diagnosis because of lactation-associated changes of the breasts and difficulty imaging pregnant patients. These patients usually present with advanced or metastatic disease. Breast conservation can be considered provided radiation can be given postpartum without significant delay. There are no studies that show the safety of lymphatic mapping during pregnancy. Blue dye should not be used in pregnant patients. Systemic chemotherapy can be safely administered after the first trimester of pregnancy.[64] For patients who present with large lesions, or present in the first trimester of pregnancy, ALND is recommended as standard of care for axillary staging, and the extent of breast surgery (ie, breast conservation versus simple mastectomy) is based on the timing of radiation. At present, ASCO guidelines list pregnancy as a contraindication to SLNB.

Inflammatory Breast Cancer

SLNB is not recommended for patients with inflammatory breast cancer because of tumor cells invading and obstructing dermal lymphatics. Unacceptably high false-negative rates have been reported for patients who underwent SLNB for inflammatory breast cancer.[65] ALND should be performed for all patients with this form of breast cancer.

OCCULT METASTASES

The accuracy of SLNB depends on intensive histologic evaluation with serial sectioning of lymph nodes, as well as IHC to enhance detection of micrometastases that may be missed on routine HE staining. The definition of micrometastases has not always been consistent, and some reports have included isolated tumor cells.

The significance of isolated tumor cells as they relate to the risk of additional metastases in nonsentinel nodes, as well as prognosis, remains unclear; however, SLNB is considered adequate surgery for control of locoregional disease. Current ASCO as well as National Comprehensive Cancer Network guidelines recommend completion ALND when micrometastatic disease is found in the SLN. Nodal micrometastases have been used clinically in treatment decisions, by identifying high-risk patients who may be candidates for systemic therapy.

The recent publication of 2 large randomized controlled trials has also changed the perspective on occult metastases in axillary lymph nodes detected by IHC. The multicenter ACOSOG Z0010 trial was designed to determine the association between survival and metastases detected by IHC staining of SLNs and bone marrow specimens from patients with early-stage breast cancer.[66] The study enrolled 5538 patients who underwent lumpectomy and sentinel node biopsy with bilateral iliac crest bone marrow aspiration. Both the bone marrow and histologically negative sentinel nodes were evaluated with IHC in a central laboratory for the presence of micrometastases. The SLN was successfully identified in 5485 women, and histologic sentinel node metastases were found in 1239 (23.9%). IHC identified an additional 349 (10.5%) patients with occult metastases that were negative on HE. Bone marrow metastases were identified by immunocytochemistry in 105 of 3491 (3%) specimens examined. At 5 years, overall survival was 92.8% among women with positive SLN histology and 95.6% with negative histology. By IHC, overall 5-year survival was 95.1% for IHC-positive SLN and 95.8% for IHC-negative SLN. This study showed that the detection of occult micrometastases for T1 to T2 N0M0 disease did not help predict overall survival; however, bone marrow status by IHC significantly predicted decreased 5-year overall survival: 90.2% for positive bone marrow biopsies and 95.1% for those that were negative. The routine examination of an SLN by IHC was not supported in this study.

NSABP B-32 was a prospectively randomized trial designed to compare SLNB with ALND in clinically node-negative patients.[67] In this trial, 5611 patients were randomized to SLNB with immediate axillary dissection (2807 patients) or SNB alone (2804 patients). This trial was designed to evaluate regional control of the axilla, and compared disease-free and overall survival. The technical success rate for identifying the sentinel nodes was reported at 96.2% and there was a false-negative rate of 6.7%. In the SLNB with immediate axillary dissection group, 1978 (70%) patients were SLN negative. Of these patients, 316 (16%) showed occult metastases on further IHC staining. In the SLNB-only group, 2011 (72%) patients were SLN negative. On further IHC staining, 300 (15%) patients showed occult metastases. Five-year Kaplan-Meier estimates of overall survival among patients in whom occult metastases were detected and those without detectable metastases were 94.6% and 95.8%, respectively. Although occult metastasis was an independent prognostic variable in patients with sentinel nodes that were negative on initial examination, the difference in outcome at 5 years was clinically insignificant. These observations are congruent with the conclusions made by the investigators of the ACOSOG Z0010 study.

POSITIVE SLN: COMPLETION ALND?

The necessity of ALND in all patients with metastatic disease to the SLN has been also been questioned. NSABP B-04 randomized clinically node-negative patients to modified radical mastectomy, total mastectomy with axillary irradiation, or total mastectomy without axillary treatment.[68] Of the patients who underwent ALND, 38% had axillary metastases. Of these women, less than 50% developed clinically evident axillary recurrences. In this study, women did not receive adjuvant systemic therapy, thus negating the theory that adjuvant treatment accounted for the lack of progression of disease.

Giuliano and colleagues[69,70] recently performed a multicenter randomized trial (ACOSOG Z0011) to answer this question. Women with T1 to T2 breast cancer with no palpable axillary lymphadenopathy were randomized after a breast conservation with 1 to 2 SLNBs that showed metastatic disease by HE to completion ALND (445 patients) followed by tangential whole-breast radiation with no axillary radiation or no further axillary surgery (446 patients) and tangential whole-breast radiation (Fig. 1). Most of the women in this study received whole-breast radiation (89.6% SLNB, 88.9% ALND), and adjuvant systemic therapy was given at the discretion of the treating physician, with 97% of patients in the SLNB group and 96% in the ALND group receiving adjuvant treatment. The median number of lymph nodes removed was 2 in the SLNB group and 17 in the ALND group. In the group that underwent completion ALND, 27% of patients had additional nodal metastases.

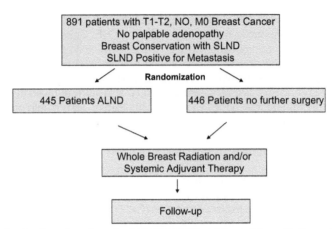

Fig. 1. Randomization of patients in ACOSOG Z0011. (*Adapted from* Giuliano AE, Hunt KK, Ballman KV, et al. Axillary dissection vs no axillary dissection in women with invasive breast cancer and sentinel node metastasis: a randomized clinical trial. JAMA 2011;305:569–75; with permission.)

With a median follow-up of 6 years, the study reported no survival advantage with the use of ALND compared with SLNB alone. Five-year survival overall was 91.8% for women who underwent ALND versus 92.5% for those who had SLNB alone (**Fig. 2**). There was also no statistically significant difference in axillary recurrence between the two groups (0.5% in the ALND group and 0.9% in the SLNB group). In addition, the disease-free survival did not differ significantly between the groups (**Fig. 3**). On multivariate analysis, only older age, estrogen-receptor status, and lack of adjuvant systemic therapy were associated with worse overall survival. This study showed that SLNB alone was not inferior to SLNB followed by ALND for women with HE-detected SLN metastases. These results indicate that women with 1 to 2 SLNs with metastatic disease who undergo breast conservation with radiation therapy followed by systemic therapy do not benefit from further axillary surgery with regard to local control, disease-free survival, or overall survival. These findings are not

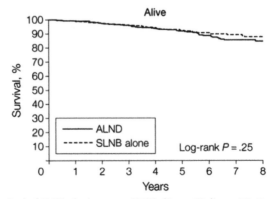

Fig. 2. Overall survival of SLNB alone versus ALND. (*From* Giuliano AE, Hunt KK, Ballman KV, et al. Axillary dissection vs no axillary dissection in women with invasive breast cancer and sentinel node metastasis: a randomized clinical trial. JAMA 2011;305:569–75; with permission.)

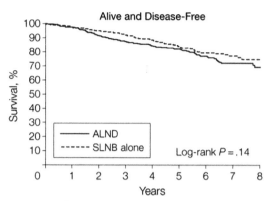

Fig. 3. Disease-free survival of SLNB alone versus ALND. (*From* Giuliano AE, Hunt KK, Ballman KV, et al. Axillary dissection vs no axillary dissection in women with invasive breast cancer and sentinel node metastasis: a randomized clinical trial. JAMA 2011;305:569–75; with permission.)

applicable to women undergoing mastectomy, partial breast radiation, radiation in the prone position, or T3 cancers.

SUMMARY

The development and wide acceptance of SLNB has profoundly affected the management of breast cancer. The technique of SLNB has spared the additional morbidity of ALND without compromising diagnostic accuracy and prognostic information in patients with clinically node-negative early-stage breast cancer. It has become an invaluable tool to clinicians to guide decisions regarding adjuvant treatment. For patients with SLNs who do not have metastatic disease, further axillary surgery is not warranted. In patients who undergo breast conservation, whole-breast irradiation, and systemic treatment and have 1 to 2 SLNs with metastatic disease, completion ALND is now thought to offer prognostic information only, and prevent future axillary recurrence. With the design and development of randomized controlled trials involving the SLNB technique, the management of breast cancer continues to advance to more minimally invasive approaches, and the role of ALND is likely to become less important in the future.

REFERENCES

1. Carter CL, Allen C, Henson DE, et al. Relation of tumor size, lymph node status, and survival in 24,270 breast cancer cases. Cancer 1989;63:181–7.
2. Beenken SW, Urist MM, Zhang Y, et al. Axillary lymph node status, but not tumor size predicts locoregional recurrence and overall survival after mastectomy for breast cancer. Ann Surg 2003;237(5):732–8.
3. Kurtz JM, Kinkel K. Breast conservation in the 21st century. Eur J Cancer 2000; 36(15):1919–24.
4. Huston TL, Simmons RM. Locally recurrent breast cancer after conservation therapy. Am J Surg 2005;189(2):229–35.
5. Fortin A, Larochelle M, Laverdiere J, et al. Local failure is responsible for the decrease in survival for patients with breast cancer treated with conservative surgery and postoperative radiotherapy. J Clin Oncol 1999;17(1):101–9.

6. Fisher B, Jeong H, Anderson S, et al. Twenty-five-year follow-up of a randomized trial comparing radical mastectomy, total mastectomy, and total mastectomy followed by irradiation. N Engl J Med 2002;347(8):567–75.

7. Sosa JA, Diener-West M, Gusev V, et al. Association between extent of axillary lymph node dissection and survival in patients with stage I breast cancer. Ann Surg Oncol 1998;5(2):140–9.

8. Schijven MP, Vingerhoets AJ, Rutten HJ, et al. Comparison of morbidity between axillary lymph node dissection and sentinel node biopsy. Eur J Surg Oncol 2003; 29(4):341–50.

9. Burak WE, Hollenbeck ST, Zervos EE, et al. Sentinel lymph node biopsy results in less postoperative morbidity compared with axillary lymph node dissection for breast cancer. Am J Surg 2002;183(1):23–7.

10. Swenson KK, Nissen MJ, Ceronsky C, et al. Comparison of side effects between sentinel lymph node and axillary lymph node dissection for breast cancer. Ann Surg Oncol 2002;9(8):745–53.

11. Gilchrist RK. Fundamental factors governing lymphatic spread of carcinoma. Ann Surg 1940;111:630–9.

12. Zeidman I, Buss JM. Experimental studies on the spread of cancer in the lymphatic system. Effectiveness of the lymph node as a barrier to the passage of embolic tumor cells. Cancer Res 1954;14:403–5.

13. Morganstern L. The Virchow-Troisier node: a historical note. Am J Surg 1979; 138(5):703.

14. Schnipper EF, Nissenblatt MJ, Schwartz M, et al. Sister Mary Joseph Node-a clue to internal malignancy. J Med Soc N J 1981;78(6):453–4.

15. Olsen KD, DeSanto LW, Pearson BW. Positive Delphian lymph node; clinical significance in laryngeal cancer. Laryngoscope 1987;97(9):1033–7.

16. Gould EA, Winship T, Philbin PH, et al. Observations of a 'sentinel node' in cancer of the parotid. Cancer 1960;13:77–8.

17. Cabanas RM. An approach for the treatment of penile carcinoma. Cancer 1977; 39:456–66.

18. Chiappa S, Uslenghi C, Bonadonna G, et al. Combined testicular and foot lymph-angiography in testicular carcinomas. Surg Gynecol Obstet 1966;123:10–4.

19. Morton DL, Wen DR, Wong JH, et al. Technical details of intraoperative lymphatic mapping for early stage melanoma. Arch Surg 1992;127(4):392–9.

20. Giuliano AE, Kirgan DM, Guenther JM, et al. Lymphatic mapping and sentinel lymphadenectomy for breast cancer. Ann Surg 1994;220(3):391–8.

21. Giuliano AE, Dale PS, Turner RR, et al. Improved axillary staging of breast cancer with sentinel lymphadenectomy. Ann Surg 1995;222:394–401.

22. Albertini JJ, Lyman GH, Cox C, et al. Lymphatic mapping and sentinel node biopsy in the patient with breast cancer. JAMA 1996;276(22):1818–22.

23. Veronesi U, Paganelli G, Galimberti V, et al. Sentinel-node biopsy to avoid axillary dissection in breast cancer with clinically negative lymph nodes. Lancet 1997;349:1864–7.

24. Krag DN, Weaver DL, Alex JC, et al. Surgical resection and radiolocalization of the sentinel node in breast cancer using gamma probe. Surg Oncol 1993;2: 335–40.

25. Miltenberg DM, Miller C, Karamlou TB, et al. Meta-analysis of sentinel lymph node biopsy in breast cancer. J Surg Res 1999;84(2):138–42.

26. Veronesi U, Viale G, Paganelli G, et al. Sentinel lymph node biopsy in breast cancer: ten-year results of a randomized controlled study. Ann Surg 2010; 251:595–600.

27. Park C, Seid P, Morita E, et al. Internal mammary sentinel lymph node mapping for invasive breast cancer: implications for staging and treatment. Breast J 2005;11(1):29–33.
28. Farrus B, Vidal-Sicart S, Velasco M, et al. Incidence of internal mammary node metastases after a sentinel lymph node technique in breast cancer and its implication in the radiotherapy plan. Int J Radiat Oncol Biol Phys 2004;60(3):715–21.
29. Estourgie SH, Nieweg OE, Olmos RA, et al. Lymphatic drainage patterns from the breast. Ann Surg 2004;239(2):232–7.
30. Derossis AM, Fey J, Yeung H, et al. A trend analysis of the relative value of blue dye and isotope localization in 2,000 consecutive cases of sentinel node biopsy for breast cancer. J Am Coll Surg 2001;193:473–8.
31. Cox CE, Salud CJ, Cantor A, et al. Learning curves for breast cancer sentinel lymph node mapping based on surgical volume analysis. J Am Coll Surg 2001;193:593–600.
32. Morrow M, Rademaker AW, Bethke KP, et al. Learning sentinel node biopsy: results of a prospective randomized trial of two techniques. Surgery 1999;126(4): 714–20.
33. Sener SF, Winchester DJ, Brinkmann E, et al. Failure of sentinel lymph node mapping in patients with breast cancer. J Am Coll Surg 2004;198(5):732–6.
34. Leppanen E, Leidenius M, Krogerus L, et al. The effect of patient and tumour characteristics on visualization of sentinel nodes after a single intratumoural injection of Tc 99m labelled human albumin colloid in breast cancer. Eur J Surg Oncol 2002;28(8):821–6.
35. Derossis AM, Fey JV, Cody HS, et al. Obesity influences outcome of sentinel lymph node biopsy in early-stage breast cancer. J Am Coll Surg 2003;197(6): 896–901.
36. Reitsamer R, Peintinger F, Rettenbacher L, et al. Subareolar subcutaneous injection of blue dye versus peritumoral injection of technetium-labeled human albumin to identify sentinel lymph nodes in breast cancer patients. World J Surg 2003;27(12):1291–4.
37. Cserni G, Rajtar M, Boross G, et al. Comparison of vital dye-guided lymphatic mapping and dye plus gamma probe-guided sentinel node biopsy in breast cancer. World J Surg 2002;26(5):592–7.
38. McMasters KM, Wong SL, Martin RC, et al. Dermal injection of radioactive colloid is superior to peritumoral injection for breast cancer sentinel lymph node biopsy: results of a multiinstitutional study. Ann Surg 2001;233(5):676–87.
39. Hartmann LC, Schaid DJ, Woods JE, et al. Efficacy of bilateral prophylactic mastectomy in women with a family history of breast cancer. N Engl J Med 1999;340(2):77–84.
40. Herrinton LJ, Barlow WE, Yu O, et al. Efficacy of prophylactic mastectomy in women with unilateral breast cancer: a cancer research network project. J Clin Oncol 2005;23(19):4275–86.
41. King TA, Ganaraj A, Fey JV, et al. Cytokeratin-positive cells in sentinel lymph nodes in breast cancer are not random events: experience in patients undergoing prophylactic mastectomy. Cancer 2004;101:926–33.
42. Zhou WB, Liu XA, Dai JC, et al. Meta-analysis of sentinel lymph node biopsy at the time of prophylactic mastectomy of the breast. Can J Surg 2011;54: 300–6.
43. Veronesi U, Galimberti V, Zurrida S, et al. Sentinel lymph node biopsy as an indicator for axillary dissection in early breast cancer. Eur J Cancer 2001;37(4): 454–8.

44. Viale G, Zurrida S, Mairoano E, et al. Predicting the status of axillary sentinel lymph nodes in 4351 patients with invasive breast carcinoma treated in a single institution. Cancer 2005;103(3):492–500.
45. Heuts EM, van der Ent FW, Kengen RA, et al. Results of sentinel node biopsy not affected by previous excisional biopsy. Eur J Surg Oncol 2006;32(3):278–81.
46. Dinan D, Cagle CE, Pettinga J. Lymphatic mapping and sentinel node biopsy in women with an ipsilateral second breast carcinoma and a history of breast and axillary surgery. Am J Surg 2005;190(4):614–7.
47. Intra M, Trifiro G, Viale G, et al. Second biopsy of axillary sentinel lymph node for reappearing breast cancer after previous sentinel lymph node biopsy. Ann Surg Oncol 2005;12(11):895–9.
48. Yen TW, Hunt KK, Ross MI, et al. Predictors of invasive breast cancer in patients with an initial diagnosis of ductal carcinoma in situ: a guide to selective use of sentinel lymph node biopsy in management of ductal carcinoma in situ. J Am Coll Surg 2005;200:516–26.
49. Jin Kim H, Heerdt AS, Cody HS, et al. Sentinel lymph node drainage in multicentric breast cancers. Breast J 2002;8(6):356–61.
50. Kumar R, Jana S, Heiba SI, et al. Retrospective analysis of sentinel node localization in multifocal, multicentric, palpable, or nonpalpable breast cancer. J Nucl Med 2003;44(1):7–10.
51. Tousimis E, Van Zee KJ, Fey JV, et al. The accuracy of sentinel lymph node biopsy in multicentric and multifocal invasive breast cancers. J Am Coll Surg 2003;197(4):529–35.
52. Goyal A, Newcombe RG, Mansel RE, et al. Sentinel lymph node biopsy in patients with multifocal breast cancer. Eur J Surg Oncol 2004;30(5):475–9.
53. Gentilini O, Veronesi P, Botteri E, et al. Sentinel lymph node biopsy in multicentric breast cancer: five-year results in a large series from a single institution. Ann Surg Oncol 2011;18(10):2879–84.
54. Fisher B, Wolmark N, Banes M. The accuracy of clinical nodal staging and of limited axillary dissection as a determinant of histologic nodal status in carcinoma of the breast. Gynecol Obstet 1981;152:765–72.
55. De Freitas R Jr, Costa MV, Schneider SV, et al. Accuracy of ultrasound and clinical examination in the diagnosis of axillary lymph node metastases in breast cancer. Eur J Surg Oncol 1991;17:240–4.
56. Cutler SJ, Axtell LM, Schottenfeld D, et al. Clinical assessment of lymph nodes in carcinoma of the breast. Surg Gynecol Obstet 1970;131:41–52.
57. Vlastos G, Mirza NQ, Lenert JT, et al. The feasibility of minimally invasive surgery for stage IIA, IIB, and IIIA breast carcinoma patients after tumor downstaging with induction chemotherapy. Cancer 2000;88(6):1417–24.
58. Cance WG, Carey LA, Calvo BF, et al. Long-term outcome of neoadjuvant therapy for locally advanced breast carcinoma: effective clinical downstaging allows breast preservation and predicts outstanding local control and survival. Ann Surg 2002;236(3):295–302.
59. Rajan R, Esteva FJ, Symmans WF. Pathologic changes in breast cancer following neoadjuvant chemotherapy: implications for the assessment of response. Clin Breast Cancer 2004;5(3):235–8.
60. Patel NA, Piper G, Patel JA, et al. Accurate axillary nodal staging can be achieved after neoadjuvant therapy for locally advanced breast cancer. Am Surg 2004;70(8):696–9.
61. Kang SH, Kang JH, Choi EA, et al. Sentinel lymph node biopsy after neoadjuvant chemotherapy. Breast Cancer 2004;11(3):233–41.

62. Abrial C, Van Praagh I, Delva R, et al. Pathological and clinical response of a primary chemotherapy regimen combining vinorelbine, epirubicin, and paclitaxel as neoadjuvant treatment in patients with operable breast cancer. Oncologist 2005;10(4):242–9.

63. Mamounas EP, Brown A, Anderson S, et al. Sentinel node biopsy after neoadjuvant chemotherapy in breast cancer: results from National Surgical Adjuvant Breast and Bowel Project Protocol B-27. J Clin Oncol 2005;23(12):2694–702.

64. Hahn KM, Johnson PH, Gordon N, et al. Treatment of pregnant breast cancer patients and outcomes of children exposed to chemotherapy in utero. Cancer 2006;107(6):1219–26.

65. Stearns V, Ewing CA, Slack R, et al. Sentinel lymphadenectomy after neoadjuvant chemotherapy for breast cancer may reliably represent the axilla except for inflammatory breast cancer. Ann Surg Oncol 2002;9(3):235–42.

66. Giuliano AE, Hawes D, Ballman KV, et al. Association of occult metastases in sentinel lymph nodes and bone marrow with survival among women with early-stage invasive breast cancer. JAMA 2011;306:385–93.

67. Weaver DL, Ashikaga T, Krag DN, et al. Effect of occult metastases on survival in node-negative breast cancer. N Engl J Med 2011;364:412–21.

68. Fisher B, Anderson S, Bryant J, et al. Twenty-year follow-up of a randomized trial comparing total mastectomy, lumpectomy, and lumpectomy plus irradiation for the treatment of invasive breast cancer. N Engl J Med 2002;347(16):1233–41.

69. Giuliano AE, Hunt KK, Ballman KV, et al. Axillary dissection vs no axillary dissection in women with invasive breast cancer and sentinel node metastasis: a randomized clinical trial. JAMA 2011;305:569–75.

70. Lyman GH, Giuliano AE, Somerfield MR, et al. American Society of Clinical Oncology guideline recommendations for sentinel lymph node biopsy in early-stage breast cancer. J Clin Oncol 2005;23(30):7703–20.

71. Nason KS, Anderson BO, Byrd DR, et al. Increased false negative sentinel node biopsy rates after preoperative chemotherapy for invasive breast carcinoma. Cancer 2000;89(11):2187–94.

72. Tafra L, Verbanac KM, Lanin DR. Preoperative chemotherapy and sentinel lymphadenectomy for breast cancer. Am J Surg 2001;182(4):312–5.

73. Fernandez A, Cortes M, Benito A, et al. Gamma probe sentinel node localization and biopsy in breast cancer patients treated with a neoadjuvant chemotherapy scheme. Nucl Med Commun 2001;22(4):361–6.

74. Haid A, Tausch C, Lang A, et al. Is sentinel lymph node biopsy reliable and indicated after preoperative chemotherapy in patients with breast carcinoma? Cancer 2001;92(5):1080–4.

75. Julian TB, Dusi D, Wolmark N. Sentinel node biopsy after neoadjuvant chemotherapy for breast cancer. Am J Surg 2002;184(4):315–7.

76. Miller AR, Thomason VE, Yeh IT, et al. Analysis of sentinel lymph node mapping with immediate pathologic review in patients receiving preoperative chemotherapy for breast carcinoma. Ann Surg Oncol 2002;9(3):243–7.

77. Piato JR, Barros AC, Pincerato AM, et al. Sentinel lymph node biopsy in breast cancer after neoadjuvant chemotherapy. A pilot study. Eur J Surg Oncol 2003; 29(2):118–20.

78. Jones JL, Zabicki K, Christian RL, et al. A comparison of sentinel node biopsy before and after neoadjuvant chemotherapy: timing is important. Am J Surg 2005;190(4):517–20.

79. Tanaka Y, Maeda H, Ogawa Y, et al. Sentinel node biopsy in breast cancer patients treated with neoadjuvant chemotherapy. Oncol Rep 2006;15(4):927–31.

80. Lee S, Kim EY, Kang SH, et al. Sentinel node identification rate, but not accuracy, is significantly decreased after pre-operative chemotherapy in axillary node-positive breast cancer patients. Breast Cancer Res Treat 2007;102(3): 283–8.
81. Gimbergues P, Abrial C, Durando X, et al. Sentinel lymph node biopsy after neoadjuvant chemotherapy is accurate in breast cancer patients with a clinically negative axillary nodal status at presentation. Ann Surg Oncol 2008;15(5): 1316–21.
82. Hunt KK, Yi M, Mittendorf EA, et al. Sentinel lymph node surgery after neoadjuvant chemotherapy is accurate and reduces the need for axillary dissection in breast cancer patients. Ann Surg Oncol 2009;250(4):558–66.
83. Classe JM, Bordes V, Campion L, et al. Sentinel lymph node biopsy after neoadjuvant chemotherapy for advanced breast cancer: results of Ganglion Sentinelle et Chimiotherapie Neoadjuvante, a French prospective multicentric study. J Clin Oncol 2009;27(5):726–32.

Tailoring Adjuvant Treatments for the Individual Patient with Luminal Breast Cancer

Elisabetta Munzone, MD[a],*, Giuseppe Curigliano, MD, PhD[b],
Marco Colleoni, MD[a]

KEYWORDS

- Breast cancer • Luminal A • Luminal B • Adjuvant therapy • Endocrine therapy
- Gene assay

KEY POINTS

- Luminal breast cancers are the most frequent subtypes; they are heterogeneous, with a large variation in clinical presentation.
- Luminal A tumors are characterized by estrogen-regulated genes and better outcomes, whereas luminal B tumors are characterized by a higher genomic grade and poorer outcomes.
- Subsets of patients with high levels of expression of estrogen receptor (ER) with low proliferation (luminal A) are commonly cured with endocrine therapy alone; subsets with doubtful endocrine responsiveness and/or with high proliferation index (luminal B) require the addition of chemotherapy.
- Recent recommendations suggest the use of standard pathology reports based on the immunohistochemical (IHC) measurements of ER, progesterone receptor (PgR), Ki67, and HER2 as a surrogate molecular classification to identify subgroups of patients who might avoid/receive chemotherapy.
- Great advances have been made in the development of multigene prognostic signatures for gene expression patterns to identify subset of patients with luminal breast cancers who benefit from adding chemotherapy to endocrine therapy.
- Much attention should be paid to the identification of biomarkers in addition to hormone receptor expression and proliferation indexes to better select those patients who would benefit from endocrine therapy.

INTRODUCTION

Luminal breast cancers are traditionally the most frequent subtypes of breast cancer, representing a heterogeneous group of tumors with a large variation in clinical

[a] Division of Medical Senology, European Institute of Oncology, Via Ripamonti 435, Milan 20141, Italy; [b] Division of Early Drug Development, European Institute of Oncology, Via Ripamonti 435, Milan 20141, Italy
* Corresponding author.
E-mail address: elisabetta.munzone@ieo.it

Hematol Oncol Clin N Am 27 (2013) 703–714
http://dx.doi.org/10.1016/j.hoc.2013.05.012
0889-8588/13/$ – see front matter © 2013 Elsevier Inc. All rights reserved.

presentation. Selection of patients who might forego chemotherapy within these sub-groups represents a major question.

Controversies concern groups with bulky tumors and/or positive nodes who present with favorable biology (ideally luminal A) versus patients with small and node-negative tumors but with an unfavorable biology (ideally biologically aggressive luminal B). Among smaller tumors traditionally judged as low risk and not requiring chemotherapy, there is a not negligible subgroup with adverse tumor biology that should be considered for a combined chemoendocrine therapeutic approach. Within this subgroup, the cross talk with other pathways should be also considered and new strategies to escape multipathway drivers of tumor growth and progression should be implemented. Novel agents to be added to endocrine therapy are under investigation to shut down bypass signaling pathways that drive tumor growth.

Similarly, among subsets defined by high levels of expression of ER along with low proliferation, commonly cured with endocrine therapy alone, there is a subgroup presenting with very large tumor burden and a related dismal prognosis that might require the addition of chemotherapy.[1,2]

Care for patients through a personalized approach remains a central issue, and clinicians are currently more likely to give selective interventions to minimize acute and late toxicity without compromising efficacy. In particular, for the subgroup of patients with ER-positive disease, appropriate adjuvant systemic therapy involves choosing treatments tailored to individual patients according to biologic features and assessments of patient risk but also according to comorbidities, desire to preserve fertility, and patient preference.[1]

Recommendations from the St. Gallen consensus panel suggested the use of standard pathology reports based on IHC measurements of ER, PgR, Ki67, and HER2 as a surrogate molecular classification to identify subgroup of patients who might avoid/receive chemotherapy.[1,2] Common features that might indicate increased response to endocrine therapy include high expression of ER and PgR.[1,2] Conversely, the presence of high proliferation index and/or lower expression of steroid hormone receptors might identify a subgroup of patients with luminal disease at higher probability of response to chemotherapy.[3]

This clinicopathologic classification requires the availability of reliable measurements of its individual components, therefore guidelines have been published for ER and PgR determination[4] and for the proper evaluation of Ki67.[5]

In parallel with clinicopathologic classification, a great advance was reached in the development of multigene prognostic signatures for gene expression patterns to identify a subset of patients with luminal breast cancers who benefit from adding chemotherapy to endocrine therapy.[3,6]

In particular, the fine tuning for prediction of which groups may benefit from endocrine therapy alone has been possible with the advent of multigene assays, such as the 21-gene recurrence score (RS) and 70-gene assays,[6] because the findings from the retrospective analysis of 2 large trials (SWOG S8814 and NSABP [National Surgical Adjuvant Breast and Bowel Project] B-20) have shown that patients with low RS may be sufficiently treated with endocrine therapy alone.[3,6] A popular method for assessing the magnitude of benefit of endocrine therapy and chemotherapy in luminal breast cancer is Adjuvant! Online (**Fig. 1**). The algorithm used, however, is based on historical trials with biologic features evaluated in an older fashion, in which the comparator groups may not have received adequate endocrine therapy.

Prospective validation of these multigene signatures is under way. Specifically, the Trial Assigning Individualized Options for treatment (Rx) (TAILORx) (ClinicalTrials.gov

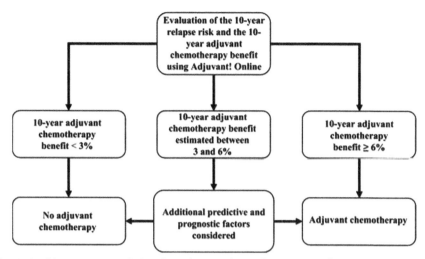

Fig. 1. Decision recommendation for adjuvant chemotherapy in early-stage breast cancer patients. (*From* Jacot W, Gutowski M, Azria D, et al. Adjuvant early breast cancer systemic therapies according to daily used technologies. Crit Rev Oncol Hematol 2012;82(3):361–9; with permission.)

identifier NCT00310180) is studying the utility of the Oncotype DX score to predict chemotherapy benefit in the intermediate score subgroup.

The Microarray in Node-negative and 1 to 3 Positive Lymph Node Disease May Avoid Chemotherapy Trial (MINDACT) (ClinicalTrials.gov identifier NCT00433589) is studying the outcomes of patients with discordant risk assessments using the 70-gene expression signature of MammaPrint compared with clinicopathologic features with the Adjuvant! Online program.[7] The RxPONDER ([Rx for Positive Node, Endocrine Responsive Breast Cancer] ClinicalTrials.gov identifier NCT01272037) is a large prospective trial designed to determine the benefit of chemotherapy among women with hormone receptor–positive breast cancer, 1 to 3 positive nodes, and an RS less than or equal to 25, as determined by Oncotype DX testing. The results from these large, prospective studies are eagerly awaited and will hopefully shed light on the best strategies to personalize adjuvant treatment in patients with luminal breast cancer.

This article discusses the evolving knowledge of adjuvant treatments in order to define reasonable but also novel treatment strategies in patients with ER-positive/HER2-negative (luminal A and luminal B) breast cancer.

SPECIFIC CONSIDERATION FOR ADJUVANT TREATMENT CHOICE IN LUMINAL A TUMORS

Based on retrospective analysis of past trials, prospectively stratified for the degree of ER expression, the effect of chemoendocrine therapy on luminal A patients compared with endocrine therapy alone is unclear. The evidence in node-negative disease comes from the International Breast Cancer Study Group (IBCSG) trial IX for postmenopausal women and from IBCSG trial VIII for premenopausal patients.[8–10]

The trials compared 3 or 6 courses of adjuvant classical cyclophosphamide, methotrexate, and fluorouracil (CMF) with or without endocrine therapy versus endocrine therapy alone. No clear chemotherapy benefit was observed in ER-positive/HER2-negative disease (hazard ratio [HR] 0.90; 95% CI, 0.74–1.11). Moreover, these 2 trials showed no benefit of chemotherapy in the subset of ER positive, HER2 negative, and low Ki67, corresponding to the surrogate definition of luminal A disease.[10]

In a retrospective analysis of the NSABP B-20 trial, the Oncotype Dx RS was used to predict CMF chemotherapy benefit. It was demonstrated that patients with ER-positive/node-negative breast cancer treated with tamoxifen and with a low RS did not benefit from the addition of chemotherapy.[6] Analogous findings were reported by Albain and colleagues,[3] in a retrospective analysis of the SWOG 8814 trial, where patients with ER-positive/node-positive disease had no benefit from adding cyclophosphamide, doxorubicin, and fluorouracil regimen to tamoxifen if low to intermediate RS was demonstrated. Clinicians in favor of the inclusion of chemotherapy might argue, however, against these conclusions, considering the retrospective nature of the studies, the small number of cases that were available for inclusion, and the lack of a taxane in the delivered chemotherapy.[11]

According to the recent St Gallen consensus conferences, the intrinsic luminal A subtype corresponds to the clinicopathologic surrogate definition as luminal A–like. These luminal A tumors are characterized by high expression of steroid hormone receptors and are HER2 negative and Ki67 low. The optimal cutpoint between high and low values for Ki67 has not been established, given the potential variability of assessment among different laboratories.

A level of Ki67 less than 14% best correlated with gene array definition of luminal A, based on results in a single reference laboratory.[12] Recent data support a threshold of 20% or higher as potentially indicative of high Ki67 status.[13,14]

Literature data recently also sustain the introduction of PgR to optimally distinguish between luminal A and luminal B tumors. The value of PgR suggested for categorizing luminal A and luminal B subtypes is proposed as more than 20%, according to a recent report, where the fine tuning was done by comparing the multigene expression–based assays across 5 independent cohorts and the IHC-based definition of luminal A and luminal B.[15]

In conclusion, the threshold for the definition of luminal disease remains a matter of debate.

Tailored Treatments of Luminal A Disease

The role of endocrine therapy in luminal A breast cancer is well consolidated.[1,2]

Tamoxifen for 5 years can be considered the default adjuvant endocrine therapy for premenopausal patients.[16]

Recently, there is evidence that extension of endocrine treatment beyond 5 years or even 10 years might be beneficial (as reported by the Adjuvant Tamoxifen—Longer Against Shorter [ATLAS] study,[17] which suggested a significant benefit for extending tamoxifen to 10 years rather than 5 years), although not required, in a large group of luminal A patients. Adding ovarian suppression to tamoxifen is a matter of controversy, especially for younger patients (<40 years), and results from the recently concluded Suppression of Ovarian Function with Triptorelin (SOFT) trial will add some information to this issue.[18] Ovarian suppression alone without tamoxifen, as well as its combination with aromatase inhibitors, should not be routinely considered unless tamoxifen is contraindicated.

Aromatase inhibitors for 5 years should be considered the mainstay of treatment for the vast majority of postmenopausal women with luminal A disease, although this strategy should be preferred for patients at high risk, such as those with luminal B disease.

There are some postmenopausal women with luminal A disease who could be treated with tamoxifen alone. Extension of aromatase inhibitor therapy beyond the first 5 years for patients with node-positive disease can be considered for patients whose initial treatment was tamoxifen or whose initial therapy was less than 5 years of an aromatase inhibitor.[19]

Multigene assays might be used in the future to select patient candidates for extending adjuvant endocrine therapies. Recently, the PAM50 signature was tested on 1478 tissue samples derived from a large cohort of endocrine-responsive breast cancer enrolled in the *Austrian Breast and Colorectal Cancer Study Group (ABCSG) 8 study.* The estimated percentage without recurrence at 15 years assessed by PAM50 was 95.6% for low risk of recurrence, 87.3% for intermediate risk of recurrence, and 72.1% for high risk of recurrence.[20]

Based on available data, it might be argued that luminal A cancers are resistant to chemotherapy, even if they have some adverse prognostic features, such as multiple positive nodes. As discussed previously, however, the best evidence supporting the theory of chemotherapy resistance in luminal A cancers is based on 2 retrospective, unplanned subgroup analyses of clinical trials performed some years ago.[3,6]

Evidence from an Early Breast Cancer Trialists' Collaborative Group (EBCTCG) overview is that cytotoxic chemotherapy is, on average, beneficial in delaying relapse and prolonging survival for women with early breast cancer[16] and, therefore, recommended for the treatment of patients with node-positive disease, irrespective of the tumor biology. It may, therefore, be concluded that because even a few patients may benefit, all should receive chemotherapy. This ignores, however, the potential harm of delaying effective endocrine therapy to those who most need it as well as the obvious harm of exposing a large majority to the toxic (occasionally fatal) adverse effects of chemotherapy.

In the few cases of luminal A disease and large tumor burden (eg, multiple positive nodes), it seems reasonable to offer chemotherapy, although benefit remains uncertain, because lymph node status is not predictive to sensitivity for either endocrine treatment or chemotherapy.

When controversies remain for deciding to give chemotherapy in ER-positive and HER2-negative cases, the use of gene array analysis might be useful for the selection of patients who might forego chemotherapy. The 21-gene RS that was demonstrated as predictive of chemotherapy responsiveness should be considered for this analysis when indicated.[6]

If given, chemotherapy for such patients could comprise less-intensive regimens, such as Adriamycin (doxorubicin) and cyclophosphamide (AC) ×4, CMF ×6, or Taxotere (docetaxel) and cyclophosphamide (TC) ×4, that demonstrated activity in luminal disease in previous studies.[1]

In the decision of whether to introduce adjuvant chemotherapy, the presence of special types should be taken into consideration. Little attention has been dedicated in the past to identification of special types of breast cancer, that is, those displaying a distinct morphology might exhibit a distinct prognostic and predictive profile compared with invasive ductal carcinomas of no special type or not otherwise specified.[21]

Within luminal A breast cancer, several special types display an extremely good prognosis, often approaching or equaling that of the general population. In particular, pure tubular and cribriform carcinomas represent a rare histologic type, correlated with a favorable prognosis.[22] Current published data indicate that, compared with grade 1 ductal carcinomas, tubular carcinoma is associated with longer disease-free survival and breast cancer–specific survival close to normal life expectancy.[23]

In locally advanced invasive lobular carcinomas, response to primary chemotherapy seemed lower in terms of pathologic complete response (0%–3%) compared with invasive ductal carcinoma.[24,25]

Lobular carcinomas are characterized by a significantly higher expression of steroid hormone receptors compared with the ductal ones, which might contribute to the lower response to preoperative chemotherapy. In addition, a large retrospective study identified 981 patients with lobular disease who had no benefit from the addition of adjuvant chemotherapy, whereas poorer disease-free survival was observed for patients with endocrine-responsive tumors who did not receive any adjuvant hormonal therapy (HR 2.35; 95% CI, 1.05–5.23).[26]

These results indicate that a tailored approach should be considered in classical lobular carcinoma, based on proper adjuvant endocrine therapy administered for perhaps a prolonged period of time.

SPECIFIC CONSIDERATION FOR ADJUVANT TREATMENT CHOICE IN LUMINAL B TUMORS

Although proper identification of intrinsic subtypes is more precise using molecular technologies, clinically useful surrogate definition of luminal B can be routinely obtained by IHC measurements of ER, PgR, Ki67, and HER2. In summary, luminal B disease comprises those luminal cases that lack the characteristics (discussed previously) for luminal A disease. Thus, either a high Ki67 or a low PgR may be used to distinguish between luminal A and luminal B/HER2 negative.

The absence of PgR may be a marker of aberrant growth factor signaling and, thus, a mechanism for antiestrogen resistance.[27,28] ER-positive/PgR-negative tumors, as defined by RNA profiling, represent a distinct subset of breast cancer with aggressive features and poor outcome despite being clinically ER positive.[29]

The prognostic value of PgR expression has been already reported in several studies. In a previous publication from the authors' group, a significant correlation between absence of PgR expression and poorer outcome in luminal breast cancer was shown.[30] Other studies in the past evaluated the impact in recurrence and mortality risks for the PgR status.[31–34] In particular, one trial reported that women with PgR-negative tumors had a higher risk of mortality independent of the different demographic and clinical characteristics compared with women with both ER-positive and PgR-positive tumors.[32]

Evidence from another study indicated that patients with ER-positive/PgR-negative tumors benefit less from adjuvant endocrine therapy, so additional or better treatments of this subset may be necessary.[35]

Luminal B tumors, being highly proliferative, are also distinguished by having higher levels of Ki67 proliferation index.

Recent meta-analyses reported that high Ki67 expression is associated with increased risk of breast cancer relapse and death.[14,36] A study by Cheang and colleagues[12] demonstrated that Ki67 determined with IHC can differentiate between luminal A and luminal B tumors. In particular, the best Ki67 index cutpoint to distinguish luminal B from luminal A tumors was 13.25%. Within this study, luminal B and luminal B HER2-positive breast cancers were statistically significantly associated with poor breast cancer recurrence-free survival and disease-specific survival in all adjuvant systemic treatment categories.

Tailored Treatments of Luminal B Disease

The question of adjuvant chemotherapy in luminal breast cancer has been directly addressed in well-conducted phase III trials.[16] An advantage was observed for chemoendocrine therapies compared with endocrine therapies alone, on average, in several of the studies.[3,6] In particular, the most recent published EBCTCG overview of chemotherapy concluded that proportional risk reductions from chemotherapy were little affected by ER status or tamoxifen use as well as by age, nodal status, tumor diameter, or differentiation.[37]

Data from past series include information on several aspects of the disease collected in the earlier period, when the various prognostic and predictive factors were not available as they are today. Mature studies were designed in an era when adjuvant therapies were selected according to the stage of the disease and where factors predictive of response (ie, hormone receptor expression and HER2 overexpression/amplification) were uncommonly taken into consideration. The correlation between chemotherapy effect and outcome may be confounded in retrospective analyses by the inclusion of both endocrine-responsive and endocrine-nonresponsive disease. The results of subgroup analyses should be treated with caution, however, especially because some of the subgroups had small sample sizes.

Moreover, in premenopausal women, cytotoxic therapy is thought to exert its effects both by direct tumor cell kill and by an endocrine effect secondary to suppression of ovarian function.[38] The extent to which chemotherapy may exert such an endocrine effect depends on the type of chemotherapy; the age of the patient, which is known to influence the probability of chemotherapy-induced amenorrhea[38,39]; and the hormone receptor expression of the tumor.[40]

Also, incremental chemotherapy strategies compared with less-extensive therapies were more effective across several trials in patients with luminal disease, although at the price of additional toxicity, inconvenience, and economical cost. For example, the NSABP B-30 evaluated patients with operable, node-positive breast cancer randomized to receive 4 courses of AC (doxorubicin and cyclophosphamide) followed by 4 courses of docetaxel, 4 courses of doxorubicin and docetaxel, or 4 courses of concurrent doxorubicin, cyclophosphamide, and docetaxel. Patients treated with sequential chemotherapy had a significant reduction in relapse or death compared with those who received a shorter duration of therapy. Prolonged chemotherapy seemed more efficacious in all subgroups, including ER-positive disease.[41] Similar results in terms of significant reduction in risk of recurrence for extended chemotherapy in luminal disease were observed in the NSABP B-28, comparing 4 courses of AC followed by 4 courses of paclitaxel with 4 courses of AC alone.[42]

The US Intergroup performed a trial where the addition of 4 cycles of paclitaxel after 4 cycles of AC demonstrated a small but significant improvement disease-free survival and overall survival using the longer, different regimen.[43] This improvement was seen mainly among patients with ER-negative tumors who did not receive tamoxifen.

In conclusion, it is generally agreed that chemotherapy is indicated for the majority of patients with luminal B (HER2-negative) disease and that chemotherapy regimens should contain anthracyclines and, for most patients, taxanes.[2]

The optimal duration is not yet been established, but it seems reasonable that 4 to 6 months of adjuvant chemotherapy is appropriate.[1,2]

The use of gene expression profiles might be useful in the future to further identify groups who do not benefit from the addition of chemotherapy in luminal B disease. Recently, the PAM50 classification showed no benefit of anthracycline-based chemotherapy compared with CMF chemotherapy in patients with either luminal A or luminal B disease.[44]

Novel Strategies to Overcome Endocrine Resistance

Among luminal B breast cancer patients, there are also subgroups characterized by a degree of endocrine resistance. Earlier studies showed that approximately 30% of ER-positive breast cancers had no benefit from endocrine therapy.[45]

In endocrine-resistant breast cancer, there is a reciprocal cross talk between ER and other signal transduction pathways, including those involving receptor tyrosine kinases and insulinlike growth factor (IGF).[46–48] As a consequence, in ER-positive/HER2-positive breast cancers, targeting both the ER and HER2 pathways is a clinically reasonable approach.

For instance, tamoxifen resistance may rely on the cross talk between ER and IGF-1 receptor (IGF-1R).[49] In addition, the activation of the IGF-1R signaling is associated with PgR loss, which is characteristic of highly proliferative luminal B subtypes resistant to tamoxifen.[50] Despite this background, however, the result of a randomized phase II trial investigating exemestane or fulvestrant plus ganitumumab (monoclonal IgG1 antibody that blocks IGF-1R) or matching placebo was recently published. This study failed to meet its endpoint, because the addition to ganitumumab to endocrine therapy did not improve outcomes of women with hormone receptor–positive locally advanced or metastatic breast cancer.[51]

The PI3K pathway is frequently hyperactivated in ER-positive breast cancers and has been recognized as involved in antiestrogen resistance.[52] In the metastatic setting, one phase II clinical trial demonstrated a promising efficacy with the combination of the mTOR inhibitor, everolimus, plus tamoxifen.[53] The combination of everolimus plus letrozole showed activity in either the metastatic[54] or the neoajuvant setting.[55] In the BOLERO-2 trial, comparing exemestane plus everolimus with exemestane plus placebo, the subset of patients who had received prior nonsteroidal aromatase inhibitors in the adjuvant or metastatic setting had an advantage from the combined treatment, with a median progression-free survival of 10.6 months versus 4.1 months (HR 0.36; 95% CI, 0.27–0.47).[47] These results represent an important improvement in the treatment of antiestrogen-resistant, hormone receptor–positive breast cancer; therefore, cotargeting the PI3K pathway in the adjuvant setting represents an appealing strategy to improve outcomes.

SUMMARY

The threshold for use of adjuvant cytotoxic chemotherapy for patients with luminal A or luminal B disease is an unresolved question. Patients with luminal disease may have tumors with very low risks of recurrence, where there is little evidence supporting the use of chemotherapy added to endocrine therapy, or may have higher-risk tumors, where prolonged chemoendocrine therapy seems justified. Therefore, women with luminal breast cancer and their physicians must weigh the risks and benefits of all therapeutic options. It is necessary to take into consideration patient preferences in defining the threshold of expected benefit when choosing which treatment should be undertaken.

Based on literature data (discussed previously), endocrine therapies alone should be considered in the majority of patients with luminal A disease patients, where the benefit of adding chemotherapy is uncertain and sometimes may seem detrimental.

A combination of chemotherapy and endocrine therapies should be considered in the presence of high Ki67, low hormone receptor status, and high 21-gene RSs, mainly representing the luminal B disease, as well as in cases of large tumor burden (eg, the involvement of more than 3 lymph nodes).

Much attention should be paid as well to the identification of additional biomarkers besides hormone receptor expression and proliferation indexes to better select those patients who would benefit from endocrine therapy. Individualized predictors of responsiveness are needed to foster a personalized approach for each patient. For those patients who do not benefit from an endocrine therapy, even if extended, it is necessary to investigate novel approaches of combining endocrine therapy with targeted treatments, based on a deeper understanding of the heterogeneity of luminal breast cancers.

REFERENCES

1. Goldhirsch A, Ingle JN, Gelber RD, et al. Thresholds for therapies: highlights of the St Gallen International Expert Consensus on the Primary Therapy of Early Breast Cancer. Ann Oncol 2009;20(8):1319–29.
2. Goldhirsch A, Wood WC, Coates AS, et al. Strategies for subtypes—dealing with the diversity of breast cancer: highlights of the St. Gallen International Expert Consensus on the Primary Therapy of Early Breast Cancer 2011. Ann Oncol 2011;22(8):1736–47.
3. Albain KS, Barlow WE, Shak S, et al. Prognostic and predictive value of the 21-gene recurrence score assay in postmenopausal women with node-positive, oestrogen-receptor-positive breast cancer on chemotherapy: a retrospective analysis of a randomised trial. Lancet Oncol 2010;11(1):55–65.
4. Hammond ME, Hayes DF, Dowsett M, et al. American Society of Clinical Oncology/College Of American Pathologists guideline recommendations for immunohistochemical testing of estrogen and progesterone receptors in breast cancer. J Clin Oncol 2010;28(16):2784–95.
5. Dowsett M, Nielsen TO, A'Hern R, et al, International Ki-67 in Breast Cancer Working Group. Assessment of Ki67 in breast cancer: recommendations from the International Ki67 in Breast Cancer working group. J Natl Cancer Inst 2011;103(22):1656–64.
6. Paik S, Tang G, Shak S, et al. Gene expression and benefit of chemotherapy in women with node-negative, estrogen receptor-positive breast cancer. J Clin Oncol 2006;24(23):3726–34.
7. Cardoso F, van't Veer L, Rutgers E, et al. Clinical application of the 70-gene profile: the MINDACT trial. J Clin Oncol 2008;26:729–35.
8. Aebi S, Sun Z, Braun D, et al. Differential efficacy of three cycles of CMF followed by tamoxifen in patients with ER-positive and ER-negative tumors: long-term follow up on IBCSG Trial IX. Ann Oncol 2011;22:1981–7.
9. Viale G, Regan MM, Maiorano E, et al. Chemoendocrine compared with endocrine adjuvant therapies for node-negative breast cancer: predictive value of centrally reviewed expression of estrogen and progesterone receptors—International Breast Cancer Study Group. J Clin Oncol 2008;26:1404–10.
10. Colleoni M, Cole BF, Viale G, et al. Classical cyclophosphamide, methotrexate, and fluorouracil chemotherapy is more effective in triple-negative, node-negative breast cancer: results from two randomized trials of adjuvant chemoendocrine therapy for node-negative breast cancer. J Clin Oncol 2010;28:2966–73.
11. Hayes DF. Targeting adjuvant chemotherapy: a good idea that needs to be proven! J Clin Oncol 2012;30(12):1264–7.
12. Cheang MC, Chia SK, Voduc D, et al. Ki67 index, HER2 status, and prognosis of patients with luminal B breast cancer. J Natl Cancer Inst 2009;101(10):736–50.
13. Nielsen TO, Polley MY, Leung SC, et al. An international Ki-67 reproducibility study. Presented at the 35th San Antonio Breast Cancer Symposium. December 4–8, 2012 [abstract S4–6].
14. de Azambuja E, Cardoso F, de Castro G Jr, et al. Ki-67 as prognostic marker in early breast cancer: a meta-analysis of published studies involving 12,155 patients. Br J Cancer 2007;96(10):1504–13.

15. Prat A, Cheang MC, Martín M, et al. Prognostic significance of progesterone receptor-positive tumor cells within immunohistochemically defined luminal a breast cancer. J Clin Oncol 2013;31(2):203–9.
16. Early Breast Cancer Trialists' Collaborative Group. Effects of chemotherapy and hormonal therapy for early breast cancer on recurrence and 15-year survival: an overview of the randomised trials. Lancet 2005;365:1687–717.
17. Davies C, Pan H, Godwin J, et al. Long-term effects of continuing adjuvant tamoxifen to 10 years versus stopping at 5 years after diagnosis of oestrogen receptor-positive breast cancer: ATLAS, a randomised trial. Lancet 2012. pii:S0140-6736(12) 61963–1. [Epub ahead of print].
18. Zickl L, Francis P, Fleming G, et al. SOFT and TEXT: trials of tamoxifen and exemestane with and without ovarian function suppression for premenopausal women with hormone receptor-positive early breast cancer. Cancer Res 2012; 72(Suppl 24) [abstract nr OT2-2-01].
19. Goss PE, Ingle JN, Pater JL, et al. Late extended adjuvant treatment with letrozole improves outcome in women with early-stage breast cancer who complete 5 years of tamoxifen. J Clin Oncol 2008;26(12):1948–55.
20. Gnant M, Filipits M, Dubsky P, et al. Predicting risk for late metastasis: the pam50 risk of recurrence (ror) score after 5 years of endocrine therapy in postmenopausal women with hr+ early breast cancer: a study on 1,478 patients from the abcsg-8 trial. Ann Oncol 2013;24(Suppl 3):iii29–37 [Abstract 530].
21. Colleoni M, Rotmensz N, Maisonneuve P, et al. Outcome of special types of luminal breast cancer. Ann Oncol 2012;23(6):1428–36.
22. Diab SG, Clark GM, Osborne CK, et al. Tumor characteristics and clinical outcome of tubular and mucinous breast carcinomas. J Clin Oncol 1999;17: 1442–8.
23. Rakha EA, Lee AH, Evans AJ, et al. Tubular carcinoma of the breast: further evidence to support its excellent prognosis. J Clin Oncol 2010;28:99–104.
24. Cristofanilli M, Gonzalez-Angulo A, Sneige N, et al. Invasive lobular carcinoma classic type: response to primary chemotherapy and surgical outcomes. J Clin Oncol 2005;23:41–8.
25. Tubiana-Hulin M, Stevens D, Lasry S, et al. Response to neoadjuvant chemotherapy in lobular and ductal breast carcinomas: a retrospective study on 860 patients from one institution. Ann Oncol 2006;17:1228–33.
26. Iorfida M, Maiorano E, Orvieto E, et al. Invasive lobular breast cancer: subtypes and outcome. Breast Cancer Res Treat 2012;133(2):713–23.
27. Cui X, Schiff R, Arpino G, et al. Biology of progesterone receptor loss in breast cancer and its implications for endocrine therapy. J Clin Oncol 2005;23: 7721–35.
28. Rakha EA, El-Sayed ME, Green AR, et al. Biologic and clinical characteristics of breast cancer with single hormone receptor positive phenotype. J Clin Oncol 2007;25:4772–8.
29. Creighton CJ, Kent Osborne C, van de Vijver MJ, et al. Molecular profiles of progesterone receptor loss in human breast tumors. Breast Cancer Res Treat 2009;114:287–99.
30. Cancello G, Maisonneuve P, Rotmensz N, et al. Progesterone receptor loss identifies Luminal B breast cancer subgroups at higher risk of relapse. Ann Oncol 2013;24(3):661–8.
31. Bauer K, Parise C, Caggiano V. Use of ER/PR/HER2 subtypes in conjunction with the 2007 St Gallen Consensus Statement for early breast cancer. BMC Cancer 2010;10:228.

32. Dunnwald L, Rossing M, Li C. Hormone receptor status, tumor characteristics, and prognosis: a prospective cohort of breast cancer patients. Breast Cancer Res 2007;9:R6.
33. Grann VR, Troxel AB, Zojwalla NJ, et al. Hormone receptor status and survival in a population-based cohort of patients with breast carcinoma. Cancer 2005;103: 2241–51.
34. Mohsin SK, Weiss H, Havighurst T, et al. Progesterone receptor by immunohistochemistry and clinical outcome in breast cancer: a validation study. Mod Pathol 2004;17:1545–54.
35. Bardou VJ, Arpino G, Elledge RM, et al. Progesterone receptor status significantly improves outcome prediction over estrogen receptor status alone for adjuvant endocrine therapy in two large breast cancer databases. J Clin Oncol 2003;21:1973–9.
36. Stuart-Harris R, Caldas C, Pinder SE, et al. Proliferation markers and survival in early breast cancer: a systematic review and meta-analysis of 85 studies in 32,825 patients. Breast 2008;17(4):323–34.
37. Early Breast Cancer Trialists' Collaborative Group (EBCTCG). Comparisons between different polychemotherapy regimens for early breast cancer: meta-analyses of long-term outcome among 100,000 women in 123 randomised trials. Lancet 2012;379(9814):432–44.
38. Pagani O, O'Neill A, Castiglione M, et al. Prognostic impact of amenorrhoea after adjuvant chemotherapy in premenopausal breast cancer patients with axillary node involvement: results of the International Breast Cancer Study Group (IBCSG) Trial VI. Eur J Cancer 1998;34:632–40.
39. Goldhirsch A, Gelber RD, Castiglione M. The magnitude of endocrine effects of adjuvant chemotherapy for premenopausal breast cancer patients. Ann Oncol 1990;1:183–8.
40. Scottish Cancer Trials Breast Group and ICRF Breast Unit. Adjuvant ovarian ablation versus CMF chemotherapy in premenopausal women with pathological stage II breast carcinoma: the Scottish trial. Lancet 1993;341: 1293–8.
41. Swain SM, Jeong JH, Geyer CE Jr, et al. Longer therapy, iatrogenic amenorrhea, and survival in early breast cancer. N Engl J Med 2010;362:2053–65.
42. Mamounas EP, Bryant J, Lembersky B, et al. Paclitaxel after doxorubicin plus cyclophosphamide as adjuvant chemotherapy for node-positive breast cancer: results from NSABP B-28. J Clin Oncol 2005;23:3686–96.
43. Henderson IC, Berry DA, Demetri GD, et al. Improved outcomes from adding sequential Paclitaxel but not from escalating Doxorubicin dose in an adjuvant chemotherapy regimen for patients with node-positive primary breast cancer. J Clin Oncol 2003;21:976–83.
44. Cheang MC, Voduc KD, Tu D, et al. Responsiveness of intrinsic subtypes to adjuvant anthracycline substitution in the NCIC.CTG MA.5 randomized trial. Clin Cancer Res 2012;18:2402–12.
45. Osborne CK. Steroid hormone receptors in breast cancer management. Breast Cancer Res Treat 1998;51(3):227–38.
46. Osborne CK, Neven P, Dirix LY, et al. Gefitinib or placebo in combination with tamoxifen in patients with hormone receptor-positive metastatic breast cancer: a randomized phase II study. Clin Cancer Res 2011;17(5):1147–59.
47. Baselga J, Campone M, Piccart M, et al. Everolimus in postmenopausal hormone-receptor-positive advanced breast cancer. N Engl J Med 2012; 366(6):520–9.

48. Shou J, Massarweh S, Osborne CK, et al. Mechanisms of tamoxifen resistance: increased estrogen receptor-HER2/neu cross-talk in ER/HER2-positive breast cancer. J Natl Cancer Inst 2004;96(12):926–35.

49. Peyrat J, Louchez M, Lefebvre J, et al. Plasma insulin-like growth factor-1 (IGF-1) concentrations in human breast cancer. Eur J Cancer 1993;29:492–7.

50. Law JH, Habibi G, Hu K, et al. Phosphorylated insulin-like growth factor-I/insulin receptor is present in all breast cancer subtypes and is related to poor survival. Cancer Res 2008;68:10238–46.

51. Robertson JF, Ferrero JM, Bourgeois H, et al. Ganitumab with either exemestane or fulvestrant for postmenopausal women with advanced, hormone-receptor-positive breast cancer: a randomised, controlled, double-blind, phase 2 trial. Lancet Oncol 2013;14(3):228–35.

52. Miller TW, Balko JM, Arteaga CL. Phosphatidylinositol 3-kinase and antiestrogen resistance in breast cancer. J Clin Oncol 2011;29:4452–61.

53. Bachelot T, Bourgier C, Cropet C, et al. Randomized phase II trial of everolimus in combination with tamoxifen in patients with hormone receptor-positive, human epidermal growth factor receptor 2-negative metastatic breast cancer with prior exposure to aromatase inhibitors: a GINECO study. J Clin Oncol 2012;30(22): 2718–24.

54. Awada A, Cardoso F, Fontaine C, et al. The oral mTOR inhibitor RAD001 (everolimus) in combination with letrozole in patients with advanced breast cancer: results of a phase I study with pharmacokinetics. Eur J Cancer 2008;44: 84–91.

55. Baselga J, Semiglazov V, van Dam P, et al. Phase II randomized study of neoadjuvant everolimus plus letrozole compared with placebo plus letrozole in patients with estrogen receptor-positive breast cancer. J Clin Oncol 2009; 27(16):2630–7.

Endocrine Therapy for Advanced/ Metastatic Breast Cancer

Gaia Schiavon, MD, PhD[a,b,*], Ian E. Smith, MD, FRCP, FRCPE[a,b]

KEYWORDS

- Advanced • Breast cancer • Endocrine resistance • Endocrine therapy • Metastatic

KEY POINTS

- Estrogen receptor–positive metastatic breast cancer is still incurable but responses can be achieved with first-line endocrine therapies in around 30% and clinical benefit (response or stable disease for at least 6 months) in around 50% of patients.
- Aromatase inhibitors (AIs) are the most effective treatment in previously untreated postmenopausal women. Tamoxifen is still an effective alternative. Most of these women nowadays have received an adjuvant AI and the optimal endocrine therapy on relapse is uncertain.
- Tamoxifen and fulvestrant both achieve clinical benefit in around 50% of such patients, although objective responses are uncommon (around 10%). Exemestane after a nonsteroidal AI can also achieve clinical benefit in 30% to 50% of patients but objective responses are rare.
- In premenopausal women, tamoxifen is the treatment of choice if no previous endocrine therapy has been used (and there is some evidence that response rates may be increased with the addition of a luteinizing hormone–releasing hormone [LHRH] analogue) but this situation is now rare. Otherwise, a combination of an AI and an LHRH analogue is indicated. An AI should not be used alone in premenopausal women.
- Combined endocrine therapy and targeted therapies to overcome endocrine resistance are a major theme in current clinical research.

INTRODUCTION

Endocrine therapy for metastatic breast cancer (mBC) is the oldest effective medical treatment in cancer medicine. As long ago as 1896, Beatson[1] described clinical improvement after oophorectomy in young women affected by breast cancer, although many decades elapsed before the underlying endocrine mechanism was understood. High-dose estrogens were reported as initial treatment of large primary

[a] Breast Unit, The Royal Marsden NHS Foundation Trust, Fulham Road, London SW3 6JJ, UK;
[b] The Institute of Cancer Research, Fulham Road, London SW3 6JB, UK
* Corresponding author. The Royal Marsden NHS Foundation Trust, Fulham Road, London SW3 6JJ, UK.
E-mail address: gaia.schiavon@rmh.nhs.uk

Hematol Oncol Clin N Am 27 (2013) 715–736
http://dx.doi.org/10.1016/j.hoc.2013.05.004
0889-8588/13/$ – see front matter © 2013 Elsevier Inc. All rights reserved.

hemonc.theclinics.com

breast cancers in the 1950s[2] and were widely used for many years, despite their significant toxicities.

Surgical adrenalectomy with cortisone substitution was first described to treat advanced breast cancer in 1952[3] and became a standard form of so-called major ablative surgery for decades as second-line treatment after oophorectomy or in post-menopausal patients; it was effective in selected cases but required specialist skills, intensive support in the immediate postoperative period, and long-term steroid supplementation.[4] Hypophysectomy also had a role as second-line therapy in selected centers.[5]

Two major developments ushered in the modern era of endocrine therapy for mBC. The first was the development of the antiestrogen, tamoxifen, which rapidly established itself as an effective treatment without the significant side effects of estrogens.

The second was the discovery of the estrogen receptor (ER) in the 1960s by Jensen,[6] followed by the investigations by McGuire and colleagues,[7] which established this molecule as the first effective tumor marker for predicting response to endocrine therapy. It is now well established that the chance of response to any type of endocrine therapy is determined by whether or not the tumor is positive for ER and/or progesterone receptors (PgR).[8]

Not all ER-positive breast cancers respond to endocrine therapy. Some seem resistant from the start (de novo resistance) and many acquire resistance during the natural history of the disease, despite continuing to express ER. Overcoming endocrine resistance in ER-positive cancers is one of the great current challenges in breast cancer treatment (discussed later).

TAMOXIFEN AND OTHER ENDOCRINE THERAPIES WITHOUT PRIOR ADJUVANT AROMATASE INHIBITORS

Tamoxifen, the earliest selective ER modulator (SERM) for clinical use, was first described in the treatment of advanced/mBC in 1971 by Cole and colleagues.[9] This new antiestrogen rapidly began to replace high-dose estrogen therapy because of its efficacy and favorable toxicity profile. In a large review of 86 clinical studies involving 5353 patients, an objective response rate (ORR; complete response [CR] + partial response [PR]) of 34% was described with an additional 19% of patients achieving stable disease (SD) for at least 6 months.[10] Median response durations of up to 24 months were reported. Response rates (RRs) tended to increase with age, with a 27% response in those less than 50 years old compared with 43% in those more than 70 years old in a selective review of 60 studies involving 1282 patients in the same publication. Although early studies suggested that responses could be achieved in patients with ER-negative tumors, there is now a strong body of evidence to show that response to tamoxifen and other endocrine therapies occur only in those with ER-positive disease.[11]

Tamoxifen is generally well tolerated with a low incidence of serious side effects except for a low but significantly increased incidence of endometrial cancer and thromboembolic events.[12]

High-dose Estrogens, Progestins, Oophorectomy, and Other SERMs

Tamoxifen was compared with many other endocrine therapies in randomized trials in the early years, and although these were small and lacked statistical power by modern standards it was nevertheless consistently at least as effective or better, and often with a better toxicity profile. These findings include comparisons with high-dose estrogens,[13,14] megestrol acetate (MA), the most widely used synthetic progestin,[15–18] and oophorectomy in premenopausal women.[19,20] Tamoxifen has been shown to be as good as other SERMs, including toremifene and idoxifene, or in some cases better (eg, droloxifene, arzoxifene); all of these were phase II crossover studies showing cross-resistance between tamoxifen and other SERMs.[21–25]

AROMATASE INHIBITORS

In recent years the third-generation aromatase inhibitors (AIs) letrozole, anastrozole, and exemestane have consistently been shown to be superior to tamoxifen both in advanced/metastatic and in early breast cancer. Unlike tamoxifen they inhibit the synthesis of estrogens from androgens in postmenopausal women (they are ineffective in premenopausal women) and they have transformed endocrine therapy in this large group of women with ER-positive disease.[26]

Second-line Treatment After Tamoxifen

In a first series of randomized control trials (RCTs), each of the third-generation AIs were shown to be superior in efficacy and/or side effects to MA or to the first-generation AI aminoglutethimide as second-line therapy for postmenopausal women progressing on tamoxifen (**Table 1**).[27–34]

First-line Treatment Compared with Tamoxifen

Letrozole, anastrozole, and exemestane were subsequently compared with tamoxifen as first-line treatment of postmenopausal women with advanced/mBC. The main trials are summarized in **Table 2**.

In a North American multicenter RCT, anastrozole was as effective as tamoxifen in terms of ORR (21% vs 17% of patients, respectively) with significant advantage compared with tamoxifen in terms of clinical benefit rate (CBR) (CR + PR + SD ≥24 weeks, 59% vs 46%, respectively; 2-sided P = .0098, retrospective analysis)

Table 1

Main randomized clinical trials testing AIs as second-line treatment (after tamoxifen failure) in mBC

Study	Arms	n	ORR (%)	Median TTP or PFS (mo)	Median OS (mo)
Letrozole vs AG[33]	Letrozole 0.5 mg	192	16.7	3.3	21 (P = .04)[a]
	Letrozole 2.5 mg	185	19.5	3.4 (P = .008)[a]	28 (P = .002)[a]
	AG 250 mg × 2	178	12.4	3.2	20
Letrozole vs MA[30]	Letrozole 0.5 mg	188	12.8	5.1 (P = .02)	21.05 (P = .03)[a]
	Letrozole 2.5 mg	174	23.6 (P = .04)[a]	5.6 (P = .07)	25.3
	MA 160 mg	189	16.4	5.5	21.5
Letrozole vs MA[34]	Letrozole 0.5 mg	202	21	6.0 (P = .044)[a]	33
	Letrozole 2.5 mg	199	16	3.0	29
	MA 40 mg × 4	201	15	3.0	26
Anastrozole vs MA[29]	Anastrozole 1 mg	263	12.5	4.8	26.7 (P = .025)[a]
	Anastrozole 10 mg	248	12.5	5.3	25.5
	MA 40 mg × 4	253	12.3	4.6	22.5
Exemestane vs MA[32]	Exemestane 25 mg	366	15	4.7 (P = .037)[a]	— (P = .039)[a]
	MA 40 mg × 4	403	12.4	3.9	28.8

Abbreviations: AG, aminoglutethimide; n, number; OS, overall survival; PFS, progression-free survival; TTP, time to progression.

[a] P versus MA (or AG).

Table 2
Main randomized clinical trials testing AIs versus tamoxifen as first-line treatment in mBC

Study/Arms	n	ORR (%)	CBR (%)	Median TTP or PFS (mo)	Median OS (mo)
Anastrozole vs	171	21	59	11.1 (P = .005)	33
tamoxifen[35]	182	17	46	5.6	32
Anastrozole vs	340	33	56	8.2	38
tamoxifen[36]	328	33	55	8.3	42
Letrozole vs	453	32 (P = .0002)	50 (P = .0004)	9.4 (P<.0001)	34
tamoxifen[39]	454	21	38	6.0	30
Exemestane vs	182	46 (P = .05)	—	9.9 (P = .05)	37
tamoxifen[40]	189	31	—	5.8	43

Abbreviation: CBR, clinical benefit rate.

and time to progression (TTP) (median, 11.1 vs 5.6 months, respectively; 2-sided P = .005).[35] Almost 90% of patients enrolled in this trial were ER positive. A rest-of-the-world study (TARGET [Tamoxifen or Arimidex Randomized Group Efficacy and Tolerability] study) reported equivalence but not superiority of anastrozole compared with tamoxifen,[36] but in this trial only 45% of patients were known to have an ER-positive tumor. The pooled retrospective combined analysis of these two trials, including only the subgroup with ER-positive tumors (60% of combined trial population), showed that anastrozole was significantly superior to tamoxifen with respect to TTP (median values of 10.7 and 6.4 months) but not for overall survival (OS).[37,38]

In another large trial comparing letrozole with tamoxifen and involving 916 patients, letrozole significantly improved TTP compared with tamoxifen (median 9.4 vs 6.0 months, respectively) but no significant improvement in OS was observed.[39]

Exemestane, a steroidal AI, was compared with tamoxifen in an RCT conducted by the European Organisation for Research and Treatment of Cancer (EORTC) Breast Cancer Cooperative Group.[40] Median progression-free survival (PFS) was longer with exemestane (9.9 months; 95% confidence interval [CI], 8.7–11.8 months) than with tamoxifen (5.8 months), but these early differences (Wilcoxon P = .028) did not translate to a longer-term benefit in PFS, the primary study end point (log-rank P = .121), or OS.

A meta-analysis conducted by Ferretti and colleagues[41] on 6 phase III prospective RCTs including those described earlier and involving 2787 women treated with second-generation or third-generation AI versus tamoxifen confirmed a significant advantage in ORR, TTP, and CBR favoring AIs rather than tamoxifen detected in the fixed-effects model but not in the random-effects model, owing to the significant heterogeneity between studies. In contrast, no difference was found in OS using either model. Tamoxifen was associated with significantly more thromboembolic events and vaginal bleeding than the AIs. Hot flushes, vomiting, and musculoskeletal pain were slightly more frequent in the AI than the tamoxifen group but without reaching statistical significance.

These trials were not always conducted with the academic rigor to be expected in large modern trials, but the weight of evidence from these consistently argued in favor of the AIs having small but significant efficacy advantages compared with tamoxifen.

THE ERA OF ADJUVANT AIS

In the last 10 years the AIs letrozole, anastrozole, and exemestane have largely replaced tamoxifen as adjuvant treatment of early breast cancer in postmenopausal women, based on a series of large adjuvant trials showing their superior efficacy.

This means that much of the evidence described earlier has become redundant, given that most postmenopausal women with metastatic ER-positive breast cancer have already relapsed on or after an adjuvant AI, and there is now uncertainty about optimal further endocrine therapy in these circumstances. Several further options are available.

Tamoxifen After AIs

There are limited data about the efficacy of tamoxifen after AI failure. Retrospective crossover data for tamoxifen treatment are available from the North American and TARGET trials described earlier comparing the efficacy of tamoxifen following anastrozole with anastrozole following tamoxifen as first-line treatment of postmenopausal patients with mBC.[42] Of the 511 patients who were initially randomized to anastrozole, 137 (26.8%) received tamoxifen as second-line therapy at crossover. Among them, 40 had intervening chemotherapy and/or other hormonal therapy and therefore tamoxifen was technically third line. Overall clinical response data were available for 119 patients, with an ORR of 10.1% (12/119) and a CBR of 48.7% (58/119). Results for patients crossing directly to tamoxifen, without intervening therapy, were similar to those for all patients. ORR and CBR were 13.3% (6/45) and 48.9% (22/45) respectively in patients with visceral metastases, compared with ORR and CBR of 8.2% (6/73) and 49.3% (36/73) respectively for nonvisceral disease.

A second source of data is the TAMRAD (Tamoxifen-RAD001 vs Tamoxifen Alone in Patients With Anti-aromatase Resistant Breast Metastatic Cancer) trial, discussed further later. In this phase 2 trial, postmenopausal women with ER-positive human epidermal growth factor receptor (HER) 2–negative mBC resistant to an AI were randomized to treatment with tamoxifen in combination with the mammalian target of rapamycin (mTOR) inhibitor everolimus (n = 54) or tamoxifen alone (n = 57).[43] Patients in the tamoxifen-alone arm had an ORR of 13%, a CBR of 42%, a median TTP of 4.5 months, and a median OS of 32.9 months.

These data show that tamoxifen is of clinical benefit (CB) in almost 50% of patients relapsing on or after an AI, but only 10% or less achieve an objective response.

Exemestane After Nonsteroidal AIs

AIs can be divided into 2 classes, with different structures and mechanisms of action on the aromatase receptor site. Letrozole and anastrozole are in the first category. These AIs have a nonsteroidal structure and bind reversibly to the active site of the aromatase enzyme. In contrast, exemestane has a steroidal structure and binds irreversibly to the active site.[44] So far there is little evidence that these differences have any major clinical relevance, although there is some suggestion of a lack of complete clinical cross-resistance.[45,46]

A phase II study evaluated exemestane in 241 patients who had progressed after treatment with a nonsteroidal AI (NSAI).[47] A clinical CR was observed in 3 (1.2%) patients, and PR in 13 (5.4%), giving an ORR of 6.6%. SD for at least 6 months was seen in 101 (41.9%) patients, and the median TTP was 14.7 months.

Lack of cross-resistance between exemestane and NSAIs was also observed in an open-label, exploratory clinical trial comparing sequential treatment with exemestane and NSAIs in mBC.[46] In this study, exemestane (n = 23) showed activity in patients after relapse or lack of response to letrozole or anastrozole with an ORR of 8.7%, a CBR of 43.5%, a median TTP of 5.1 months, and a median OS of 27.2 months. Likewise letrozole (n = 17) and anastrozole (n = 1) (total n = 18) had clinical activity after failure on exemestane with an ORR of 22.2%, a CBR of 55.6%, a median TTP of 9.3 months, and a median OS of 29.7 months.

Two trials have compared exemestane with the steroidal antiestrogen fulvestrant in patients no longer responding to an NSAI. In the first, EFECT (Evaluation of the Efficacy and Tolerability of Faslodex[Fulvestrant] and Aromasin[Exemestane] in Hormone Receptor Positive Postmenopausal Women With Advanced Breast Cancer), involving 693 postmenopausal patients with ER-positive mBC, the median TTP was 3.7 months for both arms and CBR was also similar in patients treated with exemestane (31.5% for exemestane and 32.2% for fulvestrant given in a dose of 500 mg on day 0, and 250 mg on days 14 and 28 and every 28 days thereafter).[48]

The second was the SoFEA (Fulvestrant With or Without Anastrozole or Exemestane Alone in Treating Postmenopausal Women With Locally Advanced or Metastatic Breast Cancer) trial, a multicenter, randomized, partially blinded phase III study designed to investigate fulvestrant alone (n = 231) or with concomitant anastrozole (n = 243) versus exemestane (n = 249) following progression on NSAI.[49] Inclusion criteria included response to a previous NSAI in locally advanced/metastatic disease for more than 6 months (82%) or as adjuvant therapy for more than 12 months (18%). The median PFS was 4.4, 4.8, and 3.4 months for fulvestrant plus anastrozole, fulvestrant alone, and exemestane, respectively. A longer PFS was positively correlated with duration of prior AI exposure but no interaction with treatment was observed. No difference was found in ORR, CBR, or OS. The 249 patients treated with exemestane had an ORR and CBR of 2.8% and 39.8%, respectively.

Fulvestrant

The selective ER downregulator fulvestrant is a pure antiestrogen that binds to ER, inducing a conformational change that disrupts ER transcriptional activity and accelerates ER degradation. These features are unique to this agent. Initial clinical studies showed that fulvestrant 250 mg monthly by intramuscular (IM) injection (approved dose [AD]) had similar first-line efficacy to tamoxifen, with a median TTP of 6.8 and 8.3 months respectively (hazard ratio [HR], 1.18; 95% CI, 0.98–1.44; P = .088) and ORRs of 31.6% and 33.9% respectively.[50]

Fulvestrant 250 mg was likewise similar to anastrozole in 400 patients whose disease had progressed on adjuvant endocrine therapy with an antiestrogen or whose disease had progressed after first-line endocrine therapy for advanced disease.[51] Median TTP was 5.4 months with fulvestrant (n = 206) versus 3.4 months with anastrozole (n = 194) (HR, 0.92; 95% CI, 0.74–1.14; P = .43) and ORR was 17.5% in both arms. This trial was prospectively designed to be combined with a second study[52] with similar design and the combined analysis of data at a median follow-up of 15.1 months showed that fulvestrant was at least as effective as anastrozole in terms of median TTP (5.5 months vs 4.1 months, respectively) and OR (19% vs 17%, respectively).[53] In a subsequent survival analysis after a median follow-up of 27 months there was no significant difference in the median time to death between fulvestrant and anastrozole (27.4 months vs 27.7 months, respectively).[54]

As discussed earlier, the EFECT trial showed that AD fulvestrant (500 mg on day 0, 250 mg on days 14 and 28, and 250 mg every 28 days thereafter) had similar modest efficacy to exemestane after NSAI failure.[48]

Subsequent studies suggested that the AD of fulvestrant was likely not to be the optimal dose for this agent and several trials tested different doses.[55] These trials are summarized in **Table 3**.

For example, 3 different doses of fulvestrant (AD, as defined earlier; high dose [HD], 500 mg once a month plus 500 mg on day 14 and day 28 of month 1, and monthly

Table 3
Main randomized clinical trials testing fulvestrant in mBC

Study/Arms	n	ORR (%)	CBR (%)	Median TTP or PFS (mo)	Median OS (mo)
First Line					
Fulv 250 mg monthly	313	31.6	54.3	6.8	36.9
vs tamoxifen[50]	274	33.9	62	8.3	38.7
Fulv 250 mg monthly	206	17.5	42.2	5.4	—
vs anastrozole[51]	194	17.5	36.1	3.4	—
Fulv 250 mg monthly	222	20.7	44.6	5.5	—
vs anastrozole[52]	229	15.7	45.0	5.1	—
Fulv LD +	258	31.8	55.0	10.8	37.8
anastrozole vs anastrozole[62]	256	33.6	55.1	10.2	38.2
Fulv LD +	355	—	—	15 (P<.007)	47.7 (P = .049)
anastrozole vs anastrozole[61]	352	—	—	13.5	41.3
Fulv HD vs	102	36.0	72.5	23.4 (P = .01)	—
anastrozole[59]	103	35.5	67.0	13.1	—

Study	Arms	n	ORR (%)	Median TTP or PFS (mo)	Median OS (mo)
Second Line or Beyond					
CONFIRM[57,58]	Fulv HD vs	362	9.1	6.5 (P = .006)	25.2
(second line) phase III	Fulv 250 mg monthly	374	10.2	5.5	22.8
EFECT[48] (third line	Fulv LD vs	351	7.4	3.7	NR
or more) phase III	Exemestane	342	6.7	3.7	NR
SOFEA[49] (acquired AI resistance)	Fulv LD + anastrozole vs	243	7.4	4.4	20.2
phase III	Fulv LD vs	231	6.9	4.8	19.4
	Exemestane	249	3.6	3.4	21.6

Abbreviations: CONFIRM, Fulvestrant 250 mg With Fulvestrant 500 mg in Postmenopausal Women With Estrogen Receptor–positive Advanced Breast Cancer; Fulv, fulvestrant; EFECT, Evaluation of the Efficacy and Tolerability of Faslodex (Fulvestrant) and Aromasin (Exemestane) in Hormone Receptor Positive Postmenopausal Women With Advanced Breast Cancer; HD, high dose (500 mg IM at day 0 + 500 mg IM at days 14 and 28, thereafter 500 mg IM monthly until progression); LD, loading dose regimen (500 mg IM on day 0, 250 mg on days 14, 28, and 250 mg every 28 days thereafter); NR, not reported; SOFEA, Fulvestrant With or Without Anastrozole or Exemestane Alone in Treating Postmenopausal Women With Locally Advanced or Metastatic Breast Cancer.

thereafter; and loading dose [LD], 500 mg IM on day 0, 250 mg on days 14 and 28, and 250 mg every 28 days thereafter) were compared in the FINDER II trial in 144 postmenopausal women with mBC after 1 prior endocrine therapy.[56] Fulvestrant AD, HD, and LD had ORRs of 8.5%, 5.9%, and 15.2%, respectively with longer median TTP for the HD and LD arms (6.0 and 6.1 months, respectively) versus AD (3.1 months). However, limitations because of the small sample size have to be considered.

Fulvestrant AD versus HD regimens were compared in 736 patients with ER-positive mBC progressing after prior endocrine therapy in the CONFIRM trial (Fulvestrant 250 mg With Fulvestrant 500 mg in Postmenopausal Women With Estrogen Receptor–Positive Advanced Breast Cancer).[57] ORRs and CBRs were similar in both arms (ORR, 9.1% vs 10.2%; CBR, 45.6% vs 39.6% in HD and AD, respectively). However, fulvestrant HD significantly prolonged PFS compared with fulvestrant AD (6.5 vs 5.5 months, respectively; HR, 0.80; 95% CI, 0.68–0.94; P = .006). Moreover, the toxicity profile of both doses is similar and low. Fulvestrant HD has therefore become the AD for use in Europe. The recently presented final analysis showing that a median OS of 26.4 versus 22.3 months in fulvestrant HD and AD, respectively (HR, 0.81; 95% CI, 0.69, 0.96; nominal P = .016), indicates that fulvestrant 500 mg is associated with a clinically relevant 4.1 month difference in median OS and 19% reduction in risk of death compared with fulvestrant 250 mg.[58] There were no new safety concerns associated with the use of fulvestrant 500 mg.

A phase II trial compared HD fulvestrant with anastrozole as first-line treatment of hormone receptor–positive (HR+) mBC and found no significant difference in CBR between the 2 arms (72.5% and 67.0%, respectively) but significantly longer TTP with HD fulvestrant (median TTP not reached vs 12.5 months; HR, 0.63; 95% CI, 0.39–1.00; P = .0496).[59]

The final issue with fulvestrant concerns preclinical data suggesting that it may be more effective in a low estrogen environment.[60]

To test this, 2 randomized phase III trials tested the combination of anastrozole with fulvestrant versus anastrozole alone with the same dose and schedule as first-line combination endocrine therapy in postmenopausal women with mBC. The first, Southwest Oncology Group (SWOG) S0226, showed that fulvestrant plus anastrozole significantly improved median PFS (15.0 vs 13.5 months) and median OS (47.7 vs 41.3 months) compared with anastrozole alone.[61] Safety and tolerability were similar between the two arms, and discontinuation of treatment because of side effects was rare. However, the second trial, FACT (Anastrozole Monotherapy vs Maximal Oestrogen Blockade With Anastrozole and Fulvestrant Combination Therapy), did not show any difference in the median PFS or median OS between the combination and the anastrozole arm.[62] The main difference between these trials was the percentage of endocrine therapy-naive patients: 60% and 33% in the SWOG and FACT trial respectively. In an unplanned subgroup analysis of only the endocrine-naive subgroup in the SWOG trial, a significantly greater benefit was observed in the combination arm (median PFS 17.0 vs 12.6 months), although this was not observed in the FACT trial (see **Table 1**). Both trials used the fulvestrant AD, which has been shown to be less effective than the HD, as described earlier.[57]

As described earlier, the SoFEA trial showed PFSs of 4.4, 4.8, and 3.4 months for fulvestrant LD plus anastrozole (n = 243), fulvestrant LD alone (n = 231), and exemestane (n = 249), respectively, following progression on NSAI, but no difference was found in ORR, CBR, and OS (see **Table 3**).[49]

In conclusion, fulvestrant has modest clinical efficacy following failure of treatment with prior endocrine therapy. This efficacy is probably enhanced with the HD regimen, and implies that there may be a slight additional advantage when given in combination with an AI in endocrine therapy–naive patients. This possibility is being tested further in a new prospective randomized, double-blind, phase III first-line trial, FALCON (A Global Study to Compare the Effects of Fulvestrant and Arimidex in a Subset of Patients With Breast Cancer).

OTHER ENDOCRINE THERAPY OPTIONS
Progestins and Estrogens

Medroxyprogesterone and MA are progesterone derivatives commonly used as endocrine therapy in the treatment of mBC, although their exact mechanism of antitumor action is unclear. These agents suppress adrenal steroid synthesis and suppress

ER levels, altering tumor hormone metabolism and causing tumor cell death.[63,64] They may also act through the glucocorticoid receptor, androgen receptor, or PgR and activity seems to be maintained in patients who are refractory to steroidal AIs.[64,65]

Progestins have similar RRs to tamoxifen.[66,67] They represent a useful option in some patients, but are associated with significant weight gain, fluid retention, vaginal bleeding, and risk of thromboembolic events.[65,68]

The AIs anastrozole and exemestane were shown to be marginally superior to MA in terms of survival in initial trials, as shown in **Table 1**. However, a pooled analysis of 9 phase III RCTs comparing AIs (both steroidal and nonsteroidal) versus MA in second line for patients with mBC did not show any significant difference in ORR or TTP for either drug.[69]

Trials comparing steroidal AIs with MA have not used a crossover design; therefore, the activity of MA after the failure of steroidal AIs has not been systematically studied.[65]

It has been hypothesized that estrogen deprivation therapy with AIs may paradoxically sensitize HR+ breast cancer tumor cells to low-dose estradiol therapy.

In a phase II trial including 66 postmenopausal women with mBC treated with an AI with a PFS of greater than or equal to 24 weeks or relapse after greater than or equal to 2 years of an adjuvant AI were randomized to low-dose estradiol (6 mg, achieving a level similar to that found in premenopausal women) versus HD (30 mg).[70] CBR was similar in both groups (28% and 29% in the 30-mg and 6-mg groups, respectively). The 6-mg dose was associated with fewer serious adverse events (18% vs 34% toxicities of grade 3 or greater). Seven patients with estradiol-sensitive disease were retreated with AIs at estradiol progression, among which 2 had PR and 1 had SD, suggesting resensitization to estrogen deprivation. The efficacy of treatment with the lower dose should be further examined in phase III clinical trials.

OVERCOMING RESISTANCE TO ENDOCRINE THERAPY

Many patients with ER-positive breast cancer are clinically resistant to endocrine therapy either from the start (de novo) or at some later point in the natural history of the disease (acquired). One of the challenges in breast cancer is to understand the mechanisms of resistance and to devise effective strategies to overcome these.

Acquired endocrine resistance develops as a consequence of a series of complex adaptive changes occurring in breast cancer cells during the selective pressure of long-term endocrine treatment.[71] Activation of various pathways including PIK3CA, mTOR, HER, and fibroblast growth factor receptor (FGFR) can lead to endocrine resistance in preclinical models and targeting these could reverse resistance to endocrine therapy (**Fig. 1**). There are several mechanisms that can lead to kinase activation. These include (1) genomic alteration in the bulk of the tumor at baseline, (2) protein activation at baseline in the bulk of the tumor (eg, LKB1 loss), (3) kinase activation induced by endocrine manipulations as a consequence of long-term estrogen deprivation, and (4) genomic alteration acquired during the natural course of the disease.

Table 4 shows the main randomized clinical trials testing endocrine therapy in combination with anti-HER2 agents and mTOR antagonists.

Combination with mTOR Inhibitors

One of the most important changes concerns the activation of the PI3K/AKT/mTOR pathway, the most frequently affected pathway in breast cancer.[71]

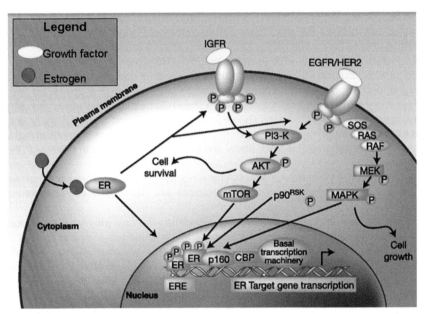

Fig. 1. Crosstalk between signal transduction pathways and ER signaling in endocrine-resistant breast cancer. Estrogen (E2)-liganded ER activates E2-regulated genes in the classic pathway. Resistance can develop after long-term endocrine therapy, with bidirectional crosstalk between ER and growth factor receptors, with association of membrane-bound ER with growth factor receptors, and/or insulin growth factor receptor (IGFR) or epidermal growth factor receptor (EGFR)/HER2 activation of ER phosphorylation. Various signal transduction inhibitors may modulate these pathways and overcome the resistance to endocrine therapy. (*Modified from* Johnston SR. New strategies in estrogen receptor-positive breast cancer. Clin Cancer Res 2010;16(7):1981; with permission.)

Preclinical data suggest a synergistic effect of the combination of mTOR antagonists with endocrine therapy,[72,73] and clinical trials investigating this are ongoing.

The earliest, a phase II study exploring the combination of temsirolimus given intravenously 10 mg daily, or 30 mg intermittently (daily for 5 days every 2 weeks), and letrozole in 104 patients with mBC showed a longer median PFS with the combination compared with letrozole alone (13.2 vs 11.6 months, respectively).[74]

A subsequent phase III randomized placebo-controlled trial (HORIZON [Letrozole Plus Oral Temsirolimus as First-Line Endocrine Therapy in Postmenopausal Women With Locally Advanced or Metastatic Breast Cancer]) tested the efficacy and safety of first-line letrozole and temsirolimus 30 mg daily (5 days every 2 weeks) versus letrozole/placebo in 1112 patients with AI-naive, HR+ advanced disease.[75] The addition of temsirolimus to letrozole did not lead to improvement in PFS as first-line therapy in patients with AI-naive advanced breast cancer. Grade 3 to 4 toxicities were more common in the temsirolimus arm versus the letrozole-alone arm, including hyperglycemia (4% vs 1%).

Everolimus, an mTOR inhibitor, has been shown experimentally and clinically to target the PI3K network in combination with endocrine treatment. A randomized phase II trial, the TAMRAD (Tamoxifen-RAD001 vs Tamoxifen Alone in Patients With Anti-aromatase Resistant Breast Metastatic Cancer) trial compared tamoxifen and everolimus with tamoxifen alone in patients with mBC resistant to an AI.[43] The everolimus combination showed an improvement in 6-month CRB (61% vs 42%), TTP (8.6 vs

Table 4
Main randomized clinical trials testing endocrine therapy in combination with anti-HER2 agents and mTOR antagonists

Study	Phase	Arms	n	ORR (%)	Median TTP or PFS (mo)	Median OS (mo)
Anti-HER2 Agents						
Cristofanilli et al,[86] 2010	II RCT	Anastrozole + placebo	50	12	8.4	NR
		Anastrozole + gefitinib	43	2	14.7	NR
Osborne et al,[85] 2011	II RCT	Tamoxifen + placebo	136	14.9	8.8	NR
		Tamoxifen + gefitinib	153	12.4	10.9	NR
TAnDEM[84]	III RCT	Anastrozole	104	6.8	2.4	23.9
		Anastrozole + trastuzumab	103	20.3[a]	4.8[a]	28.5
EGF30008[87]	III RCT	Letrozole + placebo	108	15	3	32.3
		Letrozole + lapatinib	111	28[a]	8.2[a]	33.3
eLEcTRA[88]	II RCT	Letrozole	31	13	3.3	NR
		Letrozole + trastuzumab	26	27	14.1	NR
mTOR Antagonists						
TAMRAD[43]	II RCT, with previous AI exposure[b]	Everolimus + tamoxifen	54	NR	8.6[a,d]	NR[a,d]
		Tamoxifen	57	NR	4.5	24.0
BOLERO-2[76,77]	III RCT, progressed on NSAI[c]	Everolimus + exemestane	485	9.5[a]	7.8[a]	NR
		Exemestane	239	0.4	3.2	NR
HORIZON[75]	III RCT, AI naive	Letrozole + temsirolimus	555	27	8.9	NR
		Letrozole + placebo	555	27	9.0	NR

Abbreviations: BOLERO-2, Everolimus in Combination With Exemestane in the Treatment of Post-menopausal Women With Estrogen Receptor Positive Locally Advanced or Metastatic Breast Cancer Who Are Refractory to Letrozole or Anastrozole; EGF30008, Lapatinib combined with letrozole vs letrozole alone for front line postmenopausal hormone receptor positive (HR+) metastatic breast cancer (MBC); eLEcTRA, The Study of the Efficacy and Safety of Letrozole Combined with Trastuzumab in Patients with Metastatic Breast Cancer (eLEcTRA); HORIZON, Letrozole Plus Oral Temsirolimus as First-Line Endocrine Therapy in Postmenopausal Women With Locally Advanced or Metastatic Breast Cancer; NR, not reported; TAMRAD, Tamoxifen-RAD001 vs Tamoxifen Alone in Patients With Anti-aromatase Resistant Breast Metastatic Cancer.

[a] Statistically significant difference.

[b] Stratified by primary versus secondary hormone resistance. Primary resistance is relapse during adjuvant AI therapy or progression during first 6 months of initiating AI for metastatic disease. Secondary resistance is late relapse (at or after 6 months) or previous response to AI therapy for mBC and subsequent progression.

[c] More than 50% of patients in each arm with 3 or more previous therapies, stratified by sensitivity to previous hormonal therapy and presence of visceral metastases.

[d] Exploratory analysis.

4.5 months), and median OS (not reached in the combination arm) compared with tamoxifen alone. In an exploratory subgroup analysis the CBR for the combination seemed greater (74%) in patients with acquired secondary resistance (20 of 27 patients) than in patients with primary resistance (46%, 12 of 26 patients).

This benefit with everolimus was further shown in BOLERO-2 (Everolimus in Combination With Exemestane in the Treatment of Postmenopausal Women With Estrogen Receptor Positive Locally Advanced or Metastatic Breast Cancer Who Are Refractory to Letrozole or Anastrozole), a randomized phase III trial that assigned 724 postmenopausal patients with ER-positive mBC to either exemestane alone or the combination of exemestane and everolimus.[76] All patients had progressed on an NSAI and 84% had shown prior hormone-sensitive disease. The 18-month PFS was 7.8 months for the everolimus arm compared with 3.2 months for the control arm of exemestane alone (HR = 0.45, $P<.0001$).[77] Patients with visceral metastases represented a substantial portion (n = 406) of the overall group and had a PFS benefit comparable with the overall population with CBRs in the everolimus arm, double that of the controls, and RRs 9.5% and 0.4% respectively ($P<.001$).[76] OS results were immature at the time of the interim analysis. The main disadvantage of everolimus in both trials was an increased incidence of side effects including stomatitis, fatigue, rash, diarrhea, noninfectious pneumonitis, and hyperglycemia.[43,76] This increased toxicity emphasizes the importance of research into molecular markers that might define the patients most likely to benefit from this additional treatment. So far, a biomarker to use as an indicator of mTOR activation has not been identified.

These trials differed in that HORIZON excluded patients previously exposed to AIs, whereas BOLERO-2 eligibility required progression on an NSAI during or within 12 months of completing adjuvant therapy or within 1 month if in the metastatic setting. Therefore, despite the limitations of cross-trial comparisons, this difference may explain the different PFS observed in the 2 trials, and may also explain the different RRs observed in the control arms (27% in HORIZON vs 0.4% in BOLERO-2).

Other novel drugs targeting the PI3K/AKT/mTOR pathway are currently been tested in phase I and II trials in patients who have progressed on previous hormonal treatments. These treatments include pan or specific PI3K inhibitors, dual PI3K/mTOR inhibitors, AKT inhibitors, and mTOR inhibitors.[71]

One example is BKM120, a pan-PI3K inhibitor currently undergoing phase I assessment in combination with letrozole. So far the combination has been found to be safe, and 18-fluorodeoxyglucose positron emission tomography repeated at 2 weeks after treatment seems to be a useful pharmacodynamic biomarker of PI3K inhibition.[78] The combination of BKM120 with fulvestrant is also under study.[79]

Combinations with Histone Deacetylase Inhibitors

Another approach to reversing hormone resistance is the use of histone deacetylase inhibitors (HDACI), which may resensitize cells to hormone manipulation and prevent the emergence of resistant clones. Entinostat, an HDACI, has been tested in a randomized phase II trial (ENCORE 301), with exemestane versus exemestane/placebo in patients who had received prior hormonal therapy. This trial showed prolongation of median PFS (4.3 vs 2.3 months) and extension of OS benefit (26.9 vs 19.8 months), and a randomized phase III trial is now planned.[80]

Antiandrogens

AIs are structurally related to the natural substrate androstenedione, and in postmenopausal women they inhibit aromatase without affecting adrenal biosynthesis of corticosteroids, aldosterone, or other enzymes in the steroidogenic pathway. Cytochrome P450 (CYP) 17 is upstream from aromatase in the steroid synthesis pathway and, theoretically, abiraterone acetate (AA), an irreversible inhibitor of CYP17, might provide more complete inhibition of sex steroid synthesis.

In a phase I trial, AA showed evidence of antitumor activity with manageable side effects, including hypokalemia and fluid retention.[81] A currently ongoing randomized phase II trial, BCA2001 (A Study of Abiraterone Acetate Plus Prednisone With or Without Exemestane in Postmenopausal Women With Estrogen Receptor–positive [ER+] Metastatic Breast Cancer Progressing After Letrozole or Anastrozole Therapy) is comparing AA (plus low-dose prednisone) with or without exemestane.[82] It is hypothesized that AA will reduce the production of adrenal androgens that may be converted to estrogens and therefore add to peripheral suppression of estrogen synthesis by an AI.[82] The BCA2001 study is designed to evaluate whether ER signaling remains important for breast cancer growth in the setting of AI failure in postmenopausal women with ER-positive mBC. This study also evaluates whether continued aromatase inhibition with exemestane is required to suppress estrogen biosynthesis maximally when an AA is used.

Combination Therapy with Anti-HER2 Agents in HER2-positive Breast Cancer

Preclinical studies of acquired endocrine resistance in ER-positive breast cancer have consistently shown that a functional ER signaling pathway persists that often crosstalks with enhanced peptide growth factor receptor signaling pathways including HER1 and HER2. The mitogen-activated protein kinase (MAPK) pathway mediates cell proliferation, and increased signaling of this pathway is associated with shorter duration of response to tamoxifen and with decreased survival in patients with ER-positive breast cancer.[83]

Several HER1/HER2 inhibitors are being investigated in combination with endocrine therapy for patients with mBC with the aim of overcoming or preventing endocrine resistance (see **Table 4**).[84–88]

TAnDEM (TrAstuzumab in Dual HER2 ER-Positive Metastatic breast cancer) was the first randomized phase III study to combine a hormonal agent with trastuzumab without chemotherapy in postmenopausal HR+ HER2-positive (HER2+) patients with mBC.[84] PFS was significantly longer ($P = .0016$) in patients treated with the trastuzumab plus anastrozole arm (n = 103) than anastrozole alone (n = 104). In a planned subgroup analysis in patients who were centrally confirmed as HR+, median PFS was 5.6 and 3.8 months in the trastuzumab plus anastrozole and anastrozole-alone arms, respectively ($P = .006$). OS in the overall and centrally confirmed HR+ populations showed no significant difference between the two arms. Seventy percent of patients in the anastrozole-alone arm crossed over to receive trastuzumab after progression on anastrozole alone. Grade 3 and 4 adverse events were 23% and 5% respectively in the trastuzumab plus anastrozole arm, and 15% and 1% respectively, in the anastrozole-alone arm.

In a similar phase III randomized, double-blind, multicenter trial, 1286 postmenopausal patients with HR+ mBC were randomly assigned to receive letrozole plus lapatinib, an oral dual tyrosine kinase inhibitor of HER1 and HER2, or letrozole plus placebo.[87] In the subgroup with HER2+ disease (n = 219) median PFS was 3.0 months in the letrozole/placebo arm versus 8.2 months in the combination arm ($P = .019$). In an exploratory analysis of the HER2-negative population designed to determine the influence of acquired resistance to endocrine therapy, there was no significant improvement in PFS or CBR for the combination in the population still clinically sensitive to endocrine therapy (>6 months since discontinuation of antiestrogen therapy or no prior antiestrogen therapy), whereas a trend toward a better clinical outcome was seen in the clinically resistant group (<6 months since discontinuation of tamoxifen).

These data indicate that anti-HER1/HER2 therapy may overcome resistance to endocrine treatment in patients with HR+HER2+ breast cancer, but they also suggest that there may be benefit in a subgroup of patients with ER+/HER2-negative breast cancer that has become resistant to antiestrogens through the activation of the growth factor pathway even in the absence of HER2 overexpression.

ENDOCRINE THERAPY FOR PREMENOPAUSAL PATIENTS WITH MBC

The clinical scenario of mBC in premenopausal women is becoming less common, because many premenopausal patients have already had adjuvant chemotherapy with cessation of ovarian function.

Reduction of estrogen levels by ovarian ablation using surgery or radiotherapy achieves regression of metastatic disease in about 30% of unselected premenopausal women with mBC.[8] Tamoxifen achieves similar efficacy in premenopausal women with advanced disease.[89]

A few small randomized clinical trials[19,20,90] and a meta-analysis[91] in premenopausal women with mBC confirmed that tamoxifen is of similar efficacy and it therefore became the first-line of treatment of choice in this setting, given its simplicity of administration and low incidence of significant side effects.

It was subsequently shown that the luteinizing hormone–releasing hormone (LHRH) analogues, including goserelin, can reduce estrogen levels to less than postmenopausal levels within 21 to 28 days in more than 90% of premenopausal women.[92] A phase III trial involving 136 women showed that failure-free survival (FFS) and OS were similar for goserelin and oophorectomy (FFS, 4 and 6 months, respectively; OS, 33 and 37 months, respectively).[93] Side effects including hot flushes (75% vs 46%) and tumor flare (16% vs 3%) were more common in the goserelin arm. LHRH analogues consequently also became widely used as first-line endocrine therapy in premenopausal women.

A series of small studies investigated the role of an LHRH analogue plus tamoxifen versus an LHRH analogue alone in the treatment of premenopausal women with mBC, with mixed results.[94–97] A meta-analysis of these studies showed an increase in ORR of 31%, an improvement in PFS (HR, 0.70; $P = .001$), and an improved OS (HR, 0.78; $P = .02$) in the combination group compared with the LHRH analogue alone.[98] These data suggest that the use of an LHRH analogue plus tamoxifen may therefore offer an improved clinical outcome, but there were some caveats including no formal crossover of patients who received the LHRH analogue alone to tamoxifen as second-line therapy in 3 of the 4 studies, no detailed collection of toxicity data, and a lack of quality-of-life data.[8]

AIs are inappropriate in premenopausal women because high estrogen levels render aromatase inhibition without ovarian function suppression ineffective. Their use leads to an increase in gonadotropin secretion secondary to a reduced feedback of estrogen to the hypothalamus and pituitary. AIs may therefore result in a surge of ovarian aromatase activity and higher estrogen levels. However, they could have a role in combination with an LHRH analogue. On disease progression, selected patients may be candidates for further endocrine treatment in combination with ongoing ovarian function suppression.

There are 3 short reports in the literature of the first-line use of goserelin plus anastrozole in premenopausal women with HR+ mBC. The first involved 32 patients from 2 centers (Stanford University and MD Anderson Cancer Center) and showed a 72%

CBR with a median TTP of 8 months.[99] The second was from a multicenter study in France involving 33 patients showing a CBR of 63.6% and TTP of 13 months.[100] In the third study, 36 patients with mBC were administered goserelin plus anastrozole for greater than or equal to 6 months (unless they had prior progression).[101] Thirteen received further therapy with goserelin plus exemestane. They found a CBR of 67% (5% CR, 31% PR, 31% SD for ≥6 months) with median TTP and duration of CB of 12 (2–47) months and 24+ (7–78+) months respectively. Among the 13 patients who received goserelin plus exemestane, 38% achieved CB with a mean duration of 13+ (7–32) months with minimal side effects. The combination of goserelin plus anastrozole resulted in 98% reduction (from pretreatment to 6 months) in median levels of estradiol (from 574.5 pmol/L; interquartile range [IQR], 209–1426; n = 6) to (13.45 pmol/L; IQR, 5.5–31.5; n = 4), whereas the levels of other hormones had minimal fluctuations during therapy.

A small phase II study in 16 premenopausal women with mBC showed that the combined use of goserelin and anastrozole as second-line endocrine therapy after progression on goserelin and tamoxifen achieved a CB of 75% with a median duration of remission of greater than 17 months.[102]

Therefore, there exists a high rate of CB with reasonably long duration when goserelin is used in combination with an AI, in both first-line and subsequent lines of treatment in premenopausal women with mBC that remained hormone therapy sensitive.

In another small nonrandomized study, fulvestrant 250 mg was combined with goserelin 3.6 mg every 4 weeks as first-line to fourth-line therapy, showing efficacy in 26 premenopausal patients with a CBR of 58%.[103] Median TTP was 6 months (95% CI, 2.4–9.6) and OS was 32 months (95% CI, 14.28–49.72). These results suggest that the combination of fulvestrant and goserelin offers promising activity in premenopausal patients and further investigation is warranted.

SUMMARY

First-line endocrine therapy by estrogen antagonism (eg, with tamoxifen) or suppression of estrogen (eg, AIs, LHRH analogues, or oophorectomy) achieves objective tumor responses in around 30% of patients with ER-positive mBC and CB in around 50%. In the current era of adjuvant AI therapy, the optimal endocrine therapy on relapse remains uncertain. Tamoxifen, exemestane (after prior nonsteroidal AIs), and fulvestrant have each been reported as achieving around 10% objective clinical responses and CB in around 50%.

Encouraging new evidence suggests that resistance to endocrine therapy may be overcome in a significant number of patients combining tamoxifen or an AI with the mTOR inhibitor everolimus. Likewise, in ER-positive HER2+ breast cancer the addition of an anti-HER2 agent such as trastuzumab or lapatinib to standard endocrine therapy may also improve outcome. Targeted therapies in combination with endocrine therapy are likely to become increasingly important in overcoming endocrine resistance.

ACKNOWLEDGMENTS

The authors would like to thank the Cridland Fund for supporting Dr Gaia Schiavon.

REFERENCES

1. Beatson GT. On the treatment of inoperable cases of carcinoma of the mamma: suggestions for a new method of treatment, with illustrative cases. Lancet 1896; 148(3803):104–7.

2. Kennedy BJ, Kelley RM, White G, et al. Surgery as an adjunct to hormone therapy of breast cancer. Cancer 1957;10:1055–75.

3. Huggins C, Bergenstal DM. Inhibition of human mammary and prostatic cancers by adrenalectomy. Cancer Res 1952;12:134–41.

4. Fracchia AA, Randall HT, Farrow JH. The results of adrenalectomy in advanced breast cancer in 500 consecutive patients. Surg Gynecol Obstet 1967;125:747–56.

5. Harrold BP, Cates JE, James JA. Treatment of advanced breast cancer by transsphenoidal hypophysectomy. Br J Cancer 1968;22:19–31.

6. Jensen EV, Jacobson HI, Smith S, et al. The use of estrogen antagonists in hormone receptor studies. Gynecol Invest 1972;3:108–23.

7. McGuire WL. Hormone receptors: their role in predicting prognosis and response to endocrine therapy. Semin Oncol 1978;5:428–33.

8. Pritchard KI. Endocrine therapy of advanced disease: analysis and implications of the existing data. Clin Cancer Res 2003;9:460S–7S.

9. Cole MP, Jones CT, Todd ID. A new anti-oestrogenic agent in late breast cancer. An early clinical appraisal of ICI46474. Br J Cancer 1971;25:270–5.

10. Litherland S, Jackson IM. Antioestrogens in the management of hormone-dependent cancer. Cancer Treat Rev 1988;15:183–94.

11. Effects of chemotherapy and hormonal therapy for early breast cancer on recurrence and 15-year survival: an overview of the randomised trials. Lancet 2005;365:1687–717.

12. Jordan VC. Tamoxifen: toxicities and drug resistance during the treatment and prevention of breast cancer. Annu Rev Pharmacol Toxicol 1995;35:195–211.

13. Ingle JN, Ahmann DL, Green SJ, et al. Randomized clinical trial of diethylstilbestrol versus tamoxifen in postmenopausal women with advanced breast cancer. N Engl J Med 1981;304:16–21.

14. Robertson JF. Selective oestrogen receptor modulators/new antioestrogens: a clinical perspective. Cancer Treat Rev 2004;30:695–706.

15. Gill PG, Gebski V, Snyder R, et al. Randomized comparison of the effects of tamoxifen, megestrol acetate, or tamoxifen plus megestrol acetate on treatment response and survival in patients with metastatic breast cancer. Ann Oncol 1993;4:741–4.

16. Ingle JN, Ahmann DL, Green SJ, et al. Randomized clinical trial of megestrol acetate versus tamoxifen in paramenopausal or castrated women with advanced breast cancer. Am J Clin Oncol 1982;5:155–60.

17. Morgan LR. Megestrol acetate v tamoxifen in advanced breast cancer in postmenopausal patients. Semin Oncol 1985;12:43–7.

18. Paterson AH, Hanson J, Pritchard KI, et al. Comparison of antiestrogen and progestogen therapy for initial treatment and consequences of their combination for second-line treatment of recurrent breast cancer. Semin Oncol 1990;17:52–62.

19. Buchanan RB, Blamey RW, Durrant KR, et al. A randomized comparison of tamoxifen with surgical oophorectomy in premenopausal patients with advanced breast cancer. J Clin Oncol 1986;4:1326–30.

20. Ingle JN, Krook JE, Green SJ, et al. Randomized trial of bilateral oophorectomy versus tamoxifen in premenopausal women with metastatic breast cancer. J Clin Oncol 1986;4:178–85.

21. Pyrhonen S, Ellmen J, Vuorinen J, et al. Meta-analysis of trials comparing toremifene with tamoxifen and factors predicting outcome of antiestrogen therapy in postmenopausal women with breast cancer. Breast Cancer Res Treat 1999;56:133–43.

22. Johnston SR. Endocrine manipulation in advanced breast cancer: recent advances with SERM therapies. Clin Cancer Res 2001;7:4376s–87s [discussion: 4411s–2s].

23. Buzdar A, Hayes D, El-Khoudary A, et al. Phase III randomized trial of droloxifene and tamoxifen as first-line endocrine treatment of ER/PgR-positive advanced breast cancer. Breast Cancer Res Treat 2002;73:161–75.

24. Deshmane V, Krishnamurthy S, Melemed AS, et al. Phase III double-blind trial of arzoxifene compared with tamoxifen for locally advanced or metastatic breast cancer. J Clin Oncol 2007;25:4967–73.

25. Barrios C, Forbes JF, Jonat W, et al. The sequential use of endocrine treatment for advanced breast cancer: where are we? Ann Oncol 2012;23: 1378–86.

26. Smith IE, Dowsett M. Aromatase inhibitors in breast cancer. N Engl J Med 2003; 348:2431–42.

27. Jonat W, Howell A, Blomqvist C, et al. A randomised trial comparing two doses of the new selective aromatase inhibitor anastrozole (Arimidex) with megestrol acetate in postmenopausal patients with advanced breast cancer. Eur J Cancer 1996;32A:404–12.

28. Buzdar A, Jonat W, Howell A, et al. Anastrozole, a potent and selective aromatase inhibitor, versus megestrol acetate in postmenopausal women with advanced breast cancer: results of overview analysis of two phase III trials. Arimidex Study Group. J Clin Oncol 1996;14:2000–11.

29. Buzdar AU, Jonat W, Howell A, et al. Anastrozole versus megestrol acetate in the treatment of postmenopausal women with advanced breast carcinoma: results of a survival update based on a combined analysis of data from two mature phase III trials. Arimidex Study Group. Cancer 1998;83:1142–52.

30. Dombernowsky P, Smith I, Falkson G, et al. Letrozole, a new oral aromatase inhibitor for advanced breast cancer: double-blind randomized trial showing a dose effect and improved efficacy and tolerability compared with megestrol acetate. J Clin Oncol 1998;16:453–61.

31. Goss PE, Winer EP, Tannock IF, et al. Randomized phase III trial comparing the new potent and selective third-generation aromatase inhibitor vorozole with megestrol acetate in postmenopausal advanced breast cancer patients. North American Vorozole Study Group. J Clin Oncol 1999;17:52–63.

32. Kaufmann M, Bajetta E, Dirix LY, et al. Exemestane is superior to megestrol acetate after tamoxifen failure in postmenopausal women with advanced breast cancer: results of a phase III randomized double-blind trial. The Exemestane Study Group. J Clin Oncol 2000;18:1399–411.

33. Gershanovich M, Chaudri HA, Campos D, et al. Letrozole, a new oral aromatase inhibitor: randomised trial comparing 2.5 mg daily, 0.5 mg daily and aminoglutethimide in postmenopausal women with advanced breast cancer. Letrozole International Trial Group (AR/BC3). Ann Oncol 1998;9:639–45.

34. Buzdar A, Douma J, Davidson N, et al. Phase III, multicenter, double-blind, randomized study of letrozole, an aromatase inhibitor, for advanced breast cancer versus megestrol acetate. J Clin Oncol 2001;19:3357–66.

35. Nabholtz JM, Buzdar A, Pollak M, et al. Anastrozole is superior to tamoxifen as first-line therapy for advanced breast cancer in postmenopausal women: results of a North American multicenter randomized trial. Arimidex Study Group. J Clin Oncol 2000;18:3758–67.

36. Bonneterre J, Thurlimann B, Robertson JF, et al. Anastrozole versus tamoxifen as first-line therapy for advanced breast cancer in 668 postmenopausal

women: results of the Tamoxifen or Arimidex Randomized Group Efficacy and Tolerability study. J Clin Oncol 2000;18:3748–57.

37. Bonneterre J, Buzdar A, Nabholtz JM, et al. Anastrozole is superior to tamoxifen as first-line therapy in hormone receptor positive advanced breast carcinoma. Cancer 2001;92:2247–58.

38. Nabholtz JM, Bonneterre J, Buzdar A, et al. Anastrozole (Arimidex) versus tamoxifen as first-line therapy for advanced breast cancer in postmenopausal women: survival analysis and updated safety results. Eur J Cancer 2003;39: 1684–9.

39. Mouridsen H, Gershanovich M, Sun Y, et al. Phase III study of letrozole versus tamoxifen as first-line therapy of advanced breast cancer in postmenopausal women: analysis of survival and update of efficacy from the International Letrozole Breast Cancer Group. J Clin Oncol 2003;21:2101–9.

40. Paridaens RJ, Dirix LY, Beex LV, et al. Phase III study comparing exemestane with tamoxifen as first-line hormonal treatment of metastatic breast cancer in postmenopausal women: the European Organisation for Research and Treatment of Cancer Breast Cancer Cooperative Group. J Clin Oncol 2008;26: 4883–90.

41. Ferretti G, Bria E, Giannarelli D, et al. Second- and third-generation aromatase inhibitors as first-line endocrine therapy in postmenopausal metastatic breast cancer patients: a pooled analysis of the randomised trials. Br J Cancer 2006;94:1789–96.

42. Thurlimann B, Robertson JF, Nabholtz JM, et al. Efficacy of tamoxifen following anastrozole ('Arimidex') compared with anastrozole following tamoxifen as first-line treatment for advanced breast cancer in postmenopausal women. Eur J Cancer 2003;39:2310–7.

43. Bachelot T, Bourgier C, Cropet C, et al. Randomized phase II trial of everolimus in combination with tamoxifen in patients with hormone receptor-positive, human epidermal growth factor receptor 2-negative metastatic breast cancer with prior exposure to aromatase inhibitors: a GINECO study. J Clin Oncol 2012;30: 2718–24.

44. Miller WR, Bartlett J, Brodie AM, et al. Aromatase inhibitors: are there differences between steroidal and nonsteroidal aromatase inhibitors and do they matter? Oncologist 2008;13:829–37.

45. Cardoso F, Costa A, Norton L, et al. 1st International consensus guidelines for advanced breast cancer (ABC 1). Breast 2012;21:242–52.

46. Bertelli G, Garrone O, Merlano M, et al. Sequential treatment with exemestane and non-steroidal aromatase inhibitors in advanced breast cancer. Oncology 2005;69:471–7.

47. Lonning PE, Bajetta E, Murray R, et al. Activity of exemestane in metastatic breast cancer after failure of nonsteroidal aromatase inhibitors: a phase II trial. J Clin Oncol 2000;18:2234–44.

48. Chia S, Gradishar W, Mauriac L, et al. Double-blind, randomized placebo controlled trial of fulvestrant compared with exemestane after prior nonsteroidal aromatase inhibitor therapy in postmenopausal women with hormone receptor-positive, advanced breast cancer: results from EFECT. J Clin Oncol 2008;26: 1664–70.

49. Johnston S. Fulvestrant Alone or with Concomitant Anastrozole Vs Exemestane Following Progression On Non-steroidal Aromatase Inhibitor – First Results of the SoFEa Trial (CRUKE/03/021 & CRUK/09/007) (ISRCTN44195747), European Breast Cancer Conference. Eur J Cancer 2012;(Suppl 2).

50. Howell A, Robertson JF, Abram P, et al. Comparison of fulvestrant versus tamoxifen for the treatment of advanced breast cancer in postmenopausal women previously untreated with endocrine therapy: a multinational, double-blind, randomized trial. J Clin Oncol 2004;22:1605–13.
51. Osborne CK, Pippen J, Jones SE, et al. Double-blind, randomized trial comparing the efficacy and tolerability of fulvestrant versus anastrozole in postmenopausal women with advanced breast cancer progressing on prior endocrine therapy: results of a North American trial. J Clin Oncol 2002;20: 3386–95.
52. Howell A, Robertson JF, Quaresma Albano J, et al. Fulvestrant, formerly ICI 182,780, is as effective as anastrozole in postmenopausal women with advanced breast cancer progressing after prior endocrine treatment. J Clin Oncol 2002;20:3396–403.
53. Robertson JF, Osborne CK, Howell A, et al. Fulvestrant versus anastrozole for the treatment of advanced breast carcinoma in postmenopausal women: a prospective combined analysis of two multicenter trials. Cancer 2003;98:229–38.
54. Pippen J. Fulvestrant (Faslodex) versus anastrozole (Arimidex) for the treatment of advanced breast cancer: a prospective combined survival analysis of two multicenter trials. Breast Cancer Res Treat 2003;39(9):1228–33.
55. Robertson JF. Fulvestrant (Faslodex) – how to make a good drug better. Oncologist 2007;12:774–84.
56. Pritchard KI, Rolski J, Papai Z, et al. Results of a phase II study comparing three dosing regimens of fulvestrant in postmenopausal women with advanced breast cancer (FINDER2). Breast Cancer Res Treat 2010;123:453–61.
57. Di Leo A, Jerusalem G, Petruzelka L, et al. Results of the CONFIRM phase III trial comparing fulvestrant 250 mg with fulvestrant 500 mg in postmenopausal women with estrogen receptor-positive advanced breast cancer. J Clin Oncol 2010;28:4594–600.
58. Di Leo A. Final analysis of overall survival for the phase III CONFIRM Trial: fulvestrant 500 mg versus 250 mg. San Antonio Breast Cancer Symposium. Cancer Res 2012;(Suppl 3).
59. Robertson JF, Llombart-Cussac A, Rolski J, et al. Activity of fulvestrant 500 mg versus anastrozole 1 mg as first-line treatment for advanced breast cancer: results from the FIRST study. J Clin Oncol 2009;27:4530–5.
60. Osborne CK, Coronado-Heinsohn EB, Hilsenbeck SG, et al. Comparison of the effects of a pure steroidal antiestrogen with those of tamoxifen in a model of human breast cancer. J Natl Cancer Inst 1995;87:746–50.
61. Mehta RS, Barlow WE, Albain KS, et al. Combination anastrozole and fulvestrant in metastatic breast cancer. N Engl J Med 2012;367:435–44.
62. Bergh J, Jonsson PE, Lidbrink EK, et al. FACT: an open-label randomized phase III study of fulvestrant and anastrozole in combination compared with anastrozole alone as first-line therapy for patients with receptor-positive postmenopausal breast cancer. J Clin Oncol 2012;30:1919–25.
63. Allegra JC, Kiefer SM. Mechanisms of action of progestational agents. Semin Oncol 1985;12:3–5.
64. Lonning PE. Aromatase inhibitors and inactivators for breast cancer therapy. Drugs Aging 2002;19:277–98.
65. Guerrero-Zotano A. Endocrine therapy for advanced breast cancer: beyond tamoxifen and aromatase inhibitors. Curr Cancer Ther Rev 2010;6:51–61.
66. Lundgren S. Progestins in breast cancer treatment. A review. Acta Oncol 1992; 31:709–22.

67. Sedlacek SM. An overview of megestrol acetate for the treatment of advanced breast cancer. Semin Oncol 1988;15:3–13.
68. Cruz JM, Muss HB, Brockschmidt JK, et al. Weight changes in women with metastatic breast cancer treated with megestrol acetate: a comparison of standard versus high-dose therapy. Semin Oncol 1990;17:63–7.
69. Carlini P, Bria E, Giannarelli D, et al. New aromatase inhibitors as second-line endocrine therapy in postmenopausal patients with metastatic breast carcinoma: a pooled analysis of the randomized trials. Cancer 2005;104: 1335–42.
70. Ellis MJ, Gao F, Dehdashti F, et al. Lower-dose vs high-dose oral estradiol therapy of hormone receptor-positive, aromatase inhibitor-resistant advanced breast cancer: a phase 2 randomized study. JAMA 2009;302:774–80.
71. Miller TW, Balko JM, Arteaga CL. Phosphatidylinositol 3-kinase and antiestrogen resistance in breast cancer. J Clin Oncol 2011;29:4452–61.
72. Rudolf J, Boulay A, Zumstein-Mecker S, et al. The mTOR pathway in estrogen response: a potential for combining the rapamycin derivative RAD001with the aromatase inhibitor letrozole in breast carcinomas. Proc Am Assoc Cancer Res 2004.
73. deGraffenried LA, Friedrichs WE, Russell DH, et al. Inhibition of mTOR activity restores tamoxifen response in breast cancer cells with aberrant Akt Activity. Clin Cancer Res 2004;10:8059–67.
74. Baselga J, Fumoleau P, Gil M, et al. Phase II, 3 arm study of CCI-779 in combination with letrozole in postmenopausal women with locally advanced or metastatic breast cancer. Preliminary results, ASCO Annual Meeting Proceedings. J Clin Oncol 2004;22(Suppl 14):544.
75. Wolff AC, Lazar AA, Bondarenko I, et al. Randomized phase III placebo-controlled trial of letrozole plus oral temsirolimus as first-line endocrine therapy in postmenopausal women with locally advanced or metastatic breast cancer. J Clin Oncol 2013;31:195–202.
76. Baselga J, Campone M, Piccart M, et al. Everolimus in postmenopausal hormone-receptor-positive advanced breast cancer. N Engl J Med 2012;366: 520–9.
77. Piccart M, Baselga J, Noguchi S, et al. Final progression-free survival analysis of BOLERO-2: a Phase III trial of everolimus for postmenopausal women with advanced breast cancer, San Antonio Breast Cancer Symposium. San Antonio, TX, December 4–8, 2012.
78. Mayer I. SU2C phase Ib study of pan-PI3K inhibitor BKM120 with letrozole in ER+/HER2- metastatic breast cancer (MBC). ASCO Annual Meeting. J Clin Oncol, 2012.
79. Nagarai G. A phase I study of BKM120, a novel oral selective phosphatidylinositol-3-kinase (PI3K) inhibitor, in combination with fulvestrant in postmenopausal women with estrogen receptor positive metastatic breast cancer. ASCO Annual Meeting. J Clin Oncol, 2012.
80. Klein P. Characterization of the overall survival benefit in ENCORE 301, a randomized placebo-controlled phase II study of exemestane with and without entinostat in ER+ postmenopausal women with metastatic breast cancer, ASCO Annual Meeting. J Clin Oncol. 2012.
81. Basu B. Phase I study of abiraterone acetate (AA) in patients (pts) with estrogen receptor– (ER) or androgen receptor (AR) –positive advanced breast carcinoma resistant to standard endocrine therapies, ASCO Annual Meeting. J Clin Oncol 2011.

82. O'Shaughnessy J: Randomized phase II open-label study of abiraterone acetate (AA) plus low-dose prednisone (P) with or without exemestane (E) in postmenopausal women with ER+ metastatic breast cancer (MBC) progressing after letrozole or anastrozole therapy, ASCO Annual Meeting. J Clin Oncol 2012.

83. Mueller H, Flury N, Eppenberger-Castori S, et al. Potential prognostic value of mitogen-activated protein kinase activity for disease-free survival of primary breast cancer patients. Int J Cancer 2000;89:384–8.

84. Kaufman B, Mackey JR, Clemens MR, et al. Trastuzumab plus anastrozole versus anastrozole alone for the treatment of postmenopausal women with human epidermal growth factor receptor 2-positive, hormone receptor-positive metastatic breast cancer: results from the randomized phase III TAnDEM study. J Clin Oncol 2009;27:5529–37.

85. Osborne CK, Neven P, Dirix LY, et al. Gefitinib or placebo in combination with tamoxifen in patients with hormone receptor-positive metastatic breast cancer: a randomized phase II study. Clin Cancer Res 2011;17:1147–59.

86. Cristofanilli M, Valero V, Mangalik A, et al. Phase II, randomized trial to compare anastrozole combined with gefitinib or placebo in postmenopausal women with hormone receptor-positive metastatic breast cancer. Clin Cancer Res 2010;16: 1904–14.

87. Johnston S, Pippen J Jr, Pivot X, et al. Lapatinib combined with letrozole versus letrozole and placebo as first-line therapy for postmenopausal hormone receptor-positive metastatic breast cancer. J Clin Oncol 2009;27:5538–46.

88. Huober J, Fasching PA, Barsoum M, et al. Higher efficacy of letrozole in combination with trastuzumab compared to letrozole monotherapy as first-line treatment in patients with HER2-positive, hormone-receptor-positive metastatic breast cancer - results of the eLEcTRA trial. Breast 2012;21:27–33.

89. Pritchard KI, Thomson DB, Myers RE, et al. Tamoxifen therapy in premenopausal patients with metastatic breast cancer. Cancer Treat Rep 1980;64: 787–96.

90. Sawka CA, Pritchard KI, Shelley W, et al. A randomized crossover trial of tamoxifen versus ovarian ablation for metastatic breast cancer in premenopausal women: a report of the National Cancer Institute of Canada Clinical Trials Group (NCIC CTG) trial MA.1. Breast Cancer Res Treat 1997;44:211–5.

91. Crump M, Sawka CA, DeBoer G, et al. An individual patient-based meta-analysis of tamoxifen versus ovarian ablation as first line endocrine therapy for premenopausal women with metastatic breast cancer. Breast Cancer Res Treat 1997;44:201–10.

92. Burger CW, Prinssen HM, Kenemans P. LHRH agonist treatment of breast cancer and gynecological malignancies: a review. Eur J Obstet Gynecol Reprod Biol 1996;67:27–33.

93. Taylor CW, Green S, Dalton WS, et al. Multicenter randomized clinical trial of goserelin versus surgical ovariectomy in premenopausal patients with receptor-positive metastatic breast cancer: an intergroup study. J Clin Oncol 1998;16: 994–9.

94. Klijn JG, Seynaeve C, Beex L, et al. Combined treatment with buserelin (LHRH A) and tamoxifen (TAM) vs single treatment with each drug alone in premenopausal metastatic breast cancer: preliminary results of EORTC study 10881. Proc Am Soc Clin Oncol 1996.

95. Klijn J, Seynaeve C, Beex L, et al. Combined estrogen suppression and receptor blockade by buserelin and tamoxifen in premenopausal metastatic breast

cancer: preliminary results of a 3-arm randomized study (EORTC 10881). Eur J Cancer 1996;32A:49.

96. Jonat W, Kaufmann M, Blamey RW, et al. A randomised study to compare the effect of the luteinising hormone releasing hormone (LHRH) analogue goserelin with or without tamoxifen in pre- and perimenopausal patients with advanced breast cancer. Eur J Cancer 1995;31A:137–42.

97. Boccardo F, Rubagotti A, Perrotta A, et al. Ovarian ablation versus goserelin with or without tamoxifen in pre-perimenopausal patients with advanced breast cancer: results of a multicentric Italian study. Ann Oncol 1994;5:337–42.

98. Klijn J, Blamey R, Boccardo F, et al. A new standard treatment for advanced premenopausal breast cancer: a meta-analysis of the Combined Hormonal Agent Trialists' group (CHAT). Eur J Cancer 1998;34(Suppl 5):S90.

99. Carlson RW, Theriault R, Schurman CM, et al. Phase II trial of anastrozole plus goserelin in the treatment of hormone receptor-positive, metastatic carcinoma of the breast in premenopausal women. J Clin Oncol 2010;28:3917–21.

100. Roche H, Delozier T, Chieze S, et al. Anastrozole and goserelin combination as first treatment for premenopausal receptor positive advanced or metastatic breast cancer: a phase II trial. ASCO Ann Meeting, Proc J Clin Oncol, 2009.

101. Cheung KL, Agrawal A, Folkerd E, et al. Suppression of ovarian function in combination with an aromatase inhibitor as treatment for advanced breast cancer in pre-menopausal women. Eur J Cancer 2010;46:2936–42.

102. Forward DP, Cheung KL, Jackson L, et al. Clinical and endocrine data for goserelin plus anastrozole as second-line endocrine therapy for premenopausal advanced breast cancer. Br J Cancer 2004;90:590–4.

103. Bartsch R, Bago-Horvath Z, Berghoff A, et al. Ovarian function suppression and fulvestrant as endocrine therapy in premenopausal women with metastatic breast cancer. Eur J Cancer 2012;48:1932–8.

The Management of Early-Stage and Metastatic Triple-Negative Breast Cancer: A Review

Carey K. Anders, MD[a],*, Timothy M. Zagar, MD[b],
Lisa A. Carey, MD[a]

KEYWORDS

- Breast cancer • Triple negative • Chemotherapy • Targeted agents • Radiation
- BRCA mutation

KEY POINTS

- Triple-negative breast cancer (TNBC) lacks expression of the estrogen receptor (ER), progesterone receptor (PR), and HER2 by clinical assays.
- Although more commonly associated with the basal-like subtype of breast cancer, research assays have further dissected the biology of TNBC and have identified 6 subtypes thus far.
- The incidence of *BRCA* mutations is higher among patients with TNBC (approximately 20%) compared with those with breast cancer across all subtypes (approximately 5%).
- Local and systemic therapy approaches to early-stage TNBC should be similar to those of non-TNBC; however, endocrine and HER2-directed therapies are not prescribed.
- In the metastatic setting, the mainstay of systemic therapy to treat TNBC is cytotoxic chemotherapy; targetable pathways are currently under investigation in the preclinical setting and early-phase clinical trials.
- A coordinated effort between scientists and clinicians is required to develop novel therapies to treat TNBC most effectively.

INTRODUCTION: OVERVIEW AND SCOPE OF THE PROBLEM

The management of TNBC, a disease that affects approximately 180,000 women worldwide, is challenging.[1] Clinically defined as lacking expression of the ER, the

[a] Division of Hematology-Oncology, Department of Medicine, Lineberger Comprehensive Cancer Center, University of North Carolina at Chapel Hill, 170 Manning Drive, Chapel Hill, NC 27599, USA; [b] Department of Radiation Oncology, Lineberger Comprehensive Cancer Center, University of North Carolina at Chapel Hill, 170 Manning Drive, Chapel Hill, NC 27599, USA
* Corresponding author. Division of Hematology-Oncology, Lineberger Comprehensive Cancer Center, University of North Carolina at Chapel Hill, 170 Manning Drive, Campus Box 7305, Chapel Hill, NC 27599.
E-mail address: carey_anders@med.unc.edu

Hematol Oncol Clin N Am 27 (2013) 737–749
http://dx.doi.org/10.1016/j.hoc.2013.05.003
0889-8588/13/$ – see front matter © 2013 Elsevier Inc. All rights reserved.

PR, and HER2 by immunohistochemistry (IHC), TNBC comprises approximately 15% of incident breast cancers and is over-represented among those with metastatic disease.[2–4] TNBC is usually high grade, more often an interval breast cancer (ie, diagnosed between screening mammograms), and, when recurrent, preferentially relapses in visceral sites, such as lungs, liver, and brain.[4–6] Given the higher rates of recurrence and lack of traditional targets (such as ER and HER2), treating those with TNBC evokes anxiety on the parts of both patient and provider. This review article addresses the unique biology of TNBC, followed by a detailed discussion of state-of-the-art local and systemic treatments in the early-stage setting. Approved cytotoxics to treat advanced TNBC and the many emerging targeted agents in development to treat this aggressive disease are discussed.

UNIQUE BIOLOGY OF TRIPLE-NEGATIVE BREAST CANCER

TNBC is defined clinically as lack of ER, PR, and HER2 expression by IHC (with confirmation of HER2 status by fluorescence in situ hybridization if indeterminate [2+] by IHC). According to the most recent American Society of Clinical Oncology/College of American Pathologists guidelines,[7] ER and PR negativity is strictly defined as less than 1% expression, as opposed to older definitions allowing up to 1% to 10% borderline ER/PR expression. In an analysis of more than 1700 breast tumors, although the majority of TNBCs (as strictly defined by IHC as <1% ER/PR expression) fall into the basal-like subtype by gene expression analysis (207/283, 73%), borderline cases (n = 48) were more commonly luminal (46%) or HER2 enriched (29%).[8] Based on this observation, it is recommended that clinical trials aimed at enrolling women patients with TNBC/basal-like breast cancer should adhere to the American Society of Clinical Oncology/College of American Pathologists guideline–recommended definition of ER/PR less than 1% when developing inclusion/exclusion criteria.

Although the basal-like breast cancer subtype has been associated with TNBC for approximately a decade, newer subtypes within TNBC are emerging.[9,10] More recently, a novel molecular subtype identified as claudin-low has been characterized via gene expression of human breast tumors, a panel of breast cancer cell lines, and mouse models of breast cancer.[11] Clinically, claudin-low breast tumors are commonly ER, PR, and HER2–negative via IHC and show a high frequency of metaplastic and medullary differentiation and an intermediate response to cytotoxic chemotherapy (between that of basal-like and luminal breast tumors). Moreover, claudin-low breast tumors have been shown to exhibit stem cell characteristics, low expression of cell-cell adhesion proteins (ie, claudin 3, claudin 4, and claudin 7), high enrichment for epithelial-to-mesenchymal transition (EMT) markers, and low luminal/epithelial differentiation.

A group of investigators has further dissected the biology of TNBC, identifying 6 unique subsets of TNBC through gene expression analysis of more than 500 breast tumors from more than 20 independent data sets.[12] This analysis classified TNBCs into the following clusters: 2 basal-like (BL1 and BL2), an immunomodulatory, a mesenchymal, a mesenchymal stem–like, and a luminal androgen receptor (AR) subtype. Approximately 30 TNBC cell lines were then classified into each of these categories and pharmacologically inhibited to illustrate that classification may inform therapeutic strategies. Results showed that the BL1 and BL2 subtypes, both with higher expression of DNA damage response genes, responded to cisplatin. Response to phosphatidylinositide 3-kinase (PI3K)/mammalian target of rapamycin (mTOR) and Src inhibition was observed in the mesenchymal and mesenchymal stem–like subtypes, which are enriched for EMT and growth factor pathways. Finally, cell lines within the luminal AR subtype were preferentially responsive to the AR antagonist, bicalutamide—a concept that has borne out to a degree in the clinical arena.[13] Given the apparent heterogeneity within TNBC, a 1-size-fits-all approach is no longer appropriate because clinical trials are designed for patients with TNBC. Consideration of the distinct subsets within TNBC is paramount in aiming to improve outcomes for this aggressive disease.

Association with BRCA Mutations

In addition to advances in understanding the underlying biology of TNBC, several studies have illustrated the association of TNBC with germline *BRCA* mutations. A recent observational study was aimed at determining the incidence of germline *BRCA1* and *BRCA2* mutations in 77 patients with TNBC.[14] *BRCA* mutations were detected in 19.5% of patients: 15.6% *BRCA1* and 3.9% *BRCA2*. In this cohort of patients, outcomes were superior among *BRCA* mutation carriers compared with wild-type patients, including 5-year recurrence-free survival (RFS) (51.7% vs 86.2%, $P = .031$) and 5-year overall survival (OS) (52.8% vs 73.3%, $P = .225$). Further confirming these findings, an integrated molecular analysis of breast carcinomas in The Cancer Genome Atlas (TCGA) reports that approximately 20% of basal-like breast tumors harbored a *BRCA1* or *BRCA2* mutation, of which approximately two-thirds were germline and one-third were somatic.[15] *BRCA1* inactivation was found common among both basal-like breast cancers and serous ovarian cancers. This finding suggests shared driving events for both diseases and that therapeutic approaches (ie, use of platinums, taxanes, and inhibitors of poly-ADP-ribose polymerase [PARP]) may be guided more by molecular profile and less by tissue of origin.

THERAPEUTIC OPTIONS FOR EARLY-STAGE TRIPLE-NEGATIVE BREAST CANCER

Although the basic principles, including surgical management, radiation therapy techniques, and decisions regarding systemic therapies, are similar between stages I to III TNBC (as defined by the TNM staging system) and endocrine and/or HER2+ counterparts, there are some nuances specific to TNBC that should be considered. In addition, there have been several provocative studies in the field of radiation therapy specific to patients with TNBC that are worthy of review.

Local Therapy/Radiation Therapy

Given conflicting retrospective studies regarding whether women with TNBC are at a higher risk of local recurrence after breast-conserving therapy (BCT) and whether they might be better served by a modified radical mastectomy (MRM),[16–18] it has become accepted that either treatment paradigm is reasonable in the management of early-stage TNBC. Recent studies suggested, however, that early-stage TNBC patients may be at a higher risk for local recurrence when treated with MRM alone, omitting postmastectomy radiotherapy (RT) (ie, in T1-T2N0 patients lacking classic indications for postmastectomy RT), which warrants discussion.

In a large single-institution retrospective review of 768 women with T1-T2N0 TNBC, investigators from McGill University found a significant difference in locoregional recurrence rates (LRRs) between patients treated with BCT, MRM, or MRM plus RT.[19] Five-year LRR-free survival rates were 96% and 90% in BCT and MRM patients, respectively ($P<.03$), and MRM was the only independent prognostic factor associated with LRR (hazard ratio 2.5), suggesting that MRM alone may not be enough local therapy in these patients. A prospective trial performed in Shanghai randomized 681 women with stage I-II TNBC after MRM to chemotherapy with or without RT.[20]

Although not their primary endpoints, the investigators found a statistically significant difference in RFS and OS, favoring the group who received both adjuvant chemotherapy and post-MRM RT. Five-year RFS improved from 75% to 88% with the addition of RT, and adding RT improved 5-year OS impressively, from 79% to 90%. Although retrospective and thus subject to unintended bias, these are intriguing but hypothesis-generating data, warranting further study in a rigorous randomized controlled trial but not warranting a change in clinical practice.

Many TNBC patients receive neoadjuvant chemotherapy in hopes of becoming BCT candidates or as a means to assess in vivo response to systemic therapy. There has been a growing discussion about whether or not to omit post-MRM RT in patients with significant down-staging secondary to chemotherapy or even to modify RT field design based on response to chemotherapy. This issue is not unique to women with TNBC. Unfortunately, there are no prospective data to support this practice. Retrospective data from MD Anderson Cancer Center suggest that patients with residual nodal disease benefit from post-MRM RT, but those left with stage I/II disease after chemotherapy do not derive such a benefit.[21,22] Interpretation of these findings must acknowledge, however, the limitations of subgroup analyses of patients in whom the use of RT was left to the discretion of a physician and the absence of prospective or controlled studies. In the absence of prospective data, it remains standard of care to irradiate the same fields (ie, chest wall or supraclavicular fossa, with or without irradiation of the internal mammary chain if cT3 or node positive) after neoadjuvant chemotherapy as would be done if patients had up-front surgery.

Systemic Therapy—Neoadjuvant and Adjuvant Treatments and Ongoing Clinical Trials

The only opportunity for recurrence risk reduction to treat TNBC with curative intent is systemic chemotherapy, because there are currently no approved targeted treatments, like endocrine or HER2-directed therapy, to ameliorate baseline risk. As such and in compliance with guidelines put forth by the National Cancer Comprehensive Network (www.NCCN.org), it is common and appropriate for oncologists to prescribe anthracycline/taxane-based chemotherapy at a lower stage for TNBC compared with hormone receptor–positive counterparts. Although use of a more-aggressive regimen (ie, anthracycline/taxane as opposed to a taxane-based regimen) may be reasonable in many TNBCs, it is also true that "biology does not trump anatomy." A small node-negative TNBC carries a low (15% or less) 5-year risk of recurrence[23] and a proportionally lower benefit of treatment. Using tools, such as Adjuvant! OnLine, the mortality risk at 10 years for T1a/bN0 tumors is less than 10%. An observational study of more than 1000 T1a/bN0 TNBCs found excellent prognosis, with 95% remaining free of distant metastasis at 5 years and without a notable difference between those who did and those who did not receive chemotherapy.[24] Taking this into account, a reasonable algorithm for adjuvant chemotherapy in node-negative TNBC is to offer it if tumor size is greater than 1 cm and if it is otherwise medically appropriate; a balanced discussion for 0.6 cm to 1.0 cm tumors; and no adjuvant chemotherapy in breast tumors 0.5 cm or less (T1a). As with other subtypes of breast cancer, adjuvant anthracycline/taxane-based chemotherapy is recommended in patients with lymph node–positive disease (N1 or greater), regardless of primary tumor size (**Fig. 1**).

The principles that govern the decision to proceed with neoadjuvant versus adjuvant chemotherapy are similar between TNBC and other subtypes of breast cancer. These principles are largely driven by (1) resectability of the primary tumor and lymph nodes to achieve negative margins and (2) the ability to cytoreduce a breast cancer to facilitate breast conservation, as opposed to a mastectomy. Historically and as guided by

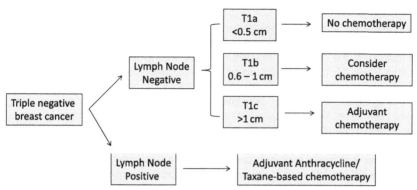

Fig. 1. General algorithm guiding adjuvant chemotherapy decisions in the treatment of early-stage triple-negative breast cancer, as adapted by www.NCCN.org, Version 1.2013, invasive breast cancer.

the landmark study National Surgical Adjuvant Breast and Bowel Project B-27,[25] chemotherapy sequenced before (as opposed to after) surgery does not seem to improve survival. Response to chemotherapy, however, in particular, achievement of pathologic complete response (pCR), can help identify those patients with better prognosis. Basal-like/TNBC has consistently been shown more sensitive to neoadjuvant chemotherapy (ie, higher pCR rates) than luminal breast cancers. Collectively, however, TNBC patients experience poorer overall outcomes compared with other breast cancer subtypes. The poorer prognosis of basal-like/TNBC has been explained by a higher likelihood of relapse in those patients in whom pCR was not achieved and has been termed, the triple-negative paradox.[26,27]

Using pCR rates for patients with TNBC as an endpoint, investigators are evaluating additional chemotherapies and targeted agents in the neoadjuvant setting. A trial of interest, Cancer and Leukemia Group B (CALGB) 40603 (NCT00861705), is evaluating the addition of a platinum (ie, carboplatin) and/or an antiangiogenesis agent (ie, bevacizumab) to standard anthracycline/taxane-based neoadjuvant chemotherapy in the setting of locally advanced TNBC. Importantly, all patients in this trial are required to undergo dedicated biopsies to identify predictive markers of response. Platinum agents have been an area of investigation in TNBC based on the hypothesis of augmented sensitivity to DNA-damaging agents in dysfunctional BRCA. Although small studies have suggested high clinical responses to cisplatin in germline BRCA mutation carriers,[28,29] whether this holds true in sporadic TNBC is uncertain; prospective data await the results of CALGB 40603. Results of neoadjuvant bevacizumab studies in TNBC have previously been mixed,[30,31] and the addition of 1 year of bevacizumab to adjuvant chemotherapy in TNBC failed to improve invasive disease-free survival in a recently reported, large (n>2500 patients), open-label, randomized, multinational phase III trial.[32] Anticipated results of CALGB 40603 will continue to add the understanding of the role of bevacizumab, if any, in the curative treatment of TNBC and to identify those patients who may benefit from these approaches.

Another area of active research pertains to those with residual disease—specifically, the group of patients with TNBC who do not achieve a pCR after neoadjuvant chemotherapy—in an effort to improve outcome for those at greatest risk for local and/or distant recurrence. Although scientists are actively analyzing the molecular changes in residual breast tumor after preoperative cytotoxic therapy,[33] an ongoing randomized phase III trial is also evaluating the benefits of an intensive diet/exercise intervention or without adjuvant metronomic chemotherapy (6 months of cyclophos-phamide/methotrexate) plus bevacizumab (12 months) in patients with residual dis-ease to determine if this strategy reduces recurrence in this high-risk group.

At this point, the choice of chemotherapy regimen does not differ between TNBC and non-TNBC. Retrospective studies have suggested that much of the benefit of adjuvant anthracyclines is in the HER2-overexpressing subset of tumors; however, this finding is not universal or definitive. More recently, molecular studies suggest that the HER2-enriched molecular subtype derived the primary benefit of an anthracy-cline regimen (cyclophosphamide, epirubicin, and 5-fluoruracil) over the classic regimen (cyclophosphamide, methotrexate, and 5-fluoruracil); in that retrospective analysis, the basal-like subtype seemed to benefit equally from both regimens.[34] Although intriguing, intrinsic subtyping for this purpose is not yet clinically available nor is it sufficiently validated for decision making. Although TNBC behaves differently from other subtypes of breast cancer, with higher local and distant metastasis rates and earlier pattern of relapse, breast conservation and multimodality options for care in the early breast cancer setting remain similar to other subtypes.

ADVANCED TRIPLE-NEGATIVE BREAST CANCER
Principles of Systemic Therapy

In spite of great excitement in the recent past with potential novel drugs, like PARP inhibitors and bevacizumab, offering a targeted option in TNBC, there remain multiple cytotoxic choices but no targeted therapy in the metastatic setting at this time. Con-ventional treatment of metastatic TNBC begins with cytotoxic chemotherapy, of which there are approximately 14 single agents and approximately 8 doublets listed in the treatment of HER2-negative, recurrent, or metastatic breast cancer acccording to the National Cancer Comprehensive Network (www.NCCN.org). Choice of palliative cytotoxic regimen is no different in TNBC than in other subtypes, with options of poly-chemotherapy generally reserved for symptomatic or rapid visceral progression and sequential single agents for asymptomatic, stage IV disease.

A recent randomized phase III study, CALGB 40502, confirms that weekly paclitaxel is the optimal first-line regimen compared with the more modern microtubule-directed agents, nab-paclitaxel or ixabepilone, including in the TNBC subset.[35] A similar subset analysis in TNBC of eribulin compared with capecitabine in the first-line to third-line setting found no difference between the 2 drugs overall, although the TNBC subset had improved progression-free survival (PFS) with eribulin compared with capecita-bine. This subset analysis, however, should be considered exploratory rather than definitive.[36] The decision of which drug to use, in this case eribulin versus capecita-bine, may reasonably be made on the basis of their different toxicity profiles. Many of the authors' patients with advanced TNBC receive a variety of cytotoxics, when still medically well enough to do so; individualizing care and selection of cytotoxic should be made on the basis of side effects, convenience, and personal choice as opposed to strictly based on subtype.

Incorporation of a platinum

As discussed in the treatment of early-stage TNBC, the question of how and when to sequence direct DNA-damaging agents in the treatment of advanced TNBC remains unknown. Platinum drugs seem to have high single-agent activity in BRCA1/2-associ-ated cancers,[28,29] but platinum agents in sporadic TNBC demonstrate reasonable yet not excessively high response rates. As an example, the Translational Breast Cancer Research Consortium (TBCRC) 009 trial found an approximately 30% response rate to cisplatin or carboplatin in the first-line or second-line treatment of advanced

TNBC[37]; in the control arm of BALI-1, first-line cisplatin alone produced responses in only 10% of advanced TNBC patients.[38] These agents are appropriate to include in the armamentarium of cytotoxic choices in TNBC but do not need to be preferentially used over other the many other available agents with different mechanisms of action in sporadic, advanced TNBC.

Targeted Agents to Treat Advanced TNBC

Given the relative paucity of available targeted agents, ongoing preclinical and clinical efforts are focused on the development of more refined strategies to control advanced TNBC beyond that of cytotoxic chemotherapy (**Table 1**). In the recently reported TCGA analysis, the most commonly mutated genes and pathways in basal-like/TNBC were the tumor suppressor gene *TP53* (approximately 80% mutated) and loss of *RB1* (tumor suppressor gene) and *BRCA1* (DNA repair gene) function as well as *PIK3CA* (approximately 9% compared with approximately 30%–49% in luminal A and B breast tumors, respectively). Comprehensive protein analysis illustrated basal-like breast cancers to have the highest relative PI3K pathway activation, likely via alternative mechanisms, such as loss of the negative regulators, phosphatase and tensin homolog (PTEN) and/or inositol polyphosphate 4-phosphatase type II (INPP4B). Other plausible drug targets identified through this comprehensive analysis included *FGFR1, FGFR2, IGFR1, KIT, MET, PDGFRA* as well as angiogenesis and/or drugs that become activated under hypoxic conditions. Large-scale, coordinated studies, such as the TCGA will only continue to foster understanding of the complex biology underlying TNBC, with the goal of translating these findings into rationally designed clinical trials; several historical trials and strategies are reviewed.

Antiangiogenic strategies

Antiangiogenic strategies seemed promising based on preclinical data in TNBC models; however, a pooled analysis, of 3 randomized first-line metastatic studies of bevacizumab added to chemotherapy (E2100, AVADO, and RIBBON-1) demonstrated improvement in PFS but no impact on OS in HER2-negative patients overall or in the TNBC subset.[39] Among approximately 2500 patients with HER2-negative metastatic breast cancer, median PFS improved from 6.7 to 9.2 months (hazard ratio 0.64, $P<.0001$) in the bevacizumab arms, and 1-year survival rates were greater in the bevacizumab plus chemotherapy arm compared with the control arms (81.6% vs 76.5%, respectively; $P = .003$). In spite of these improvements, there was no difference in OS, which was 26.4 months in the control arm and 26.7 months with the addition of bevacizumab. Based on lack of survival benefit and toxicity, bevacizumab's initial Food and Drug Administration–accelerated approval in 2008 was revoked in 2011; current

---

Table 1
Overview of targeted strategies in advanced triple-negative breast cancer

Therapeutic Target	Phase of Study	References
Angiogenesis	Phase III	38
PARP inhibition	Phase I/II	39,40
EGFR inhibition	Phase II	37,41
AR signaling	Phase II	13
PI3K inhibition	Preclinical/phase I	42
MEK inhibition	Preclinical	46,47
CHK inhibition	Preclinical	43,44
HDAC inhibition	Preclinical/phase II	48,49

use of bevaciuzmab in metastatic breast cancer is essentially restricted to clinical trials. Biomarkers predictive of response to bevacizumab have been difficult to identify; biomarker results from the neoadjuvant study CALBG 40603 are anticipated in hopes of informing future studies in the metastatic setting to augment response to antiangiogenic strategies.

Inhibitors of poly-ADP-ribose polymerase

In those patients with germline BRCA1 or BRCA2 mutations, PARP inhibition remains a promising avenue; however, this approach remains available only in clinical trials, and reports from small studies have failed to demonstrate a similar outcome in sporadic TNBC. For example, a phase II study of the PARP inhibitor, olaparib, revealed unconfirmed responses only in BRCA1/2 carriers, with no responses among patients with sporadic TNBC.[40] A phase II study of temozolomide with another PARP 1/2 inhibitor, velparib (ABT-888), enrolled 41 patients with metastatic breast cancer (approximately 50% TNBC); response rate across the entire population was 7%[41]; however, an exploratory analysis revealed that responses were essentially limited to BRCA1/2 carriers. In those 8 patients, the response rate (complete and partial responses) was 37.5% with a clinical benefit rate (defined as complete response, partial response, and stable disease >16 weeks) of 62.5%. PFS was 5.5 months for BRCA mutation carriers and 1.8 months in noncarriers, suggesting that the benefit from PARP inhibition was largely derived from those harboring mutations in DNA repair, namely through the BRCA pathway. Identifying non-BRCA–associated TNBC tumors with similar phenotype and DNA damage repair defect with potential to benefit from PARP inhibition, with or without chemotherapy, remains a subject of intense and ongoing research.

Inhibition of epithelial growth factor receptor

Although TNBC lacks ER and HER2 expression, expression of the epithelial growth factor receptor (EGFR), HER1, has been demonstrated in TNBCs at both the gene and protein level.[2,6] Several studies have evaluated the benefit of adding the EGFR-targeted monoclonal antibody, cetuximab, to platinum-based chemotherapy to treat advanced TNBC with modest results. The TBCRC 001 study evaluated treatment with cetuximab as a single agent or combined with carboplatin among 102 patients with advanced TNBC. Response rates for cetuximab as a single agent, combined with carboplatin at progression after monotherapy, or combined with cetuximab/carboplatin from the onset of treatment, were 6%, 16%, and 17%, respectively.[42] Although time to progression was short (2.1 months, 95% CI, 1.8–5.5 months), pretherapy and post-therapy biopsies evaluating dynamic changes EGFR signaling, provided further insight into possible compensatory pathways that may have been responsible for the marginal benefit observed from this novel drug combination. Dovetailing the results of TBCRC 001, the BALI-1 study reported a doubling of response rates by combining cetuximab with cisplatin compared with cisplatin alone in TNBC (response rates 20% vs 10.3%, respectively).[38] Despite improvements in response, duration of response was short; PFS was only 3.7 months after cetuximab/cisplatin versus 1.5 months after cisplatn monotherapy. Although there was initial enthusiasm and strong preclinical rationale for the incorporation of EGFR-based therapy into systemic therapy for advanced TNBC, translation of this approach clinically has resulted in only modest improvements in outcome, possibly due to heterogeneity of disease and compensatory alternate signaling in the cancer cells. Biomarkers predictive of response to this targeted therapy or combinatorial strategies may be needed to enrich for responders if this strategy is to be successful to treat advanced TNBC.

Inhibition of AR signaling

The luminal AR subtype of TNBC is sensitive to androgen deprivation in preclinical studies,[12] making AR signaling in ER-negative breast cancer an intriguing potential target. In the recent TBCRC 011 phase II trial, more than 450 hormone receptor-negative (primarily TNBC) patients were screened, of which approximately 10% had AR expression. Single-agent bicalutamide in these patients yielded a clinical benefit in 19%.[13] Continued study of AR pathway inhibition in advanced TNBC—albeit the small subset that may be driven by the AR pathway—is warranted as the era of personalized medicine is approached.

Inhibition of the PI3K, MEK, CHK, and HDAC pathways—preclinical

A tremendous amount of research is ongoing in search of targetable pathways that may be contributing to the aggressive biology of TNBC. As identified in TCGA, activation of the PI3K, either directly via PI3KCA mutations or indirectly via PTEN and/or INPP4B loss, has been identified as important in TNBC/basal-like breast cancer.[15] Preclinically, inhibition of the PI3K pathway results in TNBC cell growth arrest[43]; several small molecule inhibitors of the PI3K (and downstream mTOR pathway) are in development. Several studies, including TCGA, have identified high rates of p53 (tumor suppressor gene) mutations in TNBC/basal-like breast cancer.[15] In the absence of p53 function, cells in need of DNA damage repair rely on checkpoint kinase I (Chk1) to arrest the cell cycle and push potentially defective cells toward apoptosis; p53-deficient mouse models of breast cancer are sensitive to Chk-1 inhibition.[44,45] Chk-1 inhibitors have, therefore, become an attractive potential target for the treatment of TNBC harboring p53 mutations. In addition, inhibition of mitogen-activated protein/extracellular signal–regulated kinase (MEK), in combination with PI3K/mTOR inhibition, has shown activity in a TNBC/claudin-low genetically engineered mouse model; a window study of MEK inhibition (GSK1120212) is ongoing to evaluate dynamic reprogramming of the kinome in patients with TNBC to further identify pathways of resistance.[46,47] (NCT01467310) Finally, epigenetic regulation of gene expression has been a hot topic in TNBC for several years. An inhibitor of the histone deacetylase (HDAC) pathway (panobinostat) has been demonstrated to decrease cell growth in TNBC cell lines as well as tumorigenesis in vivo and may soon make its way into the clinic.[48] These data are in light of the randomized phase II study, TBCRC 008, where the addition of vorinostat to preoperative carboplatin and nab-paclitaxel did not seem to improve pCR rates in a TNBC, otherwise unselected, group (n = 62) of patients (vorinostat arm pCR = 27.6%; placebo arm pCR = 26.7%).[49] Biomarkers predictive of those most likely to respond to HDAC inhibition are needed.

SUMMARY AND FUTURE DIRECTIONS

In 2013, TNBC is well recognized as a distinct subset of breast cancer with a unique genomic background and characteristically aggressive clinical behavior in a relative sparse landscape of available, standard-of-care, targeted therapies. Despite this recognition, multimodality options for the care of TNBC in the early and advanced breast cancer settings remain similar (with, of course, the absence of endocrine and HER2-directed strategies) to other breast cancer subtypes. As we look ahead, we must ask ourselves, "What is the way forward?" Based on emerging understanding of the complexity of TNBC, it may be that clinician/scientist partnerships focused on comprehensive understanding of TNBC genomic, proteomic, and other biologic processes will reorient toward individualized therapy in TNBC faster than other subtypes. This shift in focus will be driven by both the heterogeneity now known to exist within TNBC and the intense need for improved treatment.

REFERENCES

1. Swain S. Triple-negative breast cancer: metastatic risk and role of platinum agents. 2008 ASCO Clinical Science Symposium. June 3, 2008.
2. Nielsen T, Hsu F, Jensen K, et al. Immunohistochemical and clinical characterization of the basal-like subtype of invasive breast carcinoma. Clin Cancer Res 2004; 10(16):5367–74.
3. Perou CM, Sorlie T, Eisen MB, et al. Molecular portraits of human breast tumours. Nature 2000;406(6797):747–52.
4. Smid M, Wang Y, Zhang Y, et al. Subtypes of breast cancer show preferential site of relapse. Cancer Res 2008;68(9):3108–14.
5. Dent R, Trudeau M, Pritchard K, et al. Triple-negative breast cancer: clinical features and patterns of recurrence. Clin Cancer Res 2007;13(15):4429–34.
6. Livasy C, Karaca G, Nanda R, et al. Phenotypic evaluation of the basal-like subtype of invasive breast carcinoma. Mod Pathol 2006;19(2):264–71.
7. Hammond ME, Hayes DF, Dowsett M, et al. American Society of Clinical Oncology/College Of American Pathologists guideline recommendations for immunohistochemical testing of estrogen and progesterone receptors in breast cancer. J Clin Oncol 2010;28(16):2784–95.
8. Cheang MC, Martin M, Nielsen TO, et al. Quantitative hormone receptors, triple-negative breast cancer (TNBC), and molecular subtypes: a collaborative effort of the BIG-NCI NABCG. J Clin Oncol 2012;30 [abstract 1008].
9. Sorlie T, Perou C, Tibshirani R, et al. Gene expression patterns of breast carcinomas distinguish tumor subclasses with clinical implications. Proc Natl Acad Sci U S A 2001;98(19):10869–74.
10. Sorlie T, Tibshirani R, Parker J, et al. Repeated observation of breast tumor subtypes in independent gene expression data sets. Proc Natl Acad Sci U S A 2003; 100(14):8418–23.
11. Prat A, Perous CM. Deconstructing the molecular portraits of breast cancer. Mol Oncol 2011;5(1):5–23.
12. Lehmann BD, Bauer JA, Chen X, et al. Identification of human triple-negative breast cancer subtypes and preclinical models for selection of targeted therapies. J Clin Invest 2011;121(7):2750–67.
13. Gucalp A, Tolaney S, Isakoff S, et al. Targeting the androgen receptor (AR) in women with AR+ ER-/PR- metastatic breast cancer TBCRC011. J Clin Oncol 2012;30 [abstract 1006].
14. Gonzalez-Angulo AM, Timms KM, Liu S, et al. Incidence and outcome of BRCA mutations in unselected patients with triple receptor-negative breast cancer. Clin Cancer Res 2011;17(5):1082–9.
15. The Cancer Genome Atlas Network. Comprehensive molecular portraits of human breast tumours. Nature 2012;490(7418):61–70.
16. Haffty BG, Yang Q, Reiss M, et al. Locoregional relapse and distant metastasis in conservatively managed triple negative early-stage breast cancer. J Clin Oncol 2006;24(36):5652–7.
17. Nguyen PL, Taghian AG, Katz MS, et al. Breast cancer subtype approximated by estrogen receptor, progesterone receptor, and HER-2 is associated with local and distant recurrence after breast-conserving therapy. J Clin Oncol 2008; 26(14):2373–8.
18. Adkins FC, Gonzalez-Angulo AM, Lei X, et al. Triple-negative breast cancer is not a contraindication for breast conservation. Ann Surg Oncol 2011;18(11): 3164–73.

19. Abdulkarim BS, Cuartero J, Hanson J, et al. Increased risk of locoregional recurrence for women with T1-2N0 triple-negative breast cancer treated with modified radical mastectomy without adjuvant radiation therapy compared with breast-conserving therapy. J Clin Oncol 2011;29(21):2852–8.

20. Wang J, Shi M, Ling R, et al. Adjuvant chemotherapy and radiotherapy in triple-negative breast carcinoma: a prospective randomized controlled multi-center trial. Radiother Oncol 2011;100(2):200–4.

21. Huang EH, Tucker SL, Strom EA, et al. Postmastectomy radiation improves local-regional control and survival for selected patients with locally advanced breast cancer treated with neoadjuvant chemotherapy and mastectomy. J Clin Oncol 2004;22(23):4691–9.

22. McGuire SE, Gonzalez-Angulo AM, Huang EH, et al. Postmastectomy radiation improves the outcome of patients with locally advanced breast cancer who achieve a pathologic complete response to neoadjuvant chemotherapy. Int J Radiat Oncol Biol Phys 2007;68(4):1004.

23. Gonzalez-Angulo AM, Litton JK, Broglio KR, et al. High risk of recurrence for patients with breast cancer who have human epidermal growth factor receptor 2–positive, node-negative tumors 1 cm or smaller. J Clin Oncol 2009;27(34):5700–6.

24. Ho AY, Gupta G, King TA, et al. Favorable prognosis in patients with T1a/T1bN0 triple-negative breast cancers treated with multimodality therapy. Cancer 2012;118(20):4944–52.

25. Bear HD, Anderson S, Smith RE, et al. Sequential preoperative or postoperative docetaxel added to preoperative doxorubicin plus cyclophosphamide for operable breast cancer: National Surgical Adjuvant Breast and Bowel Project Protocol B-27. J Clin Oncol 2006;24(13):2019–27.

26. Carey L, Dees E, Sawyer L, et al. The triple negative paradox: primary tumor chemosensitivity of breast cancer subtypes. Clin Cancer Res 2007;13(8):2329–34.

27. Liedtke C, Mazouni C, Hess K, et al. Response to neoadjuvant therapy and long-term survival in patients with triple-negative breast cancer. J Clin Oncol 2008;26(8):1275–81.

28. Silver D, Richardson A, Eklund A, et al. Efficacy of neoadjuvant Cisplatin in triple-negative breast cancer. J Clin Oncol 2010;28(7):1145–53.

29. Byrski T, Gronwald J, Huzarski T, et al. Neoadjuvant therapy with cisplatin in BRCA1-positive breast cancer patients. Hered Cancer Clin Pract 2011;9(2):A4.

30. von Minckwitz G, Eidtmann H, Rezai M, et al. Neoadjuvant Chemotherapy and Bevacizumab for HER2-Negative Breast Cancer. N Engl J Med 2012;366(4):299–309.

31. Bear HD, Tang G, Rastogi P, et al. NSABP Protocol B-40: the effect on pCR of Bevacizumab and/or antimetabolites added to standard neoadjuvant chemotherapy. J Clin Oncol 2011;29:LBA #1005.

32. Cameron D, Brown J, Dent R, et al. Primary results of BEATRICE, a randomized phase III trial evaluating adjuvant bevacizumab-containing therapy in triple-negative breast cancer. Paper presented at: Cancer Therapy and Research Center–American Association for Cancer Research San Antonio Breast Cancer Symposium, San Antonio, TX, 2012.

33. Balko JM, Wang K, Sanders ME, et al. Profiling of triple negative breast cancers after neoadjuvant chemotherapy identifies targetable molecular alterations in the treatment-refractory residual disease. Paper presented at: American Association for Cancer Research San Antonio Breast Cancer Symposium, San Antonio, TX, 2012.

34. Cheang MC, Voduc KD, Tu D, et al. Responsiveness of intrinsic subtypes to adjuvant anthracycline substitution in the NCIC. CTG MA. 5 randomized trial. Clin Cancer Res 2012;18(8):2402–12.

35. Rugo HS, Barry WT, Moreno-Aspitia A, et al. CALGB 40502/NCCTG N063H: randomized phase III trial of weekly paclitaxel (P) compared to weekly nanoparticle albumin bound nab-paclitaxel (NP) or ixabepilone (Ix) with or without bevacizumab (B) as first-line therapy for locally recurrent or metastatic breast cancer (MBC). Paper presented at: 2012 Annual ASCO Meeting, Chicago, IL, 2012.

36. Kaufmann P, Awada A, Twelves C, et al. A Phase III, open-label, randomized, multicenter study of eribulin mesylate versus capecitabine in patients with locally advanced or metastatic breast cancer previously treated with anthracyclines and taxanes. Paper presented at: San Antonio Breast Cancer Symposium, San Antonio, TX, 2012.

37. Isakoff S, Goss P, Mayer E, et al. TBCRC009: a multicenter phase II study of cisplatin or carboplatin for metastatic triple-negative breast cancer and evaluation of p63/p73 as a biomarker of response. J Clin Oncol 2011;29:Abstract 1025.

38. Baselga J, Stemmer S, Pego A, et al. Cetuximab + Cisplatin in estrogen receptor-negative, progesterone receptor-negative, HER2-negative (triple-negative) metastatic breast cancer: results of the randomized phase II BALI-1 trial. Cancer Res 2010;70(24) [abstract PD 01–10].

39. O'Shaughnessy J, Miles D, Gray RJ, et al. A meta-analysis of overall survival data from three randomized trials of bevacizumab (BV) and first-line chemotherapy as treatment for patients with metastatic breast cancer (MBC). J Clin Oncol 2010; 28(15s) [abstract 1005].

40. Gelmon KA, Tischkowitz M, Mackay H, et al. Olaparib in patients with recurrent high-grade serous or poorly differentiated ovarian carcinoma or triple-negative breast cancer: a phase 2, multicentre, open-label, non-randomised study. Lancet Oncol 2011;12(9):852–61.

41. Isakoff SJ, Overmoyer B, Tung NM, et al. A phase II trial of the PARP inhibitor veliparib (ABT888) and temozolomide for metastatic breast cancer. J Clin Oncol 2010;28(15s) [asbtract 1019].

42. Carey LA, Rugo HS, Marcom PK, et al. TBCRC 001: randomized phase II study of Cetuximab in combination with Carboplatin in stage IV triple-negative breast cancer. J Clin Oncol 2012;30(21):2615–23.

43. Marty B, Maire V, Gravier E, et al. Frequent PTEN genomic alterations and activated phosphatidylinositol 3-kinase pathway in basal-like breast cancer cells. Breast Cancer Res 2008;10(6):R101.

44. Chen M, Ryan C, Piwnica-Worms H. Chk1 kinase negatively regulates mitotic function of Cdc25A phosphatase through 14-3-3 binding. Mol Cell Biol 2003; 23(21):7488–97.

45. Ma CX, Cai S, Li S, et al. Targeting Chk1 in p53-deficient triple-negative breast cancer is therapeutically beneficial in human-in-mouse tumor models. J Clin Invest 2012;122(4):1541–52.

46. Roberts PJ, Usary J, Darr D, et al. Combined PI3K/mTOR and MEK inhibition provides broad anti-tumor activity in faithful murine cancer models. Clin Cancer Res 2012;18(19):5290–303.

47. Duncan JS, Whittle MC, Nakamura K, et al. Dynamic reprogramming of the kinome in response to targeted MEK inhibition in triple-negative breast cancer. Cell 2012; 149(2):307–21.

48. Tate CR, Rhodes L, Segar H, et al. Targeting triple-negative breast cancer cells with the HDAC inhibitor Panobinostat. Breast Cancer Res 2012;14(3):R79.

49. Connolly RM, Jeter S, Zorzi J, et al. A multi-institutional double-blind phase II study evaluating response and surrogate biomarkers to carboplatin and nab-paclitaxel (CP) with or without vorinostat as preoperative systemic therapy (PST) in HER2-negative primary operable breast cancer (TBCRC008). J Clin Oncol 2010; 28(15s) [abstract TPS111].

Treating the HER2 Pathway in Early and Advanced Breast Cancer

Mark D. Pegram, MD[a,b,c],*

KEYWORDS

- Human breast cancers • HER2 pathway • Antibody-drug conjugate

KEY POINTS

- Level I evidence from multiple large, prospective, randomized, phase III clinical trials supports the use of trastuzumab in combination with chemotherapy as treatment for early-stage ERBB2-positive breast cancer in the adjuvant or neoadjuvant settings.
- For patients with metastatic ERBB2-positive disease, there is level I evidence that pertuzumab in combination with trastuzumab and a taxane (docetaxel) yields superior progression-free and overall survival in the first-line setting compared with docetaxel plus trastuzumab alone. This regimen has secured regulatory approval and is a preferred first-line regimen according to guidelines established by the National Comprehensive Cancer Network.
- For patients with metastatic ERBB2-positive disease who have progressed following prior treatment with a taxane and trastuzumab, or relapsed within 6 months of completion of an adjuvant trastuzumab regimen, ado-trastuzumab emtansine (T-DM1) has been shown to be significantly superior (for both progression-free and overall survival) to lapatinib plus capecitabine, and is associated with fewer grade 3/4 clinical adverse events. Ado-trastuzumab emtansine was approved by the U.S. Food and Drug Administration in February 2013.

INTRODUCTION

The discovery of ERBB2 gene amplification in ~20% of human breast cancers (BC) and its association with an adverse clinical prognosis, indicating that it may be playing a critical role in disease pathogenesis, has revolutionized the diagnosis and treatment

Conflict of Interest Declaration: Consultant – Genentech/Roche, Inc.
[a] Medical Oncology, Stanford Cancer Institute, Stanford University School of Medicine, G2021B Lorry I. Lokey Building, 265 Campus Drive West, Stanford, CA 94305-5456, USA; [b] Stanford Breast Oncology Program, Stanford Cancer Institute, Stanford University School of Medicine, G2021B Lorry I. Lokey Building, 265 Campus Drive West, Stanford, CA 94305-5456, USA; [c] Molecular Therapeutics Program, Stanford Cancer Institute, Stanford University School of Medicine, G2021B Lorry I. Lokey Building, 265 Campus Drive West, Stanford, CA 94305-5456, USA
* Susy Yuan-Huey Hung Professor of Medical Oncology, Stanford Cancer Institute, Stanford University School of Medicine, G2021B Lorry I. Lokey Building, 265 Campus Drive West, Stanford, CA 94305-5456.
E-mail address: mpegram@stanford.edu

Hematol Oncol Clin N Am 27 (2013) 751–765
http://dx.doi.org/10.1016/j.hoc.2013.05.007
0889-8588/13/$ – see front matter © 2013 Elsevier Inc. All rights reserved.

of BC.[1–3] In addition to improving overall survival in ERBB2-positive advanced BC, humanized anti-ERBB2 monoclonal antibody trastuzumab, when added to standard adjuvant chemotherapy, reduces relapse risk by approximately one-half and reduces mortality by about one-third in ERBB2-amplified/overexpressed early-stage BC, and, to date, has withstood the test of time.[4,5] Trastuzumab has established a benchmark for treatment of ERBB2-positive disease and has set a high bar of efficacy to overcome for newer emerging ERBB2-targeted therapeutic approaches. However, within the past year, we have witnessed new paradigms that will challenge the chemotherapy plus trastuzumab "gold-standard" treatment for ERBB2-positive disease. These new approaches include the addition of a "second-generation" humanized anti-ERBB2 antibody (pertuzumab) in combination with trastuzumab plus chemotherapy, and the development of an antibody-drug conjugate (ADC) based on trastuzumab.[6–9] Each of these new approaches has already proven to be practice changing, once again raising the bar for clinical efficacy (and therapeutic index) against ERBB2-positive BC. Given this rapid pace of discovery research and clinical validation, the past year will likely be remembered as a golden age of ERBB2-targted therapy for BC.

INVESTIGATION OF A SECOND-GENERATION ANTI-ERBB2 ANTIBODY, PERTUZUMAB: AN ERBB2 DIMERIZATION INHIBITOR

In an early screening of a panel of murine monoclonal anti-ERBB2 antibodies, 2 antibodies stood apart from others in terms of demonstration of preclinical efficacy in cell proliferation assays in vitro, and in primary human tumor xenotransplants grown in the subrenal capsule of athymic mice in vivo (D. Slamon, personal communication, 1991). Two of the most promising murine antibodies to emerge from such screens were 4D5, which, when humanized, became trastuzumab, and 2C4, which, following humanization, is now called pertuzumab. Experimentally, it became evident that these 2 anti-ERBB2 antibodies were distinct, both functionally as well as structurally.[10,11] In contrast to trastuzumab, which binds to a juxtamembrane epitope in subdomain IV of the ERBB2 extracellular domain (ECD), pertuzumab binds to the dimerization interface contained in subdomain II of the ERBB2 ECD (**Fig. 1**). This distinction is biologically relevant in that pertuzumab disrupts the ability of ERBB2 to dimerize with any other ERBB receptor family member, thus attenuating signaling events triggered by ERBB receptor family ligands.[12] For a time it was hoped that this could set the stage for pertuzumab treatment of ERBB2 nonamplified tumor types, if their pathogenesis proved to be driven by ligand-activated heterodimeric complexes containing ERBB2 as a co-receptor.[13] Unfortunately, with the possible exception of platinum-refractory ovarian cancer,[14] this hypothesis was not supported by early clinical trial data of single-agent pertuzumab in ERBB2-negative malignancies; thus, focus returned to the development of pertuzumab in ERBB2-positive disease states, in particular, BC.[15–17] In preclinical models, a combination of trastuzumab plus pertuzumab synergistically inhibited the survival of ERBB2-amplified breast cancer cells.[18] Combination drug treatment reduced levels of total and phosphorylated ERBB2 protein and blocked receptor signaling through Akt, resulting in induction of apoptosis, but did not affect mitogen-activated protein kinase.[18] These results suggested the possibility that combining ERBB2-targeting agents may be a more effective therapeutic strategy than treating with a single ERBB2-directed antibody alone. Consequently, following phase II proof of concept clinical studies, randomized pivotal trials designed to explore the paradigm of dual antibody therapy for ERBB2-positive breast cancer ensued.[17,19] In a clinical evaluation of pertuzumab and trastuzumab (CLEOPATRA) combination in first-line metastatic disease, 808 ERBB2+ patients were randomized to receive

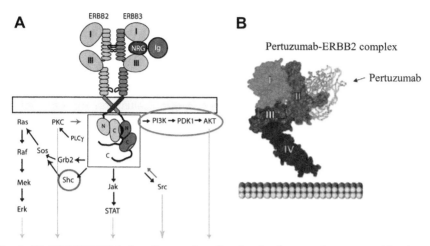

Fig. 1. (*A*) ERBB2/ERBB3 heterodimer: a functional unit of unequal partners with a broad range of signaling outcomes, including cell proliferation, enhanced cell survival, cell mobility, anoikis resistance, differentiation, and attenuation of programmed cell death. (*B*) In contrast to trastuzumab, which binds to a juxtamembrane epitope in domain IV of the ERBB2 extracellular domain (ECD), pertuzumab binds to the dimerization interface contained in domain II of the ERBB2 ECD. Pertuzumab disrupts the ability of ERBB2 to dimerize with any other ERBB receptor family member, thus attenuating signaling events triggered by ERBB receptor family ligands. In (*A*) and (*B*) the roman numerals indicate subdomains of the ERBB receptors. (*Adapted from* Landgraf R. HER2 therapy. HER2 (ERBB2): functional diversity from structurally conserved building blocks. Breast Cancer Res 2007;9(1):202 and Hubbard SR. EGF receptor inhibition: attacks on multiple fronts. Cancer Cell 2005;7:287–8; with permission.)

docetaxel plus trastuzumab and placebo versus docetaxel and trastuzumab plus pertuzumab. In an independently assessed analysis of clinical efficacy, the median progression-free survival (PFS) in the control arm was 12.4 months, compared with 18.5 months in the pertuzumab arm (hazard ratio [HR] = 0.62; $P<.001$).[8] An interim analysis of overall survival (OS) also showed a strong trend in favor of pertuzumab plus trastuzumab plus docetaxel; however, although the P value was .005, it did not cross the prespecified O'Brien-Flemming value of $P = .001$. More recently, a confirmatory OS analysis has been presented.[20] In this analysis, the hazard ratio was 0.66 (95% confidence interval [CI] = 0.52–0.84) in favor of the experimental arm, and the P-value (.0008) has achieved statistical significance. Notably, the safety profile was generally similar in the 2 treatment groups, and there was no increase in left ventricular systolic dysfunction, although the rates of febrile neutropenia and diarrhea of grade 3 or greater were higher in the pertuzumab-treated group.[8] These data suggested that further exploration of this approach in the early disease setting was warranted. Accordingly, a randomized phase II trial of pertuzumab/trastuzumab combination in the neoadjuvant setting has been conducted (NeoSphere).[6] In this multicenter, open-label, phase II study, treatment-naive women with ERBB2-positive BC were randomly assigned to receive 4 neoadjuvant cycles of trastuzumab plus docetaxel, or pertuzumab and trastuzumab plus docetaxel, or pertuzumab and trastuzumab, or pertuzumab plus docetaxel. Patients given pertuzumab and trastuzumab plus docetaxel had a significantly improved pathologic complete response (pCR) rate (45.8%) as compared with those given trastuzumab plus docetaxel (29%; $P = .0141$), without substantial differences in tolerability.[6] It should be noted, however, that the time-to-relapse event data have not yet been reported in this study; therefore, it is not yet known whether improved pCR rates for the combination arm will translate into improved relapse-free or overall survival. Therefore, in contrast to the CLEOPA-TRA study in advanced disease, the NeoSphere data cannot yet be considered to be practice changing, although under a new guidance issued recently by the US Food and Drug Administration (FDA), pertuzumab could in theory be considered for accelerated regulatory approval in the neoadjuvant setting on the basis of the NeoSphere data, coupled with the ongoing commitment to a randomized phase III adjuvant pertuzumab study. Taken together, the findings from CLEOPATRA and Neo-Sphere suggest that targeting ERBB2-positive tumors with 2 anti-ERBB2 monoclonal antibodies that have complementary mechanisms of action results in a more comprehensive blockade of ERBB2 and highlights the clinical importance of preventing the ligand-dependent formation of ERBB2-containing dimers (particularly ligand-activated heterodimers) to best silence ERBB2-driven downstream signaling events.[21] A study of pertuzumab plus trastuzumab adjuvant therapy in patients with newly diagnosed ERBB2-positive early breast cancer has been initiated and is currently underway (Adjuvant Pertuzumab and Herceptin in Initial Therapy in Breast Cancer; APHINITY; NCT01358877).

ANTIBODY-DRUG CONJUGATE ADO-TRASTUZUMAB EMTANSINE: SYNERGY BETWEEN TRASTUZUMAB AND A CYTOTOXIC VIA COVALENT CONJUGATION

Antibody-drug conjugates can be constructed by direct covalent linkage of a therapeutic drug (often a cytotoxic/chemotherapeutic species) directly to a monoclonal antibody backbone. By design, the antibody component of the ADC is merely being used as a delivery vehicle to transport a cytotoxic payload selectively to tumor cells. In ADC constructs the linker chemistry is critical to the success of the approach, because if the chemistry is too labile, the molecule will be unstable in the circulation and could lead to excessive toxicity if the cytotoxic species is liberated in normal tissue compartments. On the contrary, in theory if the linker chemistry is too stable, then the cytotoxic species may not be appropriately liberated in situ in the tumor microenvironment, thus limiting its potential for antitumor efficacy. Accordingly, fine-tuning of linker chemistry is required for optimization of ADC efficacy and may be unique to each target, especially considering pharmacologic properties of the cytotoxic moiety. For example, different results may be observed with targets that are internalized following antibody binding to tumor cells as compared with those that are not. The author previously reported preclinical efficacy of an ADC based on trastuzumab.[22] For these experiments, a bifunctional linker was used to create a targeted prodrug that links to the chemotherapeutic agent paclitaxel, via an energy-reversible ester bond. This study demonstrated in vivo efficacy of a single treatment of trastuzumab-paclitaxel ADC in decreasing tumor volume and tumor cell density of human ERBB2-positive BT-474 mammary tumor cells implanted in severe combined immunodeficiency mice. Moreover, the ADC was more effective in killing tumor cells than equivalent concentrations of coadministered trastuzumab and paclitaxel.[22] Thus the therapeutic index (efficacy ÷ toxicity) could be increased markedly by an ADC approach.

Another trastuzumab-based ADC is trastuzumab-DM1 (T-DM1; ado-trastuzumab emtansine), which is composed of a maytansinoid derivative, linked with a nonreducible thioether linker termed [N-maleimidomethyl] cyclohexane-1-carboxylate. As a result, derivatization of trastuzumab occurs predominantly on the epsilon amino groups of lysines, which are abundant (N = 91) and distributed throughout the antibody sequence.[23] Interestingly, the binding affinity, specificity, signal perturbation capability, and effector functions of trastuzumab remain intact despite DM1 conjugation.[24] Maytansinoids are natural products that are potent antimitotic agents, which, like the vinca alkaloids, prevent microtubule assembly.[23] It is postulated that following receptor-mediated endocytosis, T-DM1 undergoes intralysosomal proteolytic degradation resulting in the release of Lys-MCC-DM1 and subsequent antitubulin-associated cell death (**Fig. 2**).[23] In the phase I dose escalation study of T-DM1, thrombocytopenia was found to be a dose-limiting toxicity.[25] In 2 phase II studies in patients with heavily pretreated ERBB2-positive advanced cancers who had progressed on trastuzumab and chemotherapy, or both trastuzumab and lapatinib-based regimens in the metastatic setting, T-DM1 produced response rates between 33.8% and 41%.[9,26] In one study, higher response rates and longer response durations were seen in patients with centrally confirmed ERBB2-amplified disease, once again reinforcing the importance of accurate ERBB2 testing in patients receiving ERBB2-targeted therapies. In a randomized study in previously untreated metastatic patients with ERBB2-positive breast cancer, T-DM1 also produced higher response rates and had a favorable toxicity profile compared with free trastuzumab given in combination with free docetaxel.[27] Importantly, in terms of therapeutic index, the incidence of grade ≥3 adverse events in the T-DM1 arm was just half that observed in the trastuzumab plus docetaxel arm (37% vs 75%). No grade 3 neutropenia was observed with T-DM1, and remarkably just 1.5% of patients experienced alopecia. Fortunately, in this study trastuzumab-DM1 was not associated with an increased risk of cardiotoxicity compared with trastuzumab plus docetaxel.

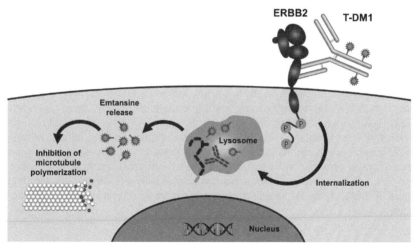

Fig. 2. Ado-trastuzumab emtansine (T-DM1): mechanism of action. Following binding of the ADC T-DM1 to the HER2 ECD, the ADC/receptor complex is internalized by receptor-mediated endocytosis. Following endocytosis, the complex enters the lysosomal compartment, whereupon the complex undergoes extensive proteolysis, which "frees" the potent emtansine moiety that then targets microtubule assembly, resulting in cytotoxicity. T-DM1 maintains trastuzumab-specific mechanisms of action: antibody-dependent cellular cytotoxicity (ADCC), Inhibition of HER2 signaling, inhibition of HER2 shedding. ADC, antibody drug conjugate. (*Data from* LoRusso PM, Weiss D, Guardino E, et al. Trastuzumab emtansine: a unique antibody-drug conjugate in development for human epidermal growth factor receptor 2-positive cancer. Clin Cancer Res 2011;17(20):6437–47.)

EMILIA (NCT00829166) is a phase 3, multinational, multicenter, open-label study evaluating the efficacy and safety of T-DM1 versus capecitabine plus lapatinib (XL), an approved combination for trastuzumab-refractory ERBB2-positive metastatic BC. Upon informed consent, patients were randomized to receive T-DM1 (3.6 mg/kg IV every 3 weeks) or X (1000 mg/m^2 twice a day, days 1–14 evert 3 weeks) + L (1250 mg PO every day, days 1–21) until disease progression. Key eligibility criteria included central confirmation of ERBB2 status (IHC 3+ or FISH-positive) and prior treatment with trastuzumab and a taxane.[28] Primary endpoints were PFS by independent review, OS, and safety. Baseline demographics, prior therapy, and disease characteristics were balanced between the T-DM1 (n = 495) and XL (n = 496) arms. Median durations of follow-up were 12.9 (T-DM1) and 12.4 (XL) months. Patients in the T-DM1 arm had significantly longer median PFS than those in the XL arm (9.6 vs 6.4 mo; HR = 0.650 [95% CI, 0.549–0.771]; P<.0001). Median OS was not reached in the T-DM1 arm versus 23.3 mo in the XL arm (HR = 0.621 [95% CI, 0.475–0.813]; P = .0005); however, the interim efficacy O'Brien-Flemming statistical boundary was not crossed. More recently, in an updated OS analysis, the O'Brien-Flemming boundary was met in this study (stratified HR = 0.682; 95% CI = 0.548–0.849, P = .0006), confirming improved OS in the T-DM1 experimental arm.[29] Moreover, in the planned analysis, 1-year (85% [95% CI, 81%–89%] vs 77% [72%–82%]) and 2-year (65% [59%–72%] vs 48% [39%–56%]) survival rates were greater with T-DM1. There were fewer grade ≥3 adverse events with T-DM1 (41% vs 57%) and fewer dose reductions (16% with T-DM1 vs 53% with X and 23% with L).[28] This impressive result from an ADC therapeutic approach offers a new paradigm for the treatment of ERBB2-positive advanced BC and suggests that further exploration of this ADC is warranted in (1) earlier lines of treatment for advanced disease, and (2) early-stage ERBB2-positive breast cancer. The Marianne study (BO22589/TDM4788g) is an ongoing randomized, phase III, placebo-controlled study in first-line ERBB2-positive metastatic BC (N = 1092) that randomizes patients to receive trastuzumab plus a taxane versus T-DM1 plus placebo versus T-DM1 plus pertuzumab.[30] Primary endpoints are PFS assessed by independent review and safety, whereas secondary endpoints include OS, patient-reported outcomes, and an exploratory biomarker analysis. It is hoped that the result of this trial will help to inform potential regimens to be considered for future adjuvant T-DM1 campaigns. Meanwhile, a randomized, multicenter, open-label phase III study is underway (NSABP B-50) to evaluate the efficacy and safety of T-DM1 versus trastuzumab as adjuvant therapy for patients with ERBB2-positive primary breast cancer whose tumors fail to achieve a pathologic complete response in the breast or axillary lymph nodes following neoadjuvant trastuzumab-based induction therapy. Such patients have a particularly high relapse risk; thus, this clinical setting is ideally suited for testing adjuvant T-DM1, because these patients have high unmet need for improved outcomes.

COMBINATIONS OF ERBB2-TARGETING AGENTS WITH ENDOCRINE THERAPY

Approximately half of ERBB2-positive breast cancers are also hormone receptor (estrogen receptor and progesterone receptor) positive.[31] Women with disease coexpressing both ERBB2 and hormone receptors may be relatively resistant to endocrine therapies compared with those with ERBB2-negative, hormone receptor-positive disease.[32] Preclinical studies suggest that there is cross-talk between cell signaling pathways activated by ERBB2 and ER. Overexpression of ERBB2 was demonstrated to cause ligand-independent down-regulation of estrogen receptor in association with suppression of ER transcripts.[33] Given this association, it was hypothesized that inhibition of ERBB2 activity may augment response to endocrine therapy by enhancing ER expression. To explore this hypothesis, the phase III TAn-DEM trial randomized ERBB2-overexpressing, HR-positive postmenopausal patients to anastrozole alone, or the combination of anastrozole and trastuzumab. Patients in the trastuzumab plus anastrozole arm experienced significant improvements in PFS compared with patients receiving anastrozole alone (HR = 0.63; 95% CI, 0.47 to 0.84; median PFS, 4.8 vs 2.4 months; log-rank P = .0016). At the time of progression, patients were given the option to begin trastuzumab therapy if they were previously randomized to the monotherapy arm. Despite the crossover allowance, a modest (statistically insignificant) trend in OS was noted from combination therapy (28.5 vs 23.9 mo; P = .325).[34] Interestingly, In a post-hoc exploratory analysis assessing the effects of crossover, median OS was significantly less in the group that received no trastuzumab therapy (ie, anastrozole alone with no crossover; median OS, 17.2 months) versus survival in groups receiving anastrozole and trastuzumab initially (median OS 28.5 months) or at the time of crossover (median OS 25.1 months).

Direct ERBB2-tyrosine kinase inhibition with the small molecule ERBB2 kinase inhibitor lapatinib in combination with endocrine therapy has also been investigated. A phase I trial using the combination of lapatinib and letrozole suggested that the combination was safe and tolerable.[35] Subsequently, a phase III trial was undertaken that compared the combination of letrozole plus lapatinib with letrozole plus placebo as first-line treatment of patients with hormone receptor-positive metastatic breast cancer, some with ERBB2-positive disease. Seventeen percent of the total study population (N = 1286) had centrally confirmed ERBB2-positive disease with roughly equal distribution in the lapatinib and placebo groups (n = 111 and n = 108, respectively). In a preplanned analysis of the ERBB2-positive population, the median PFS increased from 3 months for letrozole-placebo to 8.2 months for letrozole-lapatinib (HR = 0.71; 95% CI 0.53 to 0.96; P = .019).[36] Clinical benefit, defined as objective response or stable disease for $\geq$6 months, was also significantly improved (29%–48%; OR = 0.4; 95% CI, 0.2 to 0.8; P = .003) for the combined receptor blockade arm. There was also a (nonsignificant) trend toward improvement in OS. This regimen won regulatory approval by the US FDA in 2010. In summary, because ER signaling has been suggested as an escape mechanism causing resistance to ERBB2 targeting agents, it is important to remember that ER+ tumors in the setting of ERBB2+ disease should also be treated with ER-directed therapies. This paradigm is also suggested by recent results from the TBCRC 006 trial, in which letrozole was used in addition to trastuzumab and lapatinib in 64 evaluable patients with ERBB2+/ER+ stage II/III tumors.[37] Overall, in-breast pathologic complete response ($_{yp}T_{0-is}$) was 27% (ER+, 21%; ER−, 36%). The rate of low-volume residual disease ($_{yp}T_{1a-b}$) was 22% (ER+, 33%; ER−, 4%). Thus, in these patients with locally advanced ERBB2-positive breast cancer, this approach resulted in a high pCR rate even in the absence of chemotherapy. These data support the hypothesis that selected patients with ERBB2-positive tumors may not require chemotherapy. Consequently, multifaceted blockade of ERBB family receptors and ER is an effective strategy worthy of further study.[37]

DUAL TARGETING OF THE ERBB2 RECEPTOR: LAPATINIB PLUS TRASTUZUMAB

The rationale for dual inhibition of the ERBB2 receptor with monoclonal antibody and tyrosine kinase inhibitor treatment emerges from preclinical experiments assessing this combination in ERBB2-overexpressing BT-474 breast cancer cell lines. Treatment of BT-474 cell lines with lapatinib led to only a minimal increase in tumor cell apoptosis with an associated minimal decrease in phosphorylated ERBB2, Akt, Erk1/2, and most notably, survivin (a member of the inhibitor of apoptosis family of proteins). Similarly, treatment with trastuzumab had little effect on apoptosis or survivin concentration. However, the combination of lapatinib and trastuzumab led to markedly enhanced tumor cell apoptosis and down-regulation of survivin.[38,39] In a separate series of experiments examining a broad panel of breast cancer cell lines (including cells maintained in trastuzumab-conditioned media), synergy with concomitant trastuzumab and lapatinib treatment was observed in 4 cell lines.[40]

Data from a phase I trial showed promise for dual inhibition. This open-label trial used a 2-stage design, with the initial stage comprising lapatinib dose escalation to establish the optimally tolerated dose. The second stage included patients in an expansion cohort in which pharmacokinetic parameters were assessed. A total of 48 patients with ERBB2-overexpressing MBC were treated; among 27 evaluable patients, 1 complete response and 7 partial responses were observed—all in trastuzumab-pretreated subjects. A lapatinib dose of 1000 mg daily was identified as the optimally tolerated regimen for further trials in combination with trastuzumab.[41] A subsequent report focused on cardiac safety suggested that the combination of trastuzumab and lapatinib results in a very low frequency of symptomatic cardiac events in a large cohort of patients registered in multiple trials.[42]

Recently, overall survival benefit with lapatinib in combination with trastuzumab for patients with ERBB2-positive metastatic breast cancer was reported in the final results from the randomized, phase III EGF104900 study.[43] In this campaign, patients with ERBB2-positive MBC whose disease progressed during prior trastuzumab-based therapies were randomly assigned to receive lapatinib monotherapy or lapatinib in combination with trastuzumab. Lapatinib plus trastuzumab showed superiority to lapatinib monotherapy in PFS (HR, 0.74; 95% CI, 0.58 to 0.94; $P = .011$) and offered significant OS benefit (HR, 0.74; 95% CI, 0.57 to 0.97; $P = .026$). Multiple clinical factors, including Eastern Cooperative Oncology Group performance status 0, nonvisceral disease, <3 metastatic sites, and less time from initial diagnosis until randomization, were associated with improved OS. These data support dual ERBB2 blockade with a noncytotoxic salvage regimen in patients with heavily pretreated ERBB2-positive MBC.[43]

Combination lapatinib plus trastuzumab is also being evaluated in randomized phase III trials in the adjuvant and neoadjuvant settings. In a completed 3-arm phase III neoadjuvant trial, ERBB2-positive early-stage patients were randomized to receive lapatinib-based treatment, trastuzumab-based treatment, or a combination of both. Anti-ERBB2 therapy alone was given for the first 6 weeks; weekly paclitaxel (80 mg/m^2) was then added to the regimen for a further 12 weeks, before definitive surgery. pCR rate was significantly higher in the group given lapatinib and trastuzumab (78 of 152 patients [51·3%; 95% CI 43·1–59·5]) than in the group given trastuzumab alone (44 of 149 patients [29·5%; 95% CI 22·4–37·5]; difference 21·1%, 9·1–34·2, $P = .0001$). There was no significant difference in pCR between the lapatinib and trastuzumab groups. Time to event data for this trial have not yet been reported, although with just ~150 patients per arm the study is underpowered to expect significant differences in the secondary endpoint of disease-free survival.[7] It is interesting to speculate whether these results from the neo-ALTTO trial will foreshadow results for the large ongoing randomized phase III adjuvant ALTTO trial. The ALTTO study will compare the activity of lapatinib alone, versus trastuzumab alone, versus trastuzumab followed by lapatinib, versus lapatinib concomitantly with trastuzumab in the adjuvant treatment (following standard chemotherapy regimens) of patients with ERBB2 overexpressing and/or amplified breast cancer. On August 18, 2011, the ALTTO Independent Data Monitoring Committee (IDMC) met to review the first planned interim analysis, whereupon the IDMC reported that comparison of lapatinib alone versus trastuzumab alone crossed the futility boundary, indicating that the single-agent lapatinib arm was unlikely to meet the prespecified criteria to demonstrate noninferiority to trastuzumab with respect to the disease-free survival endpoint. The IDMC further recommended that the other 3 arms should continue as planned; thus, results from the comparison of the combination arm versus the trastuzumab-alone arm are eagerly awaited. Interestingly, in another multicenter, phase III placebo-controlled adjuvant lapatinib trial (the TEACH trial), the efficacy and safety of adjuvant lapatinib for patients with trastuzumab-naive ERBB2-positive early-stage breast cancer, started at any time after diagnosis, was assessed. In all, 3147 were assigned to lapatinib (n = 1571) or placebo (n = 1576). After a median follow-up of nearly 48 months, 210 (13%) disease-free survival events had occurred in the lapatinib group, versus 264 (17%) in the placebo group (HR $0 \cdot 83$, 95% CI $0 \cdot 70$–$1 \cdot 00$; P = .053). However, central review of ERBB2 status showed that only 2490 (79%) of the randomized women were confirmed to be ERBB2-positive. In an exploratory analysis of this subgroup, 157 (13%) of 1230 confirmed ERBB2-positive patients in the lapatinib group, and in 208 (17%) of 1260 in the placebo group had a disease-free survival event (HR $0 \cdot 82$, 95% $0 \cdot 67$–$1 \cdot 00$; P = .04), suggesting a marginal benefit for ERBB2-positive women who have not received adjuvant trastuzumab.[44]

ERBB2-POSITIVE BREAST CANCER: CURRENT DISEASE MANAGEMENT SUMMARY

- For patients with early-stage disease, there exists level I evidence to support treatment with chemotherapy plus trastuzumab combination in either the neoadjuvant or the adjuvant settings.[4,45,46] Whether the chemotherapy backbone with trastuzumab should be anthracycline-based has been extensively debated in the literature.[46,47] The only trial with both anthracycline and non-anthracycline trastuzumab-containing experimental arms (BCIRG-006) was not powered to test a hypothesis of noninferiority between the 2 experimental arms, both of which were statistically significantly superior to chemotherapy without trastuzumab control.[46] Although there is currently a trend toward fewer metastatic relapse events in favor of the anthracycline-containing experimental arm in BCIRG-006, in a post-hoc analysis, this disease-free survival trend is not statistically significant (P = .21), and therefore play of chance cannot be ruled out.[48] An event-driven, planned final efficacy analysis of this trial with longer follow-up may help to shed some light on this issue. Clearly, the anthracycline-based trastuzumab-containing regimen was associated with significantly more cardiotoxicity, including grade III/IV clinical congestive heart failure (N = 21 in the anthracycline-containing experimental arm, vs N = 4 in the nonanthracycline arm, P<.001), and late ($\geq$1 decade) cardiac effects following adjuvant anthracycline and trastuzumab exposure are unknown and merit further study.[46] In any event, the overarching principle established by multiple adjuvant and neoadjuvant trials is that chemotherapy when combined with trastuzumab is superior to chemotherapy alone, regardless of which chemotherapy base is chosen.[4,46,49] Therefore, a balanced discussion of various chemotherapy options with the patient is indicated, given the available data at present. When chemotherapy is given in conjunction with trastuzumab in the adjuvant setting, there is some evidence that concomitant drug administration may be superior to sequential chemotherapy followed by trastuzumab.[50] Whether small (T1a) lymph node-negative patients should consider ERBB2-targeted therapy in the adjuvant setting is unknown. Most authorities recommend consideration of ERBB2-directed therapy for tumors T1b and greater based on estimates of relapse risk from retrospective cohorts from the preadjuvant trastuzumab era.[51,52] In terms of optimal duration of adjuvant trastuzumab therapy, recent data have shed light on this issue. The adjuvant HERA trial compared 2 years of adjuvant trastuzumab versus 1 year. Recent presentation of this comparison showed no improvement in efficacy outcomes with longer trastuzumab exposure.[53] In another study, 6 months of adjuvant trastuzumab was compared with 12 months.[54] Although the results thus far are reported to be inconclusive, the data safety monitoring committee recommended suspension of further enrollment as there was a concerning trend toward inferiority of the shorter adjuvant trastuzumab arm.[54] Thus, at this time 1 year of adjuvant trastuzumab remains the current standard of care. Other randomized trials exploring the duration issue are forthcoming.

- For patients with metastatic ERBB2-positive disease, there is level I evidence, based on results from the CLEOPATRA trial, that pertuzumab in combination with trastuzumab and a taxane (docetaxel) yields superior progression-free and overall survival in the first-line setting compared with docetaxel plus trastuzumab. This regimen has secured regulatory approval and is a preferred first-line regimen according to guidelines established by the National Comprehensive Cancer Network.

- For ERBB2-positive patients in first line with ER-positive disease, particularly those with low volume disease burden that is asymptomatic and nonvisceral predominant, or for those who are not ideal candidates for chemotherapy-based regimens, combined receptor blockade with an anti-estrogen plus a ERBB2-targeting agent yields significantly superior progression-free survival compared with anti-estrogen alone, based on data from randomized trials (the TANDEM trial explored anastrozole plus trastuzumab, and the EGF 30008 trial tested the combination of letrozole with lapatinib, the latter garnering regulatory approval by the US FDA).

- For patients with metastatic ERBB2-positive disease who have progressed following prior treatment with a taxane and trastuzumab, or relapsed within 6 months of completion of an adjuvant trastuzumab regimen, ado-trastuzumab emtansine (T-DM1) has been shown to be significantly superior (for both progression-free and overall survival) to lapatinib plus capecitabine and is arguably better tolerated. Ado-trastuzumab emtansine also now has regulatory approval in the United States.

- Upon disease progression following a prior pertuzumab-containing regimen and prior T-DM1, lapatinib-based regimens (either lapatinib plus capecitabine or lapatinib plus trastuzumab) are a logical next choice. However, neither of these regimens have efficacy data sets yet available in the setting of prior progression after multiple ERBB2-targeting antibody (pertuzumab, T-DM1) strategies.

- In later lines of treatment, clinicians regularly default to sequential salvage chemotherapeutics given in combination with trastuzumab in multiple lines, although randomized evidence to support this practice beyond second-line treatment is lacking.

- It is important to remember that in the era of non-anthracyline-based trastzumab-containing adjuvant therapies, that anthracyclines—even as single agents—have activity against ERBB2-positive disease, particularly in those tumors (~35%) with co-amplification of the topo-isomerase IIα gene.[55] Therefore, anthracyclines should be given consideration in the salvage setting in anthracycline-naive subjects. A wash-out period from prior trastuzumab administration is advised to avoid cardiotoxicity, or anthracyclines could be used following progression on lapatinib-based regimens or T-DM1, both of which have shorter half-lives as compared with trastuzumab.

FUTURE DIRECTIONS

Despite a doubling of the number of approved ERBB2-targeting agents within the past year, there remain many new therapeutic opportunities yet to be developed. Because patients with ERBB2-positive advanced BC are only rarely cured, this disease condition will remain an unmet need pending further research to improve the efficacy and tolerability of treatment for this intrinsic BC subtype. Many new projects are currently under active investigation, including (but not limited to) study of pan-HER inhibitors (neratinib, afatinib, dacomitinib, BMS 599626, and HM781-36B), some with irreversible binding properties that distinguish them from lapatinib[56–60]; study of Fc domain-engineered antibodies with enhanced effector function (such as MGAH22) currently being studied in tumors with lower level ERBB2 (2+ IHC) expression[61]; addition of agonist antibodies directed against CD137 to augment ERBB2 antibody-induced ADCC[62]; exploration of the breast cancer stem cell paradigm targeting ERBB2-expressing cells with self-renewal properties—even in the context of ERBB2-"negative" tumors[63]; ERBB receptor aptamers with unique signal perturbation properties[64]; and finally, ERBB2 antibody fusions with other biologics (anti-angiogenic agents, NGK2D ligands).[65,66] It is hoped that further research in these areas will hasten an end to ERBB2-positive BC, with the ultimate goal of improving breast cancer survival.

REFERENCES

1. Slamon DJ, Clark GM, Wong SG, et al. Human breast cancer: correlation of relapse and survival with amplification of the HER-2/neu oncogene. Science 1987;235(4785):177–82.
2. Slamon DJ, Godolphin W, Jones LA, et al. Studies of the HER-2/neu proto-oncogene in human breast and ovarian cancer. Science 1989;244(4905): 707–12.
3. Slamon DJ, Leyland-Jones B, Shak S, et al. Use of chemotherapy plus a monoclonal antibody against HER2 for metastatic breast cancer that overexpresses HER2. N Engl J Med 2001;344(11):783–92.
4. Romond EH, Jeong JH, Rastogi P, et al. Seven-year follow-up assessment of cardiac function in NSABP B-31, a randomized trial comparing doxorubicin and cyclophosphamide followed by paclitaxel (ACP) with ACP plus trastuzumab as adjuvant therapy for patients with node-positive, human epidermal growth factor receptor 2-positive breast cancer. J Clin Oncol 2012;30(31):3792–9.
5. Perez EA, Romond EH, Suman VJ, et al. Four-year follow-up of trastuzumab plus adjuvant chemotherapy for operable human epidermal growth factor receptor 2-positive breast cancer: joint analysis of data from NCCTG N9831 and NSABP B-31. J Clin Oncol 2011;29(25):3366–73.
6. Gianni L, Pienkowski T, Im YH, et al. Efficacy and safety of neoadjuvant pertuzumab and trastuzumab in women with locally advanced, inflammatory, or early HER2-positive breast cancer (NeoSphere): a randomised multicentre, open-label, phase 2 trial. Lancet Oncol 2012;13(1):25–32.
7. Baselga J, Bradbury I, Eidtmann H, et al, NeoALTTO Study Team. Lapatinib with trastuzumab for HER2-positive early breast cancer (NeoALTTO): a randomised, open-label, multicentre, phase 3 trial. Lancet 2012;379(9816):633–40.
8. Baselga J, Cortés J, Kim SB, et al, CLEOPATRA Study Group. Pertuzumab plus trastuzumab plus docetaxel for metastatic breast cancer. N Engl J Med 2012; 366(2):109–19.
9. Burris HA 3rd, Rugo HS, Vukelja SJ, et al. Phase II study of the antibody drug conjugate trastuzumab-DM1 for the treatment of human epidermal growth factor

receptor 2 (HER2)-positive breast cancer after prior HER2-directed therapy. J Clin Oncol 2011;29(4):398–405.

10. Fendly BM, Winget M, Hudziak RM, et al. Characterization of murine monoclonal antibodies reactive to either the human epidermal growth factor receptor or HER2/neu gene product. Cancer Res 1990;50(5):1550–8.

11. Franklin MC, Carey KD, Vajdos FF, et al. Insights into ErbB signaling from the structure of the ErbB2-pertuzumab complex. Cancer Cell 2004;5(4): 317–28.

12. Adams CW, Allison DE, Flagella K, et al. Humanization of a recombinant monoclonal antibody to produce a therapeutic HER dimerization inhibitor, pertuzumab. Cancer Immunol Immunother 2006;55(6):717–27.

13. Agus DB, Akita RW, Fox WD, et al. Targeting ligand-activated ErbB2 signaling inhibits breast and prostate tumor growth. Cancer Cell 2002;2(2): 127–37.

14. Makhija S, Amler LC, Glenn D, et al. Clinical activity of gemcitabine plus pertuzumab in platinum-resistant ovarian cancer, fallopian tube cancer, or primary peritoneal cancer. J Clin Oncol 2010;28(7):1215–23.

15. Agus DB, Sweeney CJ, Morris MJ, et al. Efficacy and safety of single-agent pertuzumab (rhuMAb 2C4), a human epidermal growth factor receptor dimerization inhibitor, in castration-resistant prostate cancer after progression from taxane-based therapy. J Clin Oncol 2007;25(6):675–81.

16. Herbst RS, Davies AM, Natale RB, et al. Efficacy and safety of single-agent pertuzumab, a human epidermal receptor dimerization inhibitor, in patients with non small cell lung cancer. Clin Cancer Res 2007;13(20):6175–81.

17. Walshe JM, Denduluri N, Berman AW, et al. A phase II trial with trastuzumab and pertuzumab in patients with HER2-overexpressed locally advanced and metastatic breast cancer. Clin Breast Cancer 2006;6(6):535–9.

18. Nahta R, Hung MC, Esteva FJ. The HER-2-targeting antibodies trastuzumab and pertuzumab synergistically inhibit the survival of breast cancer cells. Cancer Res 2004;64(7):2343–6.

19. Baselga J, Gelmon KA, Verma S, et al. Phase II trial of pertuzumab and trastuzumab in patients with human epidermal growth factor receptor 2-positive metastatic breast cancer that progressed during prior trastuzumab therapy. J Clin Oncol 2010;28(7):1138–44.

20. Swain SM, Kim SB, Cortes J, et al. Confirmatory Overall Survival (OS) Analysis of CLEOPATRA: A Randomized, Double-Blind, Placebo-Controlled Phase III Study with Pertuzumab (P), Trastuzumab (T), and Docetaxel (D) in Patients (pts) with HER2-Positive First-Line (1L) Metastatic Breast Cancer (MBC) [abstract]. Cancer Res 2012;72(24 Suppl 3).

21. Arteaga CL, Sliwkowski MX, Osborne CK, et al. Treatment of HER2-positive breast cancer: current status and future perspectives. Nat Rev Clin Oncol 2011;9(1):16–32.

22. Gilbert CW, McGowan EB, Seery GB, et al. Targeted prodrug treatment of HER-2-positive breast tumor cells using trastuzumab and paclitaxel linked by A-Z-CINN Linker. J Exp Ther Oncol 2003;3(1):27–35.

23. Lewis Phillips GD, Li G, Dugger DL, et al. Targeting HER2-positive breast cancer with trastuzumab-DM1, an antibody-cytotoxic drug conjugate. Cancer Res 2008;68(22):9280–90.

24. Junttila TT, Li G, Parsons K, et al. Trastuzumab-DM1 (T-DM1) retains all the mechanisms of action of trastuzumab and efficiently inhibits growth of lapatinib insensitive breast cancer. Breast Cancer Res Treat 2011;128(2):347–56.

25. Krop IE, Beeram M, Modi S, et al. Phase I study of trastuzumab-DM1, an HER2 antibody-drug conjugate, given every 3 weeks to patients with HER2-positive metastatic breast cancer. J Clin Oncol 2010;28(16):2698–704.

26. Krop I, LoRusso P, Miller KD, et al. The Antibody-drug Conjugate Trastuzumab Emtansine (TDM-1) significantly prolongs survival in HER2 positive advanced breast cancer [abstract 2770]. Presented at: European Society for Medical Oncology Congress. Milan, October 8–12, 2010.

27. Hurvitz SA, Dirix L, Kocsis J, et al. Phase II randomized study of trastuzumab emtansine versus trastuzumab plus docetaxel in patients with human epidermal growth factor receptor 2-positive metastatic breast cancer. J Clin Oncol 2013; 31(9):1157–63.

28. Blackwell KL, Miles D, Gianni L, et al. Primary results from EMILIA, a phase 3 study of Trastuzumab Emtansine (T-DM1) vs Capecitabine and Lapatinib in HER2-positive locally advanced or metastatic breast cancer previously treated with Trastuzumab and a Taxane. Journal of Clinical Oncology, 2012 ASCO Annual Meeting Proceedings (Post-Meeting Edition) 2012;30(Suppl 18(June 20 Supplement)):LBA1.

29. Verma S, Miles D, Gianni L, et al, EMILIA Study Group. Trastuzumab emtansine for HER2-positive advanced breast cancer. N Engl J Med 2012;367(19):1783–91.

30. LoRusso PM, Weiss D, Guardino E, et al. Trastuzumab emtansine: a unique antibody-drug conjugate in development for human epidermal growth factor receptor 2-positive cancer. Clin Cancer Res 2011;17(20):6437–47.

31. Romond EH, Perez EA, Bryant J, et al. Trastuzumab plus adjuvant chemotherapy for operable HER2-positive breast cancer. N Engl J Med 2005; 353(16):1673–84.

32. Konecny G, Pauletti G, Pegram M, et al. Quantitative association between HER-2/neu and steroid hormone receptors in hormone receptor-positive primary breast cancer. J Natl Cancer Inst 2003;95(2):142–53.

33. Osborne CK, Shou J, Massarweh S, et al. Crosstalk between estrogen receptor and growth factor receptor pathways as a cause for endocrine therapy resistance in breast cancer. Clin Cancer Res 2005;11(2 Pt 2):865s–70s.

34. Kaufman B, Mackey JR, Clemens MR, et al. Trastuzumab plus anastrozole versus anastrozole alone for the treatment of postmenopausal women with human epidermal growth factor receptor 2-positive, hormone receptor-positive metastatic breast cancer: results from the randomized phase III TAnDEM study. J Clin Oncol 2009;27(33):5529–37.

35. Chu QS, Cianfrocca ME, Goldstein LJ, et al. A phase I and pharmacokinetic study of lapatinib in combination with letrozole in patients with advanced cancer. Clin Cancer Res 2008;14(14):4484–90.

36. Johnston S, Pippen J Jr, Pivot X, et al. Lapatinib combined with letrozole versus letrozole and placebo as first-line therapy for postmenopausal hormone receptor-positive metastatic breast cancer. J Clin Oncol 2009;27(33):5538–46.

37. Rimawi MF, Mayer IA, Forero A, et al. Multicenter phase II study of neoadjuvant lapatinib and trastuzumab with hormonal therapy and without chemotherapy in patients with human epidermal growth factor receptor 2-overexpressing breast cancer: TBCRC 006. J Clin Oncol 2013;31(14):1726–31.

38. Xia W, Bisi J, Strum J, et al. Regulation of surviving by ErbB2 signaling: therapeutic implications for ErbB2-overexpressing breast cancers. Cancer Res 2006;66(3):1640–7.

39. Xia W, Gerard CM, Liu L, et al. Combining lapatinib (GW572016), a small molecule inhibitor of ErbB1 and ErbB2 tyrosine kinases, with therapeutic anti-ErbB2

antibodies enhances apoptosis of ErbB2-overexpressing breast cancer cells. Oncogene 2005;24(41):6213–21.

40. Konecny GE, Pegram MD, Venkatesan N, et al. Activity of the dual kinase inhibitor lapatinib (GW572016) against HER-2-overexpressing and trastuzumab-treated breast cancer cells. Cancer Res 2006;66(3):1630–9.

41. Storniolo AM, Pegram MD, Overmoyer B, et al. Phase I dose escalation and pharmacokinetic study of lapatinib in combination with trastuzumab in patients with advanced ErbB2-positive breast cancer. J Clin Oncol 2008;26(20): 3317–23.

42. Perez EA, Byrne JA, Hammond IW, et al. Results of an analysis of cardiac function in 3558 patients treated with lapatinib. 2006 Meeting of the European Society of Medical Oncology. Istanbul, September 29–October 3, 2006.

43. Blackwell KL, Burstein HJ, Storniolo AM, et al. Randomized study of Lapatinib alone or in combination with trastuzumab in women with ErbB2-positive, trastuzumab-refractory metastatic breast cancer. J Clin Oncol 2010;28(7): 1124–30.

44. Goss PE, Smith IE, O'Shaughnessy J, et al, TEACH investigators. Adjuvant lapatinib for women with early-stage HER2-positive breast cancer: a randomised, controlled, phase 3 trial. Lancet Oncol 2013;14(1):88–96.

45. Gianni L, Eiermann W, Semiglazov V, et al. Neoadjuvant chemotherapy with trastuzumab followed by adjuvant trastuzumab versus neoadjuvant chemotherapy alone, in patients with HER2-positive locally advanced breast cancer (the NOAH trial): a randomised controlled superiority trial with a parallel HER2-negative cohort. Lancet 2010;375(9712):377–84.

46. Slamon D, Eiermann W, Robert N, et al, Breast Cancer International Research Group. Adjuvant trastuzumab in HER2-positive breast cancer. N Engl J Med 2011;365(14):1273–83.

47. Burstein HJ, Piccart-Gebhart MJ, Perez EA, et al. Choosing the best trastuzumab-based adjuvant chemotherapy regimen: should we abandon anthracyclines? J Clin Oncol 2012;30(18):2179–82.

48. Slamon D, Eiermann W, Robert N, et al. BCIRG 006 Phase III Trial Comparing AC → T with AC → TH and with TCH in the Adjuvant Treatment of HER2-Amplified Early Breast Cancer Patients: Third Planned Efficacy Analysis [abstract]. Cancer Res 2009;69(24 Suppl 3).

49. Gianni L, Dafni U, Gelber RD, et al, Herceptin Adjuvant (HERA) Trial Study Team. Herceptin Adjuvant (HERA) Trial Study Team. Treatment with trastuzumab for 1 year after adjuvant chemotherapy in patients with HER2-positive early breast cancer: a 4-year follow-up of a randomised controlled trial. Lancet Oncol 2011;12(3):236–44.

50. Perez EA, Suman VJ, Davidson NE, et al. Sequential versus concurrent trastuzumab in adjuvant chemotherapy for breast cancer. J Clin Oncol 2011;29(34): 4491–7.

51. Templeton A, Ocaña A, Seruga B, et al. Management of small HER2 overexpressing tumours. Breast Cancer Res Treat 2012;136(1):209–93.

52. Araki K, Saji S, Gallas M, et al. Possible available treatment option for early stage, small, node-negative, and HER2-overexpressing breast cancer. Breast Cancer 2012;19(2):95–103.

53. Goldhirsch A, Piccart-Gebhart MJ, Procter M, et al. HERA TRIAL: 2 years versus 1 year of trastuzumab after adjuvant chemotherapy in women with HER2-positive early breast cancer at 8 years of median follow up [abstract]. Cancer Res 2012;72(Suppl 24).

54. Pivot X, Romieu G, Bonnefoi H, et al. PHARE: Trial results comparing 6 to 12 months of trastuzumab in adjuvant early breast cancer. [abstract]. Cancer Res 2012;72(Suppl 24).

55. Press MF, Sauter G, Buyse M, et al. Alteration of topoisomerase II-alpha gene in human breast cancer: association with responsiveness to anthracycline-based chemotherapy. J Clin Oncol 2011;29(7):859–67.

56. Kalous O, Conklin D, Desai AJ, et al. Dacomitinib (PF-00299804), an irreversible Pan-HER inhibitor, inhibits proliferation of HER2-amplified breast cancer cell lines resistant to trastuzumab and lapatinib. Mol Cancer Ther 2012;11(9): 1978–87.

57. Soria JC, Cortes J, Massard C, et al. Phase I safety, pharmacokinetic and pharmacodynamic trial of BMS-599626 (AC480), an oral pan-HER receptor tyrosine kinase inhibitor, in patients with advanced solid tumors. Ann Oncol 2012;23(2): 463–71.

58. Kim HJ, Kim HP, Yoon YK, et al. Antitumor activity of HM781-36B, a pan-HER tyrosine kinase inhibitor, in HER2-amplified breast cancer cells. Anticancer Drugs 2012;23(3):288–97.

59. Chow LW, Xu B, Gupta S, et al. Combination neratinib (HKI-272) and paclitaxel therapy in patients with HER2-positive metastatic breast cancer. Br J Cancer 2013. [Epub ahead of print]. http://dx.doi.org/10.1038/bjc.2013.178.

60. Schuler M, Awada A, Harter P, et al. A phase II trial to assess efficacy and safety of afatinib in extensively pretreated patients with HER2-negative metastatic breast cancer. Breast Cancer Res Treat 2012;134(3):1149–59.

61. Nordstrom JL, Gorlatov S, Zhang W, et al. Anti-tumor activity and toxicokinetics analysis of MGAH22, an anti-HER2 monoclonal antibody with enhanced Fc receptor binding properties. Breast Cancer Res 2011;13(6):R123.

62. Kohrt HE, Houot R, Weiskopf K, et al. Stimulation of natural killer cells with a CD137-specific antibody enhances trastuzumab efficacy in xenotransplant models of breast cancer. J Clin Invest 2012;122(3):1066–75.

63. Ithimakin S, Day KC, Malik F, et al. HER2 drives luminal breast cancer stem cells in the absence of HER2 amplification: implications for efficacy of adjuvant trastuzumab. Cancer Res 2013;73(5):1635–46.

64. Zhang Q, Park E, Kani K, et al. Functional isolation of activated and unilaterally phosphorylated heterodimers of ERBB2 and ERBB3 as scaffolds in ligand-dependent signaling. Proc Natl Acad Sci U S A 2012;109(33):13237–42.

65. Shin SU, Cho HM, Merchan J, et al. Targeted delivery of an antibody-mutant human endostatin fusion protein results in enhanced antitumor efficacy. Mol Cancer Ther 2011;10(4):603–14.

66. Cho HM, Rosenblatt JD, Tolba K, et al. Delivery of NKG2D ligand using an anti-HER2 antibody-NKG2D ligand fusion protein results in an enhanced innate and adaptive antitumor response. Cancer Res 2010;70(24):10121–30.

Neoadjuvant Therapy
What are the Lessons so far?

Gunter von Minckwitz, MD[a,b,*]

KEYWORDS

- Breast cancer • Subtypes • Neoadjuvant chemotherapy
- Pathologic complete response • Surrogate marker • Postneoadjuvant treatment
- Locoregional relapse

KEY POINTS

- Recent lessons have been learned that will increase the use of neoadjuvant chemotherapy.
- With the evolving knowledge on how best to perform neoadjuvant chemotherapy in the various cancer subtypes and how to use the information gained for the individual patients, a trend toward more frequent use of this approach can be observed.
- This article provides important prognostic information for those patients with unfavorable initial prognosis for achieving a pathologic complete response and allows subsequent treatment to be adopted accordingly.
- The response-guided approach might be an option for further improving treatment, especially in hormone receptor–positive tumors.
- Neoadjuvant treatment will become standard of care when health care authorities approve the first innovative agent based on a neoadjuvant or postneoadjuvant study and patients will have to be treated neoadjuvantly to get access to the new treatment options.

INTRODUCTION

The concept of moving systemic treatment from after surgery to before surgery was first developed based on a hypothesis that the earlier disseminated single tumor cells are killed the less likely is the development of metastasis at a later stage. However, trials conducted in the 1980s and 1990s have not confirmed this concept but have found similar outcomes in patients treated with chemotherapy before or after surgery.[1] Thereafter neoadjuvant chemotherapy was mainly used to obtain a better operability of large operable or even inoperable locally advanced tumors. This approach is now

[a] German Breast Group, Martin-Behaim-Str. 12, Neu-Isenburg 63263, Germany; [b] Department of Obstetrics and Gynecology, University Women's Hospital, Theodor-Stern-Kai 5, 60590 Frankfurt, Germany
* GBG Forschungs GmbH, Martin-Behaim-Str. 12, Neu-Isenburg 63263, Germany.
E-mail address: gunter.vonminckwitz@germanbreastgroup.de

Hematol Oncol Clin N Am 27 (2013) 767–784
http://dx.doi.org/10.1016/j.hoc.2013.05.006
0889-8588/13/$ – see front matter © 2013 Elsevier Inc. All rights reserved.

considered as a model to learn not only about the biology of breast cancer in general but also about the treatment sensitivity of an individual patient's tumor (**Fig. 1**). Tumor tissue obtained by core biopsy before treatment allows biological characterization of the tumor and development of an individual treatment plan. Early assessment after the first couple of cycles allows testing for functional predictors but also the changing of treatment according to early response. After completing all neoadjuvant treatment, histologic examination of the surgically removed breast and axillary tissue allows precise assessment of tumor response and characterization of residual, treatment-resistant disease.

These arguments for neoadjuvant therapy have led to its broader use in smaller and operable disease; however, adjuvant treatment remained the first option of care in most parts of the world. This article discusses several lessons learned recently that might support the use of neoadjuvant chemotherapy as standard of care in some, mainly more aggressive, subtypes of breast cancer.

LESSON 1: DIAGNOSIS OF A PATHOLOGIC COMPLETE RESPONSE AVOID UNFAVORABLE PROGNOSIS IN PATIENTS WITH HIGH-RISK BREAST CANCER SUBTYPES

Recent results from a meta-analysis of 7 German neoadjuvant studies revealed that pathologic complete response (pCR) is not prognostic for disease-free and overall survival for all subtypes of breast cancer.[2] Subtypes were defined using estrogen and progesterone receptor status, human epidermal growth factor receptor 2 (HER2) receptor status, and tumor grade according to recent St Gallen recommendations.[3] Patients with luminal B (HER2-negative)–like (defined as hormone receptor [HR]–positive, grade 3 tumors), HER2-positive (nonluminal)–like, and triple-negative breast cancers that achieved a pCR showed a better outcome compared with those without a pCR.

However, in patients with luminal A–like (defined as HR-positive, grade 1 or 2 tumors) or luminal B (HER2-positive)–like (defined as HR-positive, HER2-positive, any grade) breast cancers, prognosis was not significantly different for patients with and without a pCR. It therefore seems that pCR as a surrogate marker for survival for patients with these two subtypes is less reliable (**Fig. 2**).

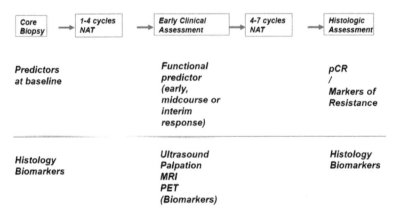

Fig. 1. The concept of neoadjuvant treatment as a model to investigate breast cancer biology and predictors of treatment efficacy. MRI, magnetic resonance imaging; NAT, neoadjuvant treatment; pCR, pathologic complete response; PET, positron emission tomography.

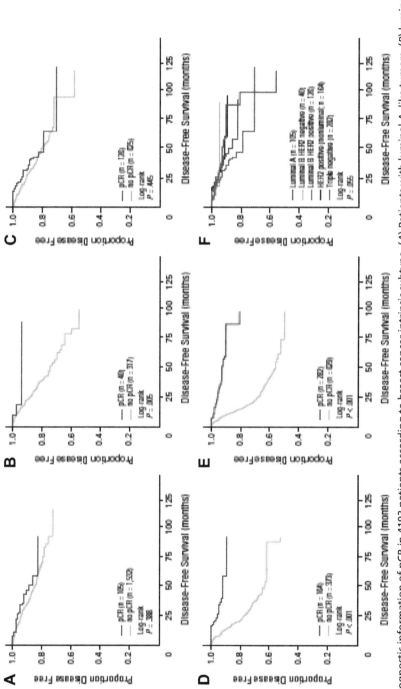

Fig. 2. Prognostic information of pCR in 4193 patients according to breast cancer intrinsic subtype. (*A*) Patients with luminal A–like tumors, (*B*) luminal B/human epidermal growth factor receptor 2 (HER2) –negative–like tumors, (*C*) luminal B/HER2-positive–like tumors, (*D*) HER2-positive (nonluminal) –like tumors, and (*E*) triple-negative tumors; (*F*) comparison of DFS in 717 patients achieving pCR according to breast cancer intrinsic subtype. (*From* von Minckwitz G, Untch M, Blohmer JU, et al. Definition and impact of pathologic complete response on prognosis after neoadjuvant chemotherapy in various intrinsic breast cancer subtypes. J Clin Oncol 2012;30:1802; with permission.)

Comparing patients with pCR of the various subtypes, it could be shown that the subtypes in which pCR showed a prognostic impact had better outcomes than the other two luminal subtypes, despite initially being considered as more aggressive. Based on these observations, patients with these three subtypes having achieved a pCR can be informed that their prognosis has turned from poor to highly favorable (see **Fig. 2**).

The Food and Drug Administration (FDA) of the United States recently gathered data not only from these German studies but also from other large-scale trials around the world.[4] A total of 12,963 patients were collected, including 2 trials from National Surgical Adjuvant Bowl and Breast Project (NSABP), 2 from European Cooperative Trials in Operable breast cancer (ECTO), and 1 from European Organization for Research and Treatment of Cancer (EORTC)/Breast International Group (BIG) groups. A similar analysis to that described earlier was conducted confirming the results for the more aggressive tumor types; however, marginal differences in favor of patients with a pCR were also observed for patients with luminal A–like ($P = .07$) and luminal B (HER2-positive)like ($P = .023$ for patients having not received trastuzumab and $P = .028$ for patients having received trastuzumab). Hazard ratios (HRs) for event-free survival between patients with and without a pCR were in the range of 0.58 and 0.63 for luminal A–like and luminal B (HER2-positive)like tumors and in the range of 0.24 to 0.27 for triple-negative, luminal B (HER2-negative)like, and HER2-positive (nonluminal)like tumors. The less extensive HRs in the first two subgroups again reflect the less favorable outcome of patients with a pCR. Outcomes of patients with a pCR in HER2-positive (nonluminal)like tumors improved substantially when trastuzumab was part of the neoadjuvant treatment.

LESSON 2: PCR SHOULD REQUEST NO INVASIVE (AND NO NONINVASIVE) RESIDUALS IN THE BREAST AND NODES; HOWEVER, SURROGACY WITH LONG-TERM SURVIVAL IS QUESTIONABLE

Two questions have to be answered: the first is regarding the optimal definition, and the second is regarding whether a change in pCR rate by, for example, a better treatment is directly associated with a change in survival time in the same direction.

Various definitions of pCR have been proposed by different groups. When systemic treatment was less effective, patients with even minimal residual invasive disease were considered as a pCR (ypT<1a ypN±); others have considered only response of the breast tumor and considered all patients without invasive tumor residuals in the breast irrespective of nodal status as a pCR (ypT0/is ypN±). With more effective treatments becoming available, definitions became more conservative, requesting either no invasive residuals in breast and nodes (ypT0/is ypN0) or even no invasive and no noninvasive residuals in all removed tissues from breast and axillary nodes (ypT0 ypN0). The comparison of these definitions was first addressed by the meta-analysis of the German studies showing that the HR between patients with and without pCR was highest for the most conservative definition ypT0 ypN0 (HR 4.04 for disease-free survival [DFS] and 7.39 for overall survival [OS]) and decreased with less conservative definitions (3.51 for DFS and 5.99 for OS for ypT0/is ypN0; 2.77 for DFS and 3.66 for OS for ypT0/is ypN±; 2.11 for DFS and 2.80 for OS for ypT<1a ypN±).[2] Again the FDA addressed the same question in their global meta-analysis and found that around 5% of patients have only in situ residuals (ypTis ypN0) and another 4% of patients have no invasive residuals in the breast but involved lymph nodes (ypT0/is ypN+), whereas 13% of patients achieved the most complete pCR (ypT0 ypN0). When plotting Kaplan-Meyer curves of patients with ypT0 ypN0, ypT0/is ypN0 and ypT0/is ypN± disease in the same diagram, no relevant difference in event-free survival and OS was observed between the first 2 curves, but the last 1 showed an inferior outcome. The conclusion therefore is that both ypT0 ypN0 as well as ypT0/is ypN0 are appropriate definitions for pCR. Because the rate of residual disease varies between tumor subtypes (highest in HER2-positive disease) the choice of the definition in clinical trials probably depends on the assumptions to be made for sample size calculation. For routine care, both definitions are suitable.

Because the FDA is currently considering accepting neoadjuvant studies as a new pathway for early drug registration,[5] an important aim of their meta-analysis concerned the second question: what magnitude of pCR improvement in a randomized trial predicts long-term clinical benefit? To answer this question, odds ratios on pCR of the randomized treatment arms were plotted against HRs of event-free survival. A straight diagonal line ideally shows that small increases in pCR rate are correlated with small improvements in event-free survival, and large increases in pCR rate are correlated with large improvements in event-free survival. However, the analysis found a horizontal line, meaning that such a correlation does not exist.

However, there are some suggestions in the literature that this might be the case, at least for patients with HER2-positive disease.

- In the NOAH (NEoAdjuvant Herceptin) study,[6] comparing patients receiving neoadjuvant chemotherapy with or without trastuzumab, it was shown that the pCR rate could be increased by 20% with the combined treatment. In addition, a significant improvement in event-free survival was reported (**Fig. 3**). This trial therefore led to the approval of trastuzumab for neoadjuvant treatment by the European Medical Agency.
- Several trials[7] have compared the tyrosine-kinase inhibitor lapatinib with trastuzumab. In all trials there was a trend toward a lower pCR rate for the combination of chemotherapy with lapatinib. The largest of these trials, the GeparQuinto study,[7] even showed a significantly inferior pCR rate for patients receiving 24 weeks of lapatinib and anthracycline-taxane–containing chemotherapy. These results are consistent with the closure of one arm of the ALTTO (adjuvant lapatinib and/or trastuzumab treatment optimazation) trial, which used lapatinib as the only adjuvant anti-HER2 treatment based on the results of an early interim efficacy analysis (**Fig. 4**).
- Another pair of trials in which a correlation of the effect of neoadjuvant treatment and outcome of adjuvant treatment may be shown is related to an antibody prohibiting the dimerization of the HER2 and the HER3 receptor, pertuzumab. The NeoSphere study[8] showed a higher pCR rate for patients receiving docetaxel chemotherapy with trastuzumab and pertuzumab. The Aphinity (BIG 4-11) study is a currently enrolling adjuvant trial testing the addition of pertuzumab to various chemotherapy-trastuzumab combinations (**Fig. 5**).

LESSON 3: TRANSLATIONAL BIOMARKER STUDIES HAVE SO FAR NOT BEEN HELPFUL IN BETTER IDENTIFYING PATIENTS WITH A HIGHER CHANCE OF TREATMENT BENEFIT

As already mentioned, the neoadjuvant approach provides various opportunities to examine the tumor in direct relationship to treatment (in contrast with the metastatic setting, in which in most cases only tumor from early disease can be examined). However, several examples show that this is not as easy as expected:

- The NeoSphere biomarker program[9] examined up to 20 markers considered as potential predictors for anti-HER2 treatment in general or specifically for

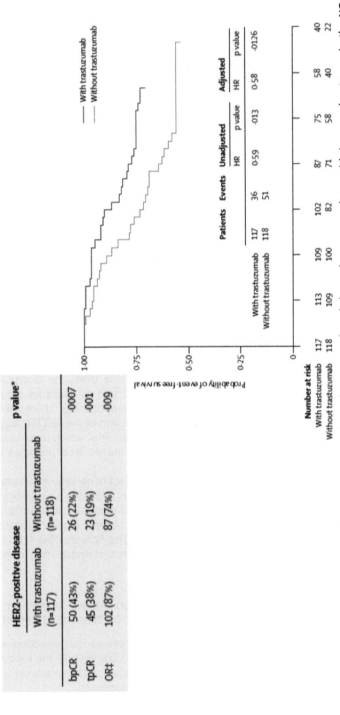

Fig. 3. Increase in pCR rates by adding trastuzumab to anthracycline–taxane–based chemotherapy correlates with improved outcome in the NOAH study. *For comparison of HER2-positive disease groups. (*Adapted from* Gianni L, Eiermann W, Semiglazov V, et al. Neoadjuvant chemotherapy with trastuzumab followed by adjuvant trastuzumab versus neoadjuvant chemotherapy alone, in patients with HER2-positive locally advanced breast cancer (the NOAH trial): a randomised controlled superiority trial with a parallel HER2-negative cohort. Lancet 2010;375(9712):377–84; with permission.)

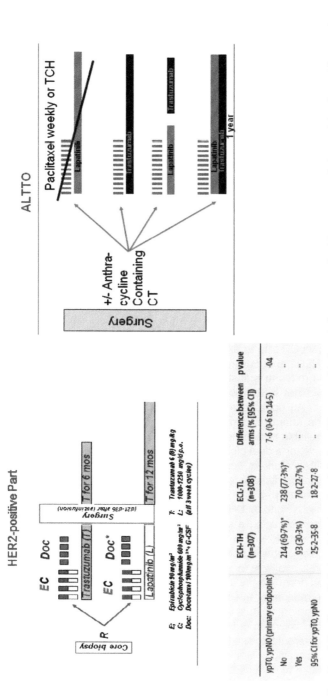

Fig. 4. Results of the GeparQuinto trials showing inferior pCR rates with lapatinib compared with neoadjuvant chemotherapy correspond with an early closure of the lapatinib-alone arm of the adjuvant ALTTO study. (*Data from* Untch M, Loibl S, Bischoff J, et al. Lapatinib versus trastuzumab in combination with neoadjuvant anthracycline-taxane-based chemotherapy (GeparQuinto, GBG 44): a randomised phase 3 trial. Lancet Oncol 2012;13(2):138.)

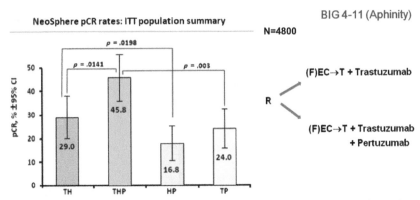

Fig. 5. Trastuzumab and pertuzumab added to docetaxel neoadjuvant chemotherapy revealed significant higher pCR rates compared with trastuzumab or pertuzumab alone added to docetaxel. These results of the NeoSphere study represent the basis of the Aphinity study exploring the combination of trastuzumab and pertuzumab versus trastuzumab alone as adjuvant treatment of HER2-positive early breast cancer. (*Data from* Gianni L, Pienkowski T, Im YH, et al. Efficacy and safety of neoadjuvant pertuzumab and trastuzumab in women with locally advanced, inflammatory, or early HER2-positive breast cancer (NeoSphere): a randomised multicentre, open-label, phase 2 trial. Lancet Oncol 2012;13(1): 25–32.)

pertuzumab. However, none of the markers could discriminate patients with a sufficiently low pCR rate to exclude them from treatment with one or the other or both anti-HER2 antibodies, or to make them exclusive candidates for such a treatment. From the statistical point of view, sample size and number of markers would not have allowed definitive conclusions because of multiple testing issues. An updated report on 5 metagenes and 5 individual markers involved in the adaptive immune system and immune checkpoints again did not reveal a reliable pattern to identify patients who require only trastuzumab, a dual blockade, or a dual blockade without chemotherapy.[10]

- Several candidate markers were investigated in participants of the GeparQuattro study for predicting resistance to trastuzumab.[11] Independent markers in multivariate analysis were p-4EBP1, an activator of the mammalian target of rapamycin (mTOR) pathways, and ALDH1, which signals stem cell properties. However, unless validated by using a separate cohort of trastuzumab-treated patients, these markers should not be considered as clinically relevant. It is therefore advisable to test promising new markers only on cohorts for which a separate second cohort is available for confirmation.

- The truncated form of the HER2-recepter, ^{p95}HER2, was considered as a discriminating marker for the effect of trastuzumab and lapatinib. Because trastuzumab is binding on the external domain of HER2, treatment effect was expected to be less in tumors showing a high percentage of ^{p95}HER2. Lapatinib, inhibiting the internal tyrosine kinase part of the receptor, was expected to work despite the truncation. However, in the GeparQuattro study, patients with ^{p95}HER2-positive tumors showed a higher pCR rate to trastuzumab compared with patients with ^{p95}HER2-negative HER2-positive tumors.[12] In the neoadjuvant Cherlob study, lapatinib showed a higher pCR rate in ^{p95}HER2-negative tumors compared with ^{p95}HER2-positive tumors.[13] Because detection of the truncated HER2-receptor by an antibody is methodologically difficult, these results are currently considered to be a result of a nonspecific antibody that might detect an even more potent form of the HER2-receptor.

- The potential of examining new potential clinically relevant markers was shown by a study investigating immunohistochemically detected Poly(adenosine diphosphate [ADP]–ribose) polymerase (PARP) on tumors from patients participating the GeparTrio study.[14] A tissue microarray including 615 tumors was stained for this marker and nuclear and cyctoplasmic PARP expression was determined. High cytoplasmic PARP expression was not only detectable in triple-negative breast cancer but also, to a lower degree, in HER2-positive and hormone receptor–positive tumors, and was associated with a higher probability for a pCR to anthracycline-taxane–containing chemotherapy as well as with a more unfavorable prognosis. This analysis was designed to provide information on how best to design a trial with a PARP inhibitor in early breast cancer.

LESSON 4: PROGNOSIS OF PATIENTS WITHOUT A PCR CAN BE ASSESSED AND PATIENTS AT HIGH RISK AND HIGH MEDICAL NEED CAN BE IDENTIFIED

Assessment of residual disease to obtain further prognostic information has recently become more interesting, especially for patients with HR-positive disease for whom not achieving a pCR is not necessarily a negative prognostic feature. This article describes 4 currently used methods:

- The ypTypN M system. It was repeatedly shown that diametric extent of residual disease as well as the number of remaining lymph nodes provides relevant prognostic information. The German metadatabase currently provides the largest set of 6619 patients after neoadjuvant anthracycline-taxane–based chemotherapy, which has shown the prognostic impact of this staging system (**Fig. 6**).[2]
- The CPS-EG score. This is a clinicopathologic score (CPS) taking into account clinical stage before neoadjuvant treatment, pathologic stage after neoadjuvant treatment, estrogen receptor content, and tumor grade (Estrogen receptor/ Grade [EG]) (**Table 1**). The score was developed and validated by the MD

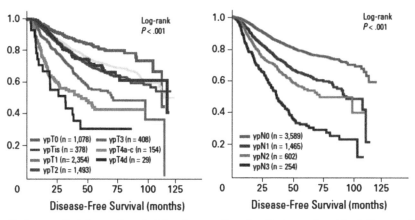

Fig. 6. Prognostic information deriving from ypT and ypN stage of residual disease after surgery in 6377 patients having received neoadjuvant anthracycline-taxane–based chemotherapy. (*From* von Minckwitz G, Untch M, Blohmer JU, et al. Definition and impact of pathologic complete response on prognosis after neoadjuvant chemotherapy in various intrinsic breast cancer subtypes. J Clin Oncol 2012;30:1799; with permission.)

Table 1
The CPS-EG scoring system

Stage	Points
Clinical Stage	
I	0
IIA	0
IIB	1
IIIA	1
IIIB	2
IIIC	2
Pathologic Stage	
0	0
I	0
IIA	1
IIB	1
IIIA	1
IIIB	1
IIIC	2
Tumor Marker	
ER negative	1
Nuclear grade 3	1

Abbreviation: ER, estrogen receptor.
Data from Mittendorf EA, Jeruss JS, Tucker SL, et al. Validation of a novel staging system for disease-specific survival in patients with breast cancer treated with neoadjuvant chemotherapy. J Clin Oncol 2011;29(15):1957.

Anderson Cancer Center.[15,16] The German Breast Group validated the score in preparation for a postneoadjuvant study using the metadatabase of the German trials and might confirm these finding; the score provided valuable prognostic information in patients with HR-positive/HER2-negative disease (**Fig. 7**) (von Minckwitz G, unpublished data).

- The residual cancer burden (RCB) score. This score is calculated as a continuous index combining pathologic measurements of primary tumor (size and cellularity) and nodal metastases (number and size) for prediction of distant relapse-free survival and was developed and validated by MD Anderson pathologists (**Fig. 8**).[17,18] Training of pathologists on how to correctly use the score is required. Detailed description of pathologic assessment and a calculator of the score are available at www.mdanderson.org/breastcancer_RCB.
- To biologically describe the proliferative capacity of residual disease, Ki-67 on the residual tumor was analyzed, including patients with a pCR in which Ki-67 was not detectable, for a total of 1150 patients from the GeparTrio study.[19] Patients were subdivided into 4 groups (pCR, Ki-67 0%–15%, Ki-67 15.1%–35%, Ki-67>35%) with significantly different DFS and OS. Posttreatment Ki-67 measurements were prognostically more relevant than pretreatment measurements or changes from before to after treatment. Patients were analyzed separately according to the hormone receptor status of their tumors and, in hormone receptor–positive disease, patients with low or moderate posttreatment Ki-67 levels had outcomes that were comparable with patients with a pCR, and only patients with high Ki-67 levels showed a high risk of relapse. However, in hormone

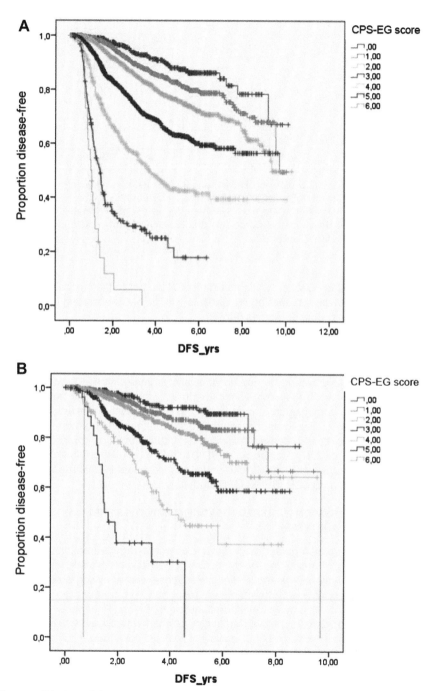

Fig. 7. Validation of the CPS-EG score in 6619 patients of all subtypes (*A*) and 2453 patients with HR-positive/HER2-negative disease (*B*) having received neoadjuvant anthracycline–taxane–based chemotherapy and conventional adjuvant endocrine treatment.

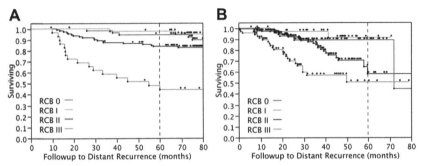

Fig. 8. Validation of the RCB score on 241 (*A*) and 323 (*B*) patients receiving neoadjuvant treatment with paclitaxel followed by 5-Fluorouracil/Epirubicin/Cyclophosphamide (FEC) at the MD Anderson Hospital. (*Data from* Symmans WF, Peintinger F, Hatzis C, et al. Measurement of residual breast cancer burden to predict survival after neoadjuvant chemotherapy. J Clin Oncol 2007;25:4414–22.)

receptor–negative disease, patients with a pCR did better than those with low or moderate Ki-67 levels, and, again, patients with highly proliferating tumors had the most unfavorable outcomes (**Fig. 9**).

At present, 2 novel compounds are in preparation to be assessed in the postneoadjuvant setting for patients not achieving a pCR after taxane-based chemotherapy. Based on new data from the phase III EMILIA study, which showed that trastuzumab emtansine (TDM-1) significantly improved survival of women with HER2-positive metastatic breast cancer,[20] postneoadjuvant treatment with TDM-1 will be randomly compared with the continuation of trastuzumab in HER2-positive patients (Katherine study; NCT01772472). Based on a randomized phase II study in hormone receptor–positive metastatic breast cancer showing an improvement of progression-free survival with a HR of 0.37,[21] palbociclib (PD-0332991), a novel cyclin-D kinase 4/6 inhibitor, is being explored in addition to endocrine treatment in patients with a high CPF-EG score[16] and no pCR (PENELOPE study).

LESSON 5: INTERIM RESPONSE-GUIDED TREATMENT IMPROVES SURVIVAL IN PATIENTS WITH LOWER RISK SUBTYPES

The concept of response-guided neoadjuvant chemotherapy was explored by the GeparTrio study.[22,23] Patients received 2 cycles of docetaxel (Taxotere), doxorubicin (Adriamycin), and cyclophosphamide (TAC). Response was assessed predominantly by sonography and patients without an early response were randomized to either 4 further cycles of TAC or 4 cycles of vinorelbine/capecitabine. Patients with an early response were considered sensitive to this type of chemotherapy and were randomized to a further 4 or 6 cycles of TAC. Analysis of pCR did not show any significant differences between the randomized groups. However, after a median of 5 years of follow-up, patients treated with the experimental treatments showed a better DFS and OS than patients treated with the conventional 6 cycles of TAC.[24] An analysis by subgroup was performed to reveal why pCR did not predict these long-term results. It could be shown that the treatment effects were restricted to patients with hormone receptor–positive tumors for whom pCR was not prognostic. However, in patients with HER2-positive (nonluminal) and triple-negative breast cancers, no difference between response-guided and conventional treatment was observed (**Fig. 10**).

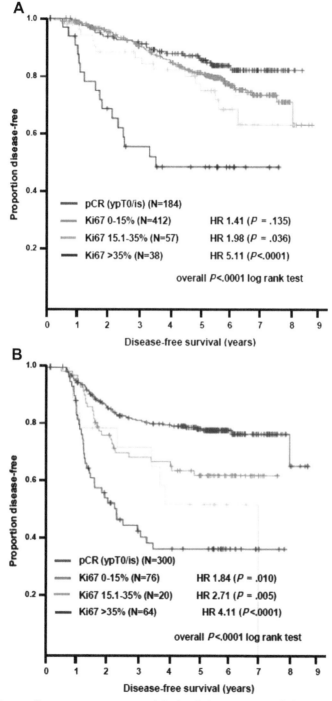

Fig. 9. DFS according to posttreatment Ki-67 levels in patients with hormone receptor–positive (*A*) and hormone receptor–negative (*B*) breast cancer. (*Data from* von Minckwitz G, Müller B, Blohmer JU, et al. Prognostic and predictive impact of Ki-67 before and after neoadjuvant chemotherapy on PCR and survival: results of the GeparTrio trial. J Clin Oncol 2012:30;15(suppl):abstract 1023.)

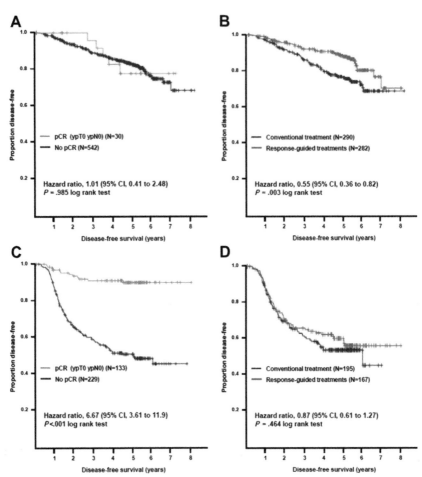

Fig. 10. Relationship of prognostic impact of pCR and effect of response-guided chemotherapy. As in patients with luminal A–like tumors, pCR was not predictive. (*A*) Superior outcome of response-guided compared with conventional chemotherapy could not be predicted (*B*). In contrast, a strong prognostic impact of pCR in patients with triple-negative disease (*C*) may have predicted differences in outcome for response-guided and conventional treatment; however, in this subtype, the response-guided approach was of no benefit (*D*). (*Data from* von Minckwitz G, Kummel S, Vogel P, et al. Intensified neoadjuvant chemotherapy in early-responding breast cancer: phase III randomized GeparTrio study. J Natl Cancer Inst 2008;100:552–62.)

Because these are the subgroups for which pCR predominantly shows its prognostic impact, the forecast of the surrogate marker was correct. It is therefore crucial to assess the relationship between the prognostic impact of pCR and the treatment effect on pCR and survival separately by subtypes (**Fig. 11**).[24]

It therefore seems that the response-guided approach should be further examined in patients with hormone receptor–positive disease. However, aggressive chemotherapy is not recommended for all kinds of luminal A–like tumors, because the GeparTrio study excluded patients with low-risk profiles. Those patients included despite a

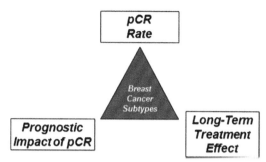

Fig. 11. The magic triangle: pCR rate, the prognostic impact of pCR, and the long-term effect of treatment varies by breast cancer subtype.

luminal A–like feature of the tumors had other clinical risk facture qualifying them for anthracycline-taxane–based chemotherapy.

LESSON 6: PATIENTS WITH PCR OF LOCALLY ADVANCED TUMORS REQUIRE LESS LOCOREGIONAL TREATMENT

The NSABP studies B-18 and B-27 were recently analyzed to identify factors predicting locoregional recurrence after neoadjuvant chemotherapy.[25] In 3088 patients, 335 locoregional recurrences occurred after 10 years of follow-up (12.3% for patients after mastectomy and 10.3% for patients after lumpectomy plus breast radiotherapy). Independent predictors of locoregional recurrence in patients after lumpectomy were age, clinical and pathologic nodal status, as well as breast tumor response; in patients after mastectomy, they were clinical tumor size, clinical nodal status, and pathologic nodal status/breast tumor response. A nomogram was developed that might help to individualize adjuvant radiotherapy (**Fig. 12**).

The database on the German neoadjuvant studies was further analyzed regarding locoregional tumor relapses[26] because early neoadjuvant trials showed a higher relapse risk for this approach. In general, patients with a pCR showed a lower locoregional relapse risk. These patients are therefore candidates to further reduce the extent of locoregional treatment. It was further shown that patients treated by breast-conserving techniques had a lower locoregional relapse risk, which was also the case for patients with locally advanced tumors before the start of treatment. Even patients with inflammatory breast cancer showed a lower locoregional relapse risk when treated with breast conservation compared with those treated with mastectomy. Because this was not a randomized comparison, it is likely that, if the investigator and the patient chose this non–state-of-the-art approach (probably because of an extensive clinical response), these were not patients at a high locoregional relapse risk. Current studies are trying to identify patients with such a high chance for a pCR that surgery might be superfluous. We therefore reanalyzed data from the GeparQuattro study to identify such a cohort. Patients with triple-negative or HER2-positive tumors showed pCR rates of 72% to 74% if they showed a complete disappearance of the breast tumor by palpation, ultrasound, mammography, and in some cases magnetic resonance imaging. In a current project, patients with such criteria undergo a second core biopsy just before surgery with the aim of finding an even higher pCR rate for patients with a core biopsy free of tumor. In 4 of the first 28 patients, residual tumor was found in the core biopsy and an additional 6 patients had tumor residuals in the surgically removed specimen. We are now trying to better standardize how such a core biopsy should be conducted to improve the results.

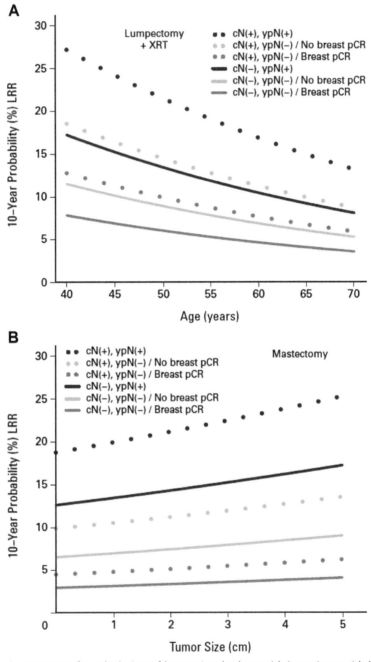

Fig. 12. A nomogram for calculation of locoregional relapse risk in patients with lumpectomy and radiotherapy or mastectomy after neoadjuvant chemotherapy. (*Data from* von Minckwitz G, Kümmel S, Vogel P, et al. Neoadjuvant vinorelbine-capecitabine versus docetaxel-doxorubicin-cyclophosphamide in early nonresponsive breast cancer: phase III randomized GeparTrio trial. J Natl Cancer Inst 2008;100:542–51.)

SUMMARY

With the evolving knowledge of how best to perform neoadjuvant chemotherapy in the various subtypes and how to use the information gained for individual patients, a trend toward more frequent use of this approach can be observed. It provides important prognostic information for those patients with unfavorable initial prognosis achieving a pCR and allows the subsequent adoption of the appropriate treatment. The response-guided approach might be an option for further improving treatment, especially in hormone receptor–positive tumors. Neoadjuvant treatment will become standard of care when authorities approve the first innovative agent based on a neoadjuvant or postneoadjuvant study, and patients will have to be treated neoadjuvantly to get access to the new treatment options.

REFERENCES

1. Fisher B, Bryant J, Wolmark N, et al. Effect of preoperative chemotherapy on the outcome of women with operable breast cancer. J Clin Oncol 1998;16:2672–85.
2. von Minckwitz G, Untch M, Blohmer JU, et al. Definition and impact of pathological complete response on prognosis after neoadjuvant chemotherapy in various intrinsic breast cancer subtypes. J Clin Oncol 2012;30:1796–804.
3. Goldhirsch A, Wood WC, Coates AS, et al. Strategies for subtypes–dealing with the diversity of breast cancer: highlights of the St. Gallen International Expert Consensus on the Primary Therapy of Early Breast Cancer 2011. Ann Oncol 2011;22:1736–47.
4. Cortazar P, Zhang L, Untch M, et al. Meta-analysis results from the Collaborative Trials in Neoadjuvant Breast Cancer (CTNeoBC). Cancer Res 2012;72(Suppl 24): 93s.
5. Prowell TM, Pazdur R. Pathological complete response and accelerated drug approval in early breast cancer. N Engl J Med 2012;366:2438–41.
6. Gianni L, Eiermann W, Semiglazov V, et al. Neoadjuvant chemotherapy with trastuzumab followed by adjuvant trastuzumab versus neoadjuvant chemotherapy alone, in patients with HER2-positive locally advanced breast cancer (the NOAH trial): a randomised controlled superiority trial with a parallel HER2-negative cohort. Lancet 2010;375(9712):377–84.
7. Untch M, Loibl S, Bischoff J, et al. Lapatinib versus trastuzumab in combination with neoadjuvant anthracycline-taxane-based chemotherapy (GeparQuinto, GBG 44): a randomised phase 3 trial. Lancet Oncol 2012;13(2):135–44.
8. Gianni L, Pienkowski T, Im YH, et al. Efficacy and safety of neoadjuvant pertuzumab and trastuzumab in women with locally advanced, inflammatory, or early HER2-positive breast cancer (NeoSphere): a randomised multicentre, open-label, phase 2 trial. Lancet Oncol 2012;13(1):25–32.
9. Gianni L, Bianchini G, Kiermaier A, et al. Neoadjuvant pertuzumab (P) and trastuzumab (H): biomarker analyses of a 4-Arm randomized phase II study (NeoSphere) in patients (pts) with HER2-positive breast cancer (BC). Cancer Res. 2011;71(Suppl 24):Abst S5-1.
10. Gianni L, Bianchini G, Valagussa P, et al. Adaptive immune system and immune checkpoints are associated with response to pertuzumab (P) and trastuzumab (H) in the NeoSphere study. Cancer Res 2011;72(Suppl 24):Abst S6-7.
11. Huober J, Loibl S, Untch M, et al. New molecular biomarkers for resistance to trastuzumab-based in primary HER2 positive breast cancer – a translational investigation from the neoadjuvant GeparQuattro study. Cancer Res 2010; 70(Suppl 24):abstract PD02–06.

12. Loibl S, Bruey JM, von Minckwitz G, et al. Validation of p95 as a predictive marker for trastuzumab-based therapy in primary HER2-positive breast cancer: a translational investigation from the neoadjuvant GeparQuattro study. J Clin Oncol 2011;29(Suppl):abstract 530.

13. Guarneri V, Frassoldati A, Bottini A, et al. Preoperative chemotherapy plus trastuzumab, lapatinib, or both in human epidermal growth factor receptor 2–positive operable breast cancer: results of the randomized phase II CHER-LOB Study. J Clin Oncol 2012. http://dx.doi.org/10.1200/JCO.2011.39.0823.

14. von Minckwitz G, Muller BM, Loibl S, et al. Cytoplasmic poly(ADP-ribose) polymerase expression is predictive and prognostic in patients with breast cancer treated with neoadjuvant chemotherapy. J Clin Oncol 2011;29:2150–7.

15. Jeruss JS, Mittendorf EA, Tucker SL, et al. Combined use of clinical and pathologic staging variables to define outcomes for breast cancer patients treated with neoadjuvant therapy. J Clin Oncol 2008;26(2):246–52.

16. Mittendorf EA, Jeruss JS, Tucker SL, et al. Validation of a novel staging system for disease-specific survival in patients with breast cancer treated with neoadjuvant chemotherapy. J Clin Oncol 2011;29(15):1956–62.

17. Symmans WF, Peintinger F, Hatzis C, et al. Measurement of residual breast cancer burden to predict survival after neoadjuvant chemotherapy. J Clin Oncol 2007;25:4414–22.

18. Chavez-Mac Gregor M, Hubbard R, Meric-Bernstam F. Residual cancer burden (RCB) in breast cancer patients treated with taxane- and anthracycline-based neoadjuvant chemotherapy: The effect of race. J Clin Oncol 2010;28:15s (suppl; abstr 607).

19. von Minckwitz G, Müller B, Blohmer JU, et al. Prognostic and predictive impact of Ki-67 before and after neoadjuvant chemotherapy on PCR and survival: results of the GeparTrio trial. J Clin Oncol 2012;30(Suppl):abstract 1023.

20. Blackwell K, Miles D, Gianni L, et al. Primary results from EMILIA, a phase III study of trastuzumab emtansine (T-DM1) versus capecitabine (X) and lapatinib (L) in HER2-positive locally advanced or metastatic breast cancer (MBC) previously treated with trastuzumab (T) and a taxane. J Clin Oncol 2012; 30(Suppl):abstract LBA1.

21. Finn RS, Crown JP, Boer K, et al. Results of a randomized phase 2 study of PD 0332991, a cyclin-dependent kinase (CDK) 4/6 inhibitor, in combination with letrozole versus letrozole alone for first-line treatment of ER+/HER2- advanced breast cancer. Ann Oncol 2012;23:ii43–5.

22. von Minckwitz G, Kummel S, Vogel P, et al. Intensified neoadjuvant chemotherapy in early-responding breast cancer: phase III randomized GeparTrio study. J Natl Cancer Inst 2008;100:552–62.

23. von Minckwitz G, Kümmel S, Vogel P, et al. Neoadjuvant vinorelbine-capecitabine versus docetaxel-doxorubicin-cyclophosphamide in early nonresponsive breast cancer: phase III randomized GeparTrio trial. J Natl Cancer Inst 2008;100:542–51.

24. von Minckwitz G, Blohmer JU, Costa SD, et al. Neoadjuvant chemotherapy adapted by interim response improves overall survival of primary breast cancer patients – results of the GeparTrio trial. Cancer Res 2011;71(24 Suppl):103s.

25. Mamounas EP, Anderson SJ, Dignam JJ, et al. Predictors of locoregional recurrence after neoadjuvant chemotherapy: results from combined analysis of National Surgical Adjuvant Breast and Bowel Project B-18 and B-27. J Clin Oncol 2012;30:3960–6.

26. von Minckwitz G, Kaufmann M, Kümmel S, et al. Local recurrence risk after neoadjuvant chemotherapy. Pooled analysis on 5477 breast cancer patients. Cancer Res 2011;71(24 Suppl):142s.

Challenges in the Treatment of Older Breast Cancer Patients

Grant R. Williams, MD[a], Ellen Jones, MD, PhD[a],
Hyman B. Muss, MD[b],*

KEYWORDS

- Breast cancer • Age • Aged • Elderly • Geriatric

KEY POINTS

- The US population is aging, and increasing age is the major risk factor for breast cancer.
- Treatment decisions are not based on age but estimated survival.
- Adjuvant therapy decisions are based on breast cancer stage and phenotype, patient goals, treatment options, potential toxicity, and estimated survival.
- All therapy is palliative in the metastatic setting, and controlling symptoms and maintaining quality of life are the key goals of treatment.
- Partnering with geriatricians, internists, and family practitioners optimizes patient management.

INTRODUCTION

In the United States and other developed nations, the incidence and mortality rates for breast cancer rise dramatically with increasing age, making aging the major risk factor for breast cancer.[1] For example, at present, the risk of developing a new breast cancer is 1 in 15 for women 70 years old as contrasted to 1 in 203 for those younger than 39 years old.[2] Moreover the current aging of the US population will compound these numbers and lead to major increases in the number of older women with breast cancer. The median age of onset of breast cancer is approximately 61 years in the United States and a majority of women who die of breast cancer are 65 years and older. Of the 130,000 estimated new breast cancers in the United States, in 2013, 40% will be in women older than 65 years.[3] In addition, of the approximately 3 million breast

Disclosures: The authors have no significant financial interest in or other relationship with the manufacturers of any products or providers of any service mentioned in this article.
[a] University of North Carolina, 170 Manning Drive, Campus Box 7305, Chapel Hill, NC 27599-7550, USA; [b] Lineberger Comprehensive Cancer Center, University of North Carolina, 170 Manning Drive, Campus Box 7305, Chapel Hill, NC 27599, USA
* Corresponding author.
E-mail address: muss@med.unc.edu

Hematol Oncol Clin N Am 27 (2013) 785–804
http://dx.doi.org/10.1016/j.hoc.2013.05.008
0889-8588/13/$ – see front matter © 2013 Elsevier Inc. All rights reserved.

cancer survivors in 2012, a majority are greater than 65 years. The challenge of caring for older women is tailoring the treatment to fit the patient. Although this is true for all patients, it is germane in elders, in whom comorbidity and functional loss can lead to undertreatment and the risk for shorter breast cancer–specific survival or to overtreatment and needless toxicity.

Most practicing oncologists have not had geriatric training but still may think they have the necessary knowledge and skills to make optimal treatment decisions; available data suggest this is not the case.[4–6] A common error is to equate chronologic age with physiologic age in making treatment decisions. There can be wide variability in estimated survival for patients of the same age, however, depending on their comorbidities and general health status. As an example, a 75-year-old woman in average health has an estimated survival of 12 more years whereas an 85-year-old woman has approximately 7 years (http://www.census.gov/compendia/statab/2012/tables/12s0105.pdf). This article focuses on issues directly related to treatment decisions for older women with breast cancer, including defining the goals of treatment, estimating survival, and selecting appropriate therapy in the adjuvant and metastatic settings. Other outstanding reviews on this topic have also been published.[7,8] **Table 1** provides a list of Web sites that are helpful resources when making treatment decisions for older patients with breast cancer and other cancers.

DEFINING THE GOALS OF TREATMENT

It is key before discussing treatment options with a patient that an oncologist makes clear to the patient the goals of therapy. Is treatment recommended to improve survival, as in the adjuvant setting, or to improve quality of life and control cancer-related symptoms, as in the venue of metastatic disease? The purposes of treatment in the adjuvant and metastatic settings are easily defined, but the functional (and today the financial) price paid to achieve them may differ greatly in older versus younger women. Treatment goals in elders are likely to differ substantially from younger women. For younger patients maintaining relationships, raising children, and being

Table 1	
Useful online resources for treating older patients with breast cancer	
Site	**Web Address**
ePrognosis • Life expectancy calculators	www.eprognosis.org
POGOe • Comprehensive Web site on geriatrics	www.pogoe.org
Adjuvant! Online • Estimates treatment benefit	www.adjuvantonline.com
PREDICT • Estimates treatment benefit and includes patients with HER2-positive tumors	www.predict.nhs.uk
Cancer and Aging Research Group • Provides toxicity calculator and other educational materials	www.mycarg.org
Moffitt Cancer Center CRASH Score • Toxicity prediction calculator	www.moffitt.org/saoptools
UNC Lineberger Geriatric Oncology • Provides other helpful links and educational material	http://unclineberger.org/geriatric
World Health Organization FRAX	www.shef.ac.uk/FRAX

gainfully employed are major issues and result in younger patients more willing to accept serious toxicities for longer survivals. Older patients frequently have different goals. In a seminal study in which older patients were offered a treatment that would improve survival, 75% would refuse treatment if it were associated with a risk of severe functional impairment whereas almost 90% would refuse for a risk of severe cognitive loss.[9] For older women living independently, not being a burden on their families is a major concern and oncologists must factor this in to their treatment recommendations. Being clear on the goals of treatment is essential in the care of all patients, but especially in elders, where a physician's preferences may not be similar to the patient's.

ESTIMATING SURVIVAL AND GERIATRIC ASSESSMENT

Once the goals of treatment are defined, a patient's estimated survival from non–breast cancer causes should be assessed. Such estimates can be obtained from Web-based calculators available on www.eprognosis.org and derived from key studies of elders.[10,11] These calculators, although not perfect, are generally better than an educated guess and rely on clinical as well as functional information that can be obtained as part of the history and physical examination and a brief geriatric assessment. An example of how these calculators can help estimate survival is shown in **Table 2**. For women with breast cancer, survival can also be estimated using the calculator in Adjuvant! Online (www.adjuvantonline.com).[12] This program uses US census data to estimate life expectancy based on age at breast cancer diagnosis and allows clinicians to provide an estimate of general health that may also influence survival and potential benefits of treatment. Such information can be of great help because for most breast cancer patients, especially elders, the likelihood of dying of a non–breast cancer cause is greater than that of breast cancer (**Fig. 1**).[13] The

Table 2
The life expectancy from non–breast cancer causes for 2 75-year-old patients with a new diagnosis of breast cancer; 5% and 9% mortality rates were calculated using the Schonberg Index (www.eprognosis.com).

Variable	Patient 1	Patient 2
Age	75	75
Gender	Female	Female
Smoking	Never	Former
BMI	30	23
History of Ca	No	No
Diabetes	No	Yes
COPD	No	Yes
Hospitalizations past year	None	Once
Self-rated health	Excellent	Fair
Dependent IADL	None	1
Difficulty walking 1/4 mile	No	Yes
5-y Mortality	6%	43%
9-y Mortality	16%	75%

This model provides estimated life expectancy exclusive of the patient's breast cancer diagnosis.
Abbreviations: BMI, body mass index; COPD, chronic obstructive pulmonary disease; IADL, dependent instrumental activities of daily living.

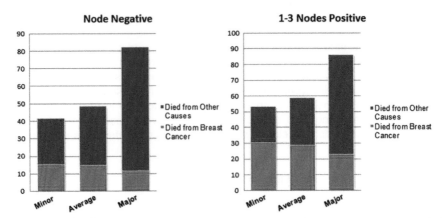

Fig. 1. Estimated 10-year mortality of 75-year-old patients with TNBC 1-cm to 2-cm grade 3 without treatment based on comorbidities and node status. Major comorbidity is defined as a history of myocardial infarction, congestive heart failure, diabetes, or vascular disease. Only in patients with 1 to 3 node-positive tumors and minor comorbidites was the risk of death from breast cancer greater than the risk of death from other causes (calculated from www.adjuvantonline.com).

likelihood of non–breast cancer–related mortality helps put the benefits of breast cancer adjuvant therapy into better perspective.

The Eastern Cooperative Oncology Group (ECOG) and Karnofsky Performance Status are commonly used by oncologists as a global assessment of function in cancer patients. Although these measures correlate well with cancer-related mortality, they are an inadequate measure of functional impairment in elders.[14,15] A comprehensive geriatric assessment (CGA) assesses functional status, comorbidity, medication use, cognition, social support, and nutritional status, all key domains related to quality of life and longevity. The CGA can help identify problems that can be improved or overcome by interventions that have been shown beneficial in improving quality of life and reducing morbidity in older patients.[16,17] Unfortunately, CGA is a time-consuming process, which, coupled with the lack of available geriatricians, makes it impractical for older cancer patients. To compensate, several validated screening tools can be used to identify vulnerable and frail patients who can then be referred for a more comprehensive assessment.[18–21]

An abbreviated geriatric assessment that evaluates key domains has also been shown feasible in the clinical trials setting.[22] This assessment takes approximately 10 minutes of professional time to perform a brief mental status evaluation and up-and-go test and approximately 20 minutes of a patient's time to provide self-reported information on other key domains, such as activities of daily living (which evaluates tasks, such as washing and dressing, that are necessary for caring for one-self), instrumental activities of daily living (tasks, such as cooking and paying bills, that allow living independently), depression and anxiety (common problems in older patients that are frequently underdiagnosed and undertreated), comorbidity, medications, nutritional status, and social support. Information from the CGA can be used to inform models that predict survival (such as the www.eprognosis.com calculator [discussed previously]) and chemotherapy-related toxicity (discussed later) as well as to identify other problems, such as poor function, lack of social support, polypharmacy, and poor nutrition—all which lend themselves to potentially beneficial interventions. The International Society of Geriatric Oncology and the National Comprehensive

Cancer Network recommend that CGA be performed on older patients with cancer.[17,23]

PREDICTING CHEMOTHERAPY TOXICITY

Toxicity is a concern of all breast cancer patients offered treatment, but especially elders, in whom side effects, such as neuropathy and fatigue, can convert an independent community living elder to someone needing institutional care. Two tools are now available that use both clinical information generally collected as part of the standard patient evaluation and items collected in a geriatric assessment.[24,25] The Chemotherapy Risk Assessment Scale for High-Age Patients (CRASH) score, available online at www.moffitt.org/saoptools, provides 2 subscores that predict the risk of grade 4 hematologic toxicity and grades 3 to 4 nonhematologic toxicity.[24] This tool assigns a toxicity risk to different chemotherapy regimens and includes diastolic blood pressure, activities of daily living, instrumental activities of daily living, ECOG performance status, mental status, and nutritional status to predict toxicity.

A second calculator has been developed by the Cancer and Aging Research Group (www.mycarg.org).[25] Like the CRASH score, this tool uses clinical and geriatric assessment data and provides a score predictive of grades 3 to 5 toxicity. The score was derived from a study of 500 patients 65 years and older who had a brief geriatric assessment prior to chemotherapy and included patients with different stages I to IV cancers; grades 3 to 5 toxicity were noted in 53% of the entire group and 2% died of treatment-related toxicity. Karnofsky Performance Status in this study was not predictive of toxicity, although the model clearly distinguished between low-risk and high-risk groups.

DUCTAL CARCINOMA IN SITU

With the advent of routine screening mammography, an increasing proportion of breast cancer patients are diagnosed with preinvasive in situ cancers. Although some patients with extensive ductal cancer in situ (DCIS) may undergo mastectomy, another proved approach to management includes lumpectomy (with re-excision if necessary to achieve negative margins) and adjuvant breast radiation. There may also be favorable subsets of patients with DCIS for whom it is reasonable to consider deferring adjuvant radiation.

In a meta-analysis incorporating individualized patient data from 4 randomized trials in patients with DCIS, the Early Breast Cancer Trialists' Collaborative Group found that adjuvant radiotherapy reduced the absolute 10-year risk of ipsilateral breast events by approximately half (28.1% with breast conservation surgery alone to 12.9% with breast conservation surgery plus RT), with an absolute reduction in breast recurrence of 15.2% at 10 years.[26] The proportional reduction in breast cancer recurrence was greater for the more advanced age cohorts. Although approximately half of recurrences were invasive cancers, the addition of radiation did not increase breast cancer–specific or overall survival.

Prospective observational studies have been performed in low-risk patients with DCIS treated with lumpectomy alone.[27,28] In one trial the 5-year ipsilateral recurrence rate was 12% in patients who did not receive tamoxifen and had tumors smaller than 2.5 cm that were low or intermediate grade, and with at least a 1-cm surgical margin. In this series, approximately half of the patients enrolled were premenopausal.[27] Another trial found an overall 6.1% 5-year ipsilateral recurrence rate in patients with tumors smaller than 2.5 cm, low or intermediate grade, and 3-mm surgical margins. The median age in that series was 60, and the median tumor size was 5 mm. There was a 15.3% recurrence rate in the subset of patients with high-grade tumors[28] and 10% of patients in this trial received tamoxifen. The investigators concluded that, for patients with low-grade or intermediate-grade tumors meeting these clinical criteria, that radiation could be omitted. A randomized trial of breast conserving surgery with or without radiation in this good-risk DCIS population (Radiation Therapy Oncology Group 9804) has been reported in abstract only. This trial closed early due to poor accrual (n = 636), but a statistically different difference in ipsilateral recurrence at 5 years was seen (3.2% no radiation vs 0.4% with radiation).[29] These data suggest that it is reasonable to omit breast radiation in elderly DCIS patients with low-grade to intermediate-grade lesions smaller than 2.5 cm with negative margins (at least 3 mm) given the low rate of in breast recurrence and lack of impact on breast cancer–specific or overall survival.

EARLY-STAGE BREAST CANCER
Selecting Systemic Adjuvant Therapy

In women 70 years and older, a majority of breast cancers are hormone receptor positive (HR+) and HER2-negative (HER2−).[30] These breast cancers have significantly different clinical courses and outcomes compared with triple-negative breast cancer (TNBC) (estrogen receptor [ER] negative, progesterone receptor negative, and HER2−) and with HR−, HER2+ cancers. For HR+, HER2− tumors, a majority of relapses for patients given adjuvant endocrine therapy are seen years after initial diagnosis, with a continued hazard for relapse of 1% to 2% per year after 5 years, and a vast majority of cancer deaths in this group are seen well after 5 years.[31] Conversely, a majority of patients with TNBC or HR−, HER2+ breast cancers relapse much earlier (generally within 5 years), with cancer deaths occurring earlier as well. This difference in clinical course, based solely on HR phenotype, has profound treatment implications, particularly for older patients with short estimated survival times.

Endocrine therapy is the linchpin of adjuvant treatment of older women with HR+, HER2− breast cancer. The major challenge in older patients with HR+, HER2− breast cancer is determining who would potentially benefit from chemotherapy. The addition of chemotherapy to endocrine therapy improves survival in some women with HR+ early-stage breast cancer but for the majority, chemotherapy provides modest or no survival benefit.[32] Unfortunately the data on chemotherapy are sparse for patients 70 years and older and the likely benefits of chemotherapy can vary greatly depending on the biologic characteristics the tumor.[33] Older patients with HR+, node-negative, 1 to 3 node-positive tumors, and a life expectancy less than 10 years are excellent candidates for endocrine therapy. Few of these patients will benefit from chemotherapy and treatment can cause substantial toxicity, including potential loss of function and diminished quality of life that are unacceptable. (See **Fig. 2** for a general algorithm to the approach of an older patient with HR+, HER2− breast cancer based on life expectancy.) Only after estimating non–breast cancer–related life expectancy can the potential benefits of chemotherapy be determined. For patients with T1 and T2 node-negative, HR+ tumors who receive adjuvant endocrine therapy, the added value of chemotherapy can be estimated by the Oncotype DX assay (Genomic Health, Redwood City, California).[34] Recent data from this assay suggest that the primary benefit of chemotherapy in this patient group is in those with high recurrence scores, with minimal value among patients with low recurrence scores, including women with 1 to 3 positive nodes.[35] The authors suggest that patients with intermediate recurrence scores also be evaluated using Adjuvant! Online to estimate the added value of chemotherapy in reducing breast cancer mortality.[12] The value of chemotherapy in patients with T1 and T2 node-negative lesions with a low-intermediate recurrence score

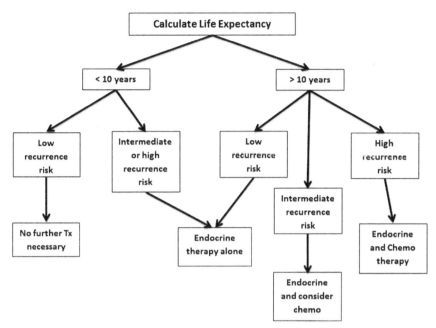

Fig. 2. General algorithm to the approach to older patients with HR+, HER2− breast cancer based on life expectancy when determining adjuvant therapy treatment. Other important factors when considering adjuvant treatment include patient goals, quality of life, comorbidities, and social support system.

is also being evaluated in a randomized clinical trial (Trial Assigning Individualized Options for Treatment [Rx]); clinicaltrials.gov identifier NCT00310180). The trial is closed to accrual, and the results are expected in 2015. A similar trial is ongoing in women with 1 to 3 positive lymph nodes.

TNBC and HER2+ breast cancers are each seen in approximately 15% of older patients.[30] For TNBC, chemotherapy is the only systemic therapy of benefit and should be considered for most fit older patients. HER2+ cancers that are HR−, the most ominous phenotype when untreated, have a better outcome than TNBC since the advent of chemotherapy and trastuzumab (Herceptin). For those patients with small HR+, HER2+ (triple-positive) lesions, who have a better short-term prognosis than those with HR−, HER2+ tumors, the decision regarding the use of chemotherapy and trastuzumab must be individualized, especially in less fit patients.[36]

Adjuvant Endocrine Therapy

Randomized trials in patients older than 70 years with HR+ tumors have shown that adjuvant tamoxifen reduces the annual risk of recurrence of breast cancer by approximately half and the annual odds of dying from breast cancer by 37%, irrespective of nodal status.[32] The absolute benefit can vary greatly, however, and is small for patients with cancers that have a low risk of recurrence. Tamoxifen is generally well tolerated in older patients and is available at a low cost. Tamoxifen can also maintain or improve bone density and lower cholesterol levels in postmenopausal women. There is, however, an approximately 1% risk of endometrial cancer and venous thrombosis associated with 5 years of use. In older patients, the requirement for a pelvic examination and Papanicolaou smear yearly can be an obstacle.

Many large clinical trials have been performed that compared tamoxifen to aromatase inhibitors (AIs) and a small improvement in relapse-free survival of a few percentage points has been shown with the use of AIs; however, there is no convincing improvement in overall survival. Updated American Society of Clinical Oncology guidelines for use of endocrine therapy are available.[37] Although there are many strategies regarding endocrine therapy, the initiation of tamoxifen and then changing to an AI 2 to 3 years later has been shown to improve survival by approximately a percentage point and may represent the best strategy.[37] Until recently, AIs were expensive, but their cost has significantly dropped since going off patent. American Society of Clinical Oncology guidelines have recommended that AIs be considered for use in all postmenopausal patients at some time during their endocrine treatment. AIs, although not associated with an increased risk of endometrial cancer or thromboembolism, can cause severe arthralgia and myalgia that can impede function, although the toxicity of AIs seems less in elders.[38] Changing to another AI can be helpful in some patients experiencing these symptoms, but, if symptoms persist, switching to tamoxifen is probably the best strategy.

AI therapy is associated with accelerated bone loss and an increased risk of fracture. Many older patients already have baseline osteopenia or osteoporosis at diagnosis, and these patients are particularly at risk from further bone loss. Older adults on AI therapy should be encouraged to exercise regularly as well as take the recommended daily doses of vitamin D and calcium. For patients with osteoporosis, treatment with either bisphosphonates or other bone-protecting agents, such as denosumab, should be considered. The World Health Organization fracture risk assessment tool, FRAX, can be used to estimate fracture risk from clinical and bone densitometry data (www.shef.ac.uk/FRAX) that can assist in decision making.

Nonadherence to medications can occur for a variety of reasons and older adults are particularly susceptible. Many are prescribed several medications for treatment of comorbidities, making for complicated medication regimens and polypharmacy.[39] Other factors related to adherence include cognitive, visual, and physical impairments. In a recent systematic review of adherence to adjuvant hormonal therapy among breast cancer survivors, adherence ranged from 41% to 72% and discontinuation ranged from 31% to 73%, with older age a risk factor for nonadherence.[40] Although the best way to improve medication adherence is unclear, educating older patients and their families about the value of treatment and possible side effects is important. Many family members and other caregivers play a vital role in assisting patients with their medications.[41] Patients should also be queried on each clinic visit as to the medications they are taking and specifically asked about their adherence to their prescribed endocrine treatment.

Adjuvant Chemotherapy

The decision to recommend chemotherapy to an older patient is complicated. The decision requires consideration of the effect of treatment on improving survival as well as balancing potential toxicity that may result in loss of function or reduced quality of life. To further complicate the decision, the social (increased need for family support) and financial costs of treatment must also be considered. Like endocrine therapy, chemotherapy results in similar proportional reductions in recurrence and survival, irrespective of nodal status. Once the decision to recommend chemotherapy is made, a second difficult decision for the medical oncologist is which chemotherapy regimen to recommend.

Adjuvant! Online is a useful tool to use when making treatment selections because it directly compares survival outcomes for different chemotherapy regimens. It categorizes regimens as to first, second, and third (the most aggressive) regimens for defining treatment benefit (**Table 3**). Older first-generation chemotherapy regimens, such as cyclophosphamide, methotrexate, and fluorouracil and doxorubicin and cyclophosphamide (AC), have been supplanted by newer, more-effective second-generation and third-generation treatments.[42] The second-generation regimen of 4 cycles of docetaxel cyclophosphamide (TC) is superior to 4 cycles of AC[43] and has been tested in large numbers of older patients and is generally well tolerated.[44] Estimates of effectiveness of second-generation and third-generation chemotherapy regimens by Adjuvant! Online for older patients have not been validated in clinical trials and it is possible that the value of such regimens is overestimated in older patients. For fit patients who are at a high risk of relapse, treatment with third-generation regimens improves survival by a few percentage points compared with first-generation or second-generation regimens. For patients who are not at high risk of relapse, the authors suggest consideration of second-generation regimens, such as TC, to avoid potential anthracycline cardiac and hematologic (myelodysplasia and acute leukemia) toxicity.[44] For those at high-risk, a third generation regimen should be considered if estimates suggest an improvement of a few percent or more in 5-year survival. These third-generation, anthracycline-containing regimens should generally be reserved for patients who are highly functional with minimal comorbidity. A large retrospective study of node-positive patients in randomized trials compared less-intense with more-intense chemotherapy and showed that treatment with more-intensive regimens in both older and younger patients resulted in a similar proportional improvement in relapse and survival rates.[45]

The potential toxicity related to chemotherapy treatment is a major concern of older patients and there is a paucity of clinical trial data on how treatment-related toxicity affects function in older women. Third-generation regimens, such as dose-dense AC and paclitaxel, AC followed by docetaxel, and TAC, are all associated with considerable toxicity, such as nausea, fatigue, and neutropenia. Concerns regarding toxicity should not, however, preclude providing adequate treatment dosing; arbitrary dose modifications of trial-defined dosages should be avoided because they can be associated with poorer outcomes.[46]

Adjuvant Anti-HER2–Directed Therapy

The HER2 protein is a unique and useful target for drug therapy and is overexpressed in 15% to 25% of all breast cancer patients,[47] although less frequently with increasing age.[48] Patients with HER2+ tumors obtain the greatest benefit from a combination of

Table 3
Commonly used adjuvant chemotherapy regimens for breast cancer.

1st Generation	CMF	Cyclophosphamide, methotrexate, fluorouracil
	AC (Adriamycin with Doxorubicin)	Doxorubicin, cyclophosphamide for 4 cycles
2nd Generation	TC	Docetaxel, cyclophosphamide
	FEC	Fluorouracil, epirubicin, cyclophosphamide
	FAC	Fluorouracil, adriamycin, cyclophosphamide
3rd Generation	AC followed by a taxane	Every 2-wk (dose dense) or 3-wk AC followed by paclitaxel (dose dense or weekly) or docetaxel (every 3 wk)
	TAC	Docetaxel, doxorubicin, cyclophosphamide

First-generation, second-generation, and third-generation regimens are defined per Adjuvant! Online (www.adjuvantonline.com).

chemotherapy and trastuzumab. Because cardiac toxicity is the major side effect of trastuzumab and the prevalence of cardiac disease increases with age, older patients are at increased risk for cardiac toxicity and require careful monitoring.[49] Measurements of left ventricular ejection fraction prior to therapy and every several months during treatment should be the norm. Combination trastuzumab regimens, such as docetaxel, carboplatin, and trastuzumab, are similar in efficacy as trastuzumab and anthracycline–containing chemotherapy, are associated with less cardiac toxicity,[50] and should be strongly considered for older patients. Although not yet confirmed in the clinical trial setting, trastuzumab alone may be considered for older frail patients with high-risk HER2+ tumors that are at significant risk of toxicity from chemotherapy. Currently Adjuvant! Online cannot directly calculate the added value of including trastuzumab with chemotherapy in patients with HER2+ tumors, but the added value of trastuzumab can probably be fairly estimated by multiplying the chemotherapy percentage in the "Adjuvant Therapy Effectiveness" box by 1.5 (based on a hazard ratio of approximately 0.5 for chemotherapy plus trastuzumab compared with chemotherapy alone). PREDICT is another an online tool for breast cancer prognostication that incorporates the added value of trastuzumab to chemotherapy in patients with HER2+ tumors; it can help in estimating the potential value of chemotherapy and trastuzumab in older patients (www.predict.nhs.uk).[51]

Radiation Therapy in Early-Stage Invasive Breast Cancer

For elderly patients with early-stage invasive breast cancer, there are randomized trials comparing tamoxifen (20 mg daily) with or without breast radiation therapy (RT) after breast conservation surgery. One randomized trial included 769 patients (age ≥50) with surgically resected T1 or T2 invasive cancers, negative margins, and pathologically negative axillary lymph nodes (except in patients 65 and older who were eligible if pathologically or clinically node negative).[52] Whole-breast irradiation was given in a hypofractionated regimen of 40 Gy (16 fractions) followed by a boost of 12.5 Gy (5 fractions) to the lumpectomy site. The 5-year local relapse rate was 0.6% in the RT plus tamoxifen group and 7.7% for those receiving tamoxifen alone (P <.05). There were no differences in distant relapse rates or overall survival, but such differences would not be expected with the short follow-up of this favorable group. A second randomized trial (Cancer and Leukemia Group B 9343) included 636 women 70 years and older with lumpectomy-treated T1, HR+, clinically or pathologically node-negative tumors. All patients received tamoxifen and were randomized to radiation or no radiation.[53] After a median follow-up of 10.5 years, the incidence of locoregional recurrence was 2% in the tamoxifen and RT group compared with 9% in the tamoxifen-alone group.[54] Breast cancer–specific survival was 98% for the tamoxifen alone group and 96% for the tamoxifen/RT group, and, although all-cause mortality was 43%, the vast majority of deaths was due to non–breast cancer causes.

The EBCTG meta-analysis compared approximately 11,000 patients with early-stage breast cancer randomized to postoperative radiation or not.[55] The RT treated group had an overall 16% absolute decrease (19% vs 35%) in the risk of breast cancer recurrence and a 4% absolute decrease (21% vs 25%) in the risk of dying from breast cancer—clearly showing good local control correlates with improved survival. This analysis stratified women by age, and although the benefit was less in those 70 and older, there was still an absolute overall reduction in the 10-year risk of a locoregional or distant recurrence of 8.9% (95% CI, 4.0%–13.8%). Given the large number of patients in this meta-analysis, data could be analyzed by age, tumor grade, receptor status, and tamoxifen use. The detailed characteristics for patients 70 and older under consideration for use or omission of radiation are summarized in **Table 4**.[55] The

Table 4
Risk of any breast cancer recurrence at 10 years for patients in randomized trials of radiation versus not and/or tamoxifen versus not

		10-Y Risk of Any Recurrence (%)		
		Grade 1	Grade 2	Grade 3
	Patient Characteristics	No RT vs RT	No RT vs RT	No RT vs RT
T1	ER positive	27 vs 15	41 vs 23	59 vs 21
	No tamoxifen			
	ER positive with tamoxifen	10 vs 5	16 vs 7	27 vs 7
	ER negative	23 vs 19	31 vs 28	40 vs 27
T2	ER positive	39 vs 24	57 vs 34	75 vs 32
	No tamoxifen			
	ER positive with tamoxifen	15 vs 7	24 vs 11	38 vs 10
	ER negative	34 vs 29	49 vs 41	56 vs 39

Modified from Darby S, McGale P, Correa C, et al. Effect of radiotherapy after breast-conserving surgery on 10-year recurrence and 15-year breast cancer death: meta-analysis of individual patient data for 10,801 women in 17 randomised trials. Lancet 2011;378(9804):1707–16.

data were reported as absolute 10-year risk (%) of any recurrence, locoregional or distant.

Based on these data, there are several potential treatment strategies. For those patients with ER-negative tumors, use of adjuvant radiation and chemotherapy for patients 70 years and older and in overall good health should be considered. Molecular profiling may provide additional useful data to guide systemic decisions.[56] For those patients with ER-positive tumors who are candidates for tamoxifen (and where compliance with therapy is mandatory), radiation might be deferred. For those patients with T1 tumors who are ER positive and who take tamoxifen, the recurrence rate approximately triples without radiation between the grade 1 (10% 10-year recurrence) and grade 3 subgroups (27% 10-year recurrence). Although a majority of elderly patients with receptor-positive tumors have lower-grade histology, for those with high-grade tumors, data from the EBCTG support the addition of adjuvant radiation irrespective of tumor size. When radiation was added to the T1 grade 3 patients who took tamoxifen, the 10-year recurrence dropped from 27% to 7%, suggesting to a large proportion of patients where local recurrence was prevented with the addition of adjuvant radiation.

When adjuvant radiation is given, there are different options for fractionation schedules (ie, standard vs hypofractionated)[57,58] and treatment volume (ie, whole breast vs accelerated partial breast).[59] Although the detailed nuances of radiation planning are beyond the scope of this review, there are expert consensus statements that provide a solid framework for clinical decision making.[58,59]

METASTATIC BREAST CANCER
Goals of Treatment

A majority of patients with metastatic disease develop metastases months to years after their initial diagnosis and treatment. Approximately 5% of new breast cancer patients present with metastases at time of diagnosis.[60] Because metastatic breast cancer (irrespective of age) is not curable, the main treatment goals are to maintain quality of life, prolong survival, and minimize symptoms.[61] Because the treatment is primarily palliative, significant toxicity should be avoided. (See **Fig. 3** for a suggested

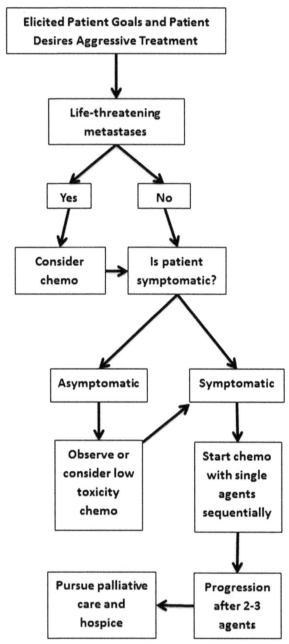

Fig. 3. Algorithm outlining the treatment of older patients with metastatic breast cancer refractory to endocrine therapy or with TNBC.

treatment algorithm for older patients with HR refractory or HR− metastatic breast cancer.)

The breast cancer phenotype can often predict the likely site of metastases and the tempo of progression. For example, patients with HR+ tumors are more likely to develop bone metastases and have a longer clinical course.[30] Conversely, patients with TNBC are more likely to lung metastases and have a shorter clinical course.[62] Additional complexity occurs in up to 30% of patients when the phenotype of the malignant cells in the metastatic sites differs from the initial phenotype.[63] This observation has led to increased use of biopsy of metastatic sites to determine if there have been any changes to the HR or HER2 status that can significantly affect treatment selection.

Radiation Therapy

RT is used to palliate localized, symptomatic sites of metastatic breast cancer. Timing of treatment is best coordinated with multidisciplinary care providers, and the overall approach is highly individualized. The location of the metastatic site, disease-free interval, tempo of progression, extent of symptoms, and patient performance status are all important considerations.

Endocrine Therapy in Metastatic Disease

Endocrine treatment should be the treatment of choice for women with HR+ tumors (ie, the ER and/or progesterone receptor is positive) who do not have life-threatening metastases.[61] Most patients with HR+ metastatic tumors should be treated with endocrine therapy until disease progression and when it is clear that the tumor is refractory to further endocrine treatment. Significant treatment benefits have been shown in older patients with endocrine therapy.[64] There is no optimal sequence of agents. For those patients who develop metastasis while taking an AI or tamoxifen in the adjuvant setting, initial endocrine therapy should consist of the alternate agent. Endocrine therapies are generally used sequentially and continued until metastases progress. Patients may be retreated with previously used endocrine agents and may respond again, as long as it has been more than a year or prior to tumor progression.[61] Patients with slow-growing tumors refractory to AI or tamoxifen can be further treated with fulvestrant, progestins (megestrol acetate, among others), estradiol, and even glucocorticoids. Using endocrine therapy until metastases are convincingly refractory to hormonal treatment allows for a delay in chemotherapy initiation and maintenance of the highest quality of life with minimal treatment-related toxicity.

Chemotherapy in Metastatic Disease

For older patients with metastatic breast cancer, the use of chemotherapy should be considered with the possible exception of frail patients. Chemotherapy is generally the only treatment available for women with tumors that are HR− or endocrine refractory. The risk of toxicity is higher with chemotherapy compared with endocrine therapy and can result in decreased function and quality of life. Palliative measures without chemotherapy may be a reasonable choice for elderly, unfit patients who are asymptomatic and/or have a low burden of disease.[65] Fit women older than 70 years of age, however, have response rates, duration of response, and overall survival rates with chemotherapy similar to their younger counterparts.[66]

The specific choice of a particular chemotherapy depends on several factors, including individual patient characteristics, physician and patient preferences, and drug availability.[61] Sequential treatment with single agents is generally preferred for older cancer patients, given the potential reduction in the risk of toxicity. There is no optimal sequence of single chemotherapy agents and starting with the least toxic agent first is a good strategy. Single-agent treatments used as first-line treatments are associated with response rates of approximately 20% to 60%. Subsequent therapies tend to only be approximately half as effective as the previous treatment, although exceptions are common. Initial responses typically last for approximately 6 months, but some patients may have prolonged periods of tumor stability. Although combination chemotherapy improves response rates and time to progression compared with single agents, there is no convincing improvement in overall survival and combination regimens usually cause greater toxicity.[67] In certain circumstances that require urgent reduction in tumor disease, combination therapy is reasonable.

Anti-HER2 Therapy

For patients with HER2 overexpressing metastatic breast cancer, the addition of tras-tuzumab to first-line chemotherapy has improved survival compared with chemo-therapy alone.[68] Elderly patients have been shown to tolerate trastuzumab, but careful management is necessary. There is an increased risk of trastuzumab-induced heart failure with increasing age.[49] Patients with a history of cardiac disease and diabetes seem at the highest risk for developing cardiotoxicity, and the increased risk may be more related to the prevalence of comorbidities than to age alone.[69] Lapa-tinib, another anti-HER2–directed small molecule, can also increase response rates and duration of response when added to chemotherapy.[70] The recent approval of trastuzumab-emtansine[71] represents a novel monotherapy option for older patients with HER2+ metastases and is likely better tolerated than combinations of standard chemotherapy agents and anti-HER2 agents.

Bone Metastases

Regardless of age, patients with lytic bone metastasis should be treated with bone resorption inhibitory drugs (eg, bisphosphonates or denosumab).[72] Although antire-sorptive therapies are generally well tolerated, there have been reports of serious adverse events, such as hypocalcemia and osteonecrosis of the jaw. Recent studies have shown that denosumab (a specific inhibitor of receptor activator of nuclear factor κ (RANK) ligand) is superior to bisphosphonates in delaying or preventing skeletal-related events in patients with breast cancer metastatic to bone.[73] For older women with painful bone metastases refractory to systemic therapies, radiopharma-ceuticals may provide meaningful palliation.[74]

PALLIATIVE CARE AND HOSPICE

Studies have shown that hospice and palliative care interventions are associated with improved quality of life and even a potential increase in survival in some cancer pa-tients.[75] Palliative care has traditionally been delivered late in the course of disease, but recent data have shown a structured palliative care program integrated early can lead to improved quality of life and survival in patients with metastatic cancer, including patients receiving chemotherapy.[75] Hospice care should be considered for patients when further cancer-directed therapy is considered ineffective. Hospice enrollment early may also improve survival and leads to improved support for patients and families.[76]

CLINICAL TRIALS

In spite of increased interest, there remains a need for clinical trials in older patients with breast cancer. Although age bias remains a major barrier in offering clinical trials to older patients, older and younger patients when offered trials have similar rates of participation.[77] Other barriers to accrual include (1) identifying older patients for tri-als, (2) physician-related barriers, (3) nursing and staff–related barriers, (4) patient-related barriers, and (5) trial-related barriers. Identifying patients for trials is a major challenge and success requires strong collaborative relationship with primary care physicians interested in elder care, including educating primary care colleagues on trial availability, treatment regimens, and potential toxicities. In the current clinic environment, irrespective of whether an academic or community setting, remembering to offer a trial to an older patient is a major challenge. Developing a reminder system for identifying patients for potential trials should be considered and optimally should include training of office staff who can screen patients and then remind physicians of available studies. Nursing and office staff, if properly educated on the importance and rationale of trials, can be a major source of recruitment.[78] Physician-related barriers remain a major challenge and, in one study, physicians thought that the 3 most cost-effective ways to increase accrual are to (1) have more personnel in clinic to explain trials to patients, (2) to have more physician education about toxicity issues, and (3) to provide transportation for older patients.[79] It is always tempting to add clinical trials responsibilities to those of busy office staff, but this is unlikely to work in the long term and adequate funding is mandatory for supporting trial commitments.

Patient-related barriers remain a major challenge. As a group, older patients are not as well educated as younger patients and require additional time for explaining the trial and obtaining consent. Healthy older patients offered trials should be reassured that they are likely to tolerate surgery, RT, and chemotherapy similar to younger patients.[80–83] Also, addressing logistics with elders and their caregivers is essential when discussing trials because many elders need help with transportation and trial logistics. Restrictive eligibility criteria, excessive testing, complex treatment regimens, and cost remain main obstacles. A study from the National Cancer Institute of cooperative group trials estimated that elderly participation would have increased by 30% if eligibility exclusions were relaxed.[84] Only organ dysfunction that may compromise safety should exclude participation. Trials are desperately needed for vulnerable and frail patients. There is also a great need to test the safety of newer agents in an adequate sample of older patients. Lastly, there remains a pressing need to test the effect of commonly used regimens in older patients using quality of life and changes in function as major endpoints.

SUMMARY

Caring for older women with breast cancer remains a challenge. As a group, older women have not shared equally in the successes due to improved treatment of early breast cancer and frequently continue to be undertreated due to age bias and lack of geriatric training of oncologists. Tools now exist to help physicians make better treatment decisions based on accurate estimations of longevity as well as potential toxicities. Such tools can prevent overtreatment, with an associated negative therapeutic index, as well as identify elders who should receive state-of-the-art treatment. Patient goals for treatment should synergize with the recommendations of the oncology team, and caregivers must be intimately involved in all aspects of care. Improving clinical trial accrual of older women with breast cancer must remain a national priority, and trials for vulnerable and frail patients should be developed. Older women with metastatic breast cancer should be managed with a focus on controlling symptoms and maintaining the highest quality of life, and oncologists should enlist the help of their palliative care colleagues to optimize management. A team approach that includes oncologists, geriatricians and primary care physicians, pharmacists, social workers, and other support staff is the ideal model for providing the best care for the elderly patients with breast cancer.

REFERENCES

1. Howlader N, Noone AM, Krapcho M, et al. SEER cancer statistics review, 1975-2008. Bethesda (MD): National Cancer Institute; 2011.
2. Siegel R, Naishadham D, Jemal A. Cancer statistics, 2012. CA Cancer J Clin 2012;62(1):10–29.
3. Siegel R, Naishadham D, Jemal A. Cancer statistics, 2013. CA Cancer J Clin 2013;63(1):11–30.
4. Bouchardy C, Rapiti E, Fioretta G, et al. Undertreatment strongly decreases prognosis of breast cancer in elderly women. J Clin Oncol 2003;21(19):3580–7.
5. Smith BD, Jiang J, McLaughlin SS, et al. Improvement in breast cancer outcomes over time: are older women missing out? J Clin Oncol 2011;29: 4647–53 Eng.
6. Owusu C, Lash TL, Silliman RA. Effect of undertreatment on the disparity in age-related breast cancer-specific survival among older women. Breast Cancer Res Treat 2007;102(2):227–36.
7. Biganzoli L, Wildiers H, Oakman C, et al. Management of elderly patients with breast cancer: updated recommendations of the International Society of Geriatric Oncology (SIOG) and European Society of Breast Cancer Specialists (EUSOMA). Lancet Oncol 2012;13(4):e148–60.
8. Jones EL, Leak A, Muss HB. Adjuvant therapy of breast cancer in women 70 years of age and older: tough decisions, high stakes. Oncology (Williston Park) 2012;26(9):793–801.
9. Fried TR, Bradley EH, Towle VR, et al. Understanding the treatment preferences of seriously ill patients. N Engl J Med 2002;346(14):1061–6.
10. Lee S, Smith AK, Widera EW, et al. ePrognosis. 2012. Available at: http://www.eprognosis.org. Accessed February 12, 2013.
11. Yourman LC, Lee SJ, Schonberg MA, et al. Prognostic indices for older adults: a systematic review. JAMA 2012;307(2):182–92.
12. Ravdin PM, Siminoff LA, Davis GJ, et al. Computer program to assist in making decisions about adjuvant therapy for women with early breast cancer. J Clin Oncol 2001;19(4):980–91.
13. Schairer C, Mink PJ, Carroll L, et al. Probabilities of death from breast cancer and other causes among female breast cancer patients. J Natl Cancer Inst 2004;96(17):1311–21.
14. Repetto L, Fratino L, Audisio RA, et al. Comprehensive geriatric assessment adds information to Eastern Cooperative Oncology Group performance status in elderly cancer patients: an Italian Group for Geriatric Oncology Study. J Clin Oncol 2002;20(2):494–502.
15. Owusu C, Koroukian SM, Schluchter M, et al. Screening older cancer patients for a Comprehensive Geriatric Assessment: a comparison of three instruments. J Geriatr Oncol 2011;2:121–9.
16. Extermann M, Hurria A. Comprehensive geriatric assessment for older patients with cancer. J Clin Oncol 2007;25(14):1824–31.
17. Extermann M, Aapro M, Bernabei R, et al. Use of comprehensive geriatric assessment in older cancer patients: recommendations from the task force on CGA of the International Society of Geriatric Oncology (SIOG). Crit Rev Oncol Hematol 2005;55(3):241–52.
18. Soubeyran P, Bellera C, Goyard J, et al. Validation of the G8 screening tool in geriatric oncology: the ONCODAGE project. J Clin Oncol 2011;29(15S): 550S.

19. Mohile SG, Bylow K, Dale W, et al. A pilot study of the vulnerable elders survey-13 compared with the comprehensive geriatric assessment for identifying disability in older patients with prostate cancer who receive androgen ablation. Cancer 2007;109(4):802–10.

20. Luciani A, Ascione G, Bertuzzi C, et al. Detecting disabilities in older patients with cancer: comparison between comprehensive geriatric assessment and vulnerable elders survey-13. J Clin Oncol 2010;28(12):2046–50.

21. Kenis C, Schuermans H, Van Custem E, et al. Screening for a geriatric risk profile in older cancer patients: a comparative study of the predictive validity of three screening tools. Crit Rev Oncol Hematol 2009;72(Suppl):22.

22. Hurria A, Cirrincione CT, Muss HB, et al. Implementing a geriatric assessment in cooperative group clinical cancer trials: CALGB 360401. J Clin Oncol 2011; 29(10):1290–6.

23. Mohile SG, Fan L, Reeve E, et al. Association of cancer with geriatric syndromes in older Medicare beneficiaries. J Clin Oncol 2011;29(11):1458–64.

24. Extermann M, Boler I, Reich RR, et al. Predicting the risk of chemotherapy toxicity in older patients: the Chemotherapy Risk Assessment Scale for High-Age Patients (CRASH) score. Cancer 2012;118(13):3377–86.

25. Hurria A, Togawa K, Mohile SG, et al. Predicting chemotherapy toxicity in older adults with cancer: a Prospective Multicenter Study. J Clin Oncol 2011;29(25): 3457–65.

26. Correa C, McGale P, Taylor C, et al. Overview of the randomized trials of radiotherapy in ductal carcinoma in situ of the breast. J Natl Cancer Inst Monographs 2010;2010(41):162–77.

27. Wong JS, Kaelin CM, Troyan SL, et al. Prospective study of wide excision alone for ductal carcinoma in situ of the breast. J Clin Oncol 2006;24(7):1031–6.

28. Hughes LL, Wang M, Page DL, et al. Local excision alone without irradiation for ductal carcinoma in situ of the breast: a trial of the Eastern Cooperative Oncology Group. J Clin Oncol 2009;27(32):5319–24.

29. McCormick B. RTOG 9804: a prospective randomized trial for "good risk" ductal carcinoma in situ (DCIS), comparing radiation (RT) to observation (OBS). Chicago (IL): 2012 ASCO Annual Meeting. J Clin Oncol 2012;30(suppl):p. abstract 1004.

30. Blows FM, Driver KE, Schmidt MK, et al. Subtyping of breast cancer by immunohistochemistry to investigate a relationship between subtype and short and long term survival: a collaborative analysis of data for 10,159 cases from 12 studies. PLoS Med 2010;7(5):e1000279.

31. Saphner T, Tormey DC, Gray R. Annual hazard rates of recurrence for breast cancer after primary therapy. J Clin Oncol 1996;14(10):2738–46.

32. Abe O, Abe R, Enomoto K, et al. Effects of chemotherapy and hormonal therapy for early breast cancer on recurrence and 15-year survival: an overview of the randomised trials. Lancet 2005;365(9472):1687–717.

33. Coates AS, Colleoni M, Goldhirsch A. Is adjuvant chemotherapy useful for women with luminal a breast cancer? J Clin Oncol 2012;30(12):1260–3.

34. Paik S, Tang G, Shak S, et al. Gene expression and benefit of chemotherapy in women with node-negative, estrogen receptor-positive breast cancer. J Clin Oncol 2006;24(23):3726–34.

35. Dowsett M, Cuzick J, Wale C, et al. Prediction of risk of distant recurrence using the 21-gene recurrence score in node-negative and node-positive postmenopausal patients with breast cancer treated with anastrozole or tamoxifen: a TransATAC study. J Clin Oncol 2010;28(11):1829–34.

36. Chia S, Norris B, Speers C, et al. Human epidermal growth factor receptor 2 overexpression as a prognostic factor in a large tissue microarray series of node-negative breast cancers. J Clin Oncol 2008;26(35):5697–704.

37. Burstein HJ, Prestrud AA, Seidenfeld J, et al. American Society of Clinical Oncology clinical practice guideline: update on adjuvant endocrine therapy for women with hormone receptor-positive breast cancer. J Clin Oncol 2010; 28(23):3784–96.

38. Muss HB, Tu D, Ingle JN, et al. Efficacy, toxicity, and quality of life in older women with early-stage breast cancer treated with letrozole or placebo after 5 years of tamoxifen: NCIC CTG intergroup trial MA.17. J Clin Oncol 2008; 26(12):1956–64.

39. Maggiore RJ, Gross CP, Hurria A. Polypharmacy in older adults with cancer. Oncologist 2010;15(5):507–22.

40. Murphy CC, Bartholomew LK, Carpentier MY, et al. Adherence to adjuvant hormonal therapy among breast cancer survivors in clinical practice: a systematic review. Breast Cancer Res Treat 2012;134(2):459–78.

41. Miaskowski C, Shockney L, Chelbowski RT. Adherence to oral endocrine therapy for breast cancer: a nursing perspective. Clin J Oncol Nurs 2008;12(2): 213–21.

42. Albain K, Anderson S, Arriagada R, et al. Comparisons between different polychemotherapy regimens for early breast cancer: meta-analyses of long-term outcome among 100 000 women in 123 randomised trials. Lancet 2012; 379(9814):432–44.

43. Jones S, Holmes FA, O'Shaughnessy J, et al. Docetaxel with cyclophosphamide is associated with an overall survival benefit compared with doxorubicin and cyclophosphamide: 7-year follow-up of US oncology research trial 9735. J Clin Oncol 2009;27(8):1177–83.

44. Freyer G, Campone M, Peron J, et al. Adjuvant docetaxel/cyclophosphamide in breast cancer patients over the age of 70: results of an observational study. Crit Rev Oncol Hematol 2011;80(3):466–73.

45. Muss HB, Woolf S, Berry D, et al. Adjuvant chemotherapy in older and younger women with lymph node-positive breast cancer. JAMA 2005;293(9): 1073–81.

46. Lyman GH. Impact of chemotherapy dose intensity on cancer patient outcomes. J Natl Compr Canc Netw 2009;7(1):99–108.

47. Slamon DJ, Clark GM, Wong SG, et al. Human breast cancer: correlation of relapse and survival with amplification of the HER-2/neu oncogene. Science 1987;235(4785):177–82.

48. Diab SG, Elledge RM, Clark GM. Tumor characteristics and clinical outcome of elderly women with breast cancer. J Natl Cancer Inst 2000;92(7):550–6.

49. Sawaki M, Mukai H, Tokudome N, et al. Safety of adjuvant trastuzumab for HER-2-overexpressing elderly breast cancer patients: a multicenter cohort study. Breast Cancer 2012;19(3):253–8.

50. Slamon D, Eiermann W, Robert N, et al. Adjuvant Trastuzumab in HER2-Positive Breast Cancer. N Engl J Med 2011;365(14):1273–83.

51. Wishart GC, Bajdik CD, Dicks E, et al. PREDICT Plus: development and validation of a prognostic model for early breast cancer that includes HER2. Br J Cancer 2012;107(5):800–7.

52. Fyles AW, McCready DR, Manchul LA, et al. Tamoxifen with or without breast irradiation in women 50 years of age or older with early breast cancer. N Engl J Med 2004;351(10):963–70.

53. Hughes KS, Schnaper LA, Berry D, et al. Lumpectomy plus tamoxifen with or without irradiation in women 70 years of age or older with early breast cancer. N Engl J Med 2004;351(10):971–7.

54. Hughes KS, Schnaper LA, Cirrincione C, et al. Lumpectomy plus tamoxifen with or without irradiation in women age 70 or older with early breast cancer. ASCO Meeting Abstracts. J Clin Oncol 2010;28(Suppl 15):abstract 507.

55. Darby S, McGale P, Correa C, et al. Effect of radiotherapy after breast-conserving surgery on 10-year recurrence and 15-year breast cancer death: meta-analysis of individual patient data for 10,801 women in 17 randomised trials. Lancet 2011;378(9804):1707–16.

56. Gokmen-Polar Y, Badve S. Molecular profiling assays in breast cancer: are we ready for prime time? Oncology 2012;26(4):350–7.

57. Whelan TJ, Pignol JP, Levine MN, et al. Long-term results of hypofractionated radiation therapy for breast cancer. N Engl J Med 2010;362(6):513–20.

58. Smith BD, Bentzen SM, Correa CR, et al. Fractionation for whole breast irradiation: an American Society for Radiation Oncology (ASTRO) evidence-based guideline. Int J Radiat Oncol Biol Phys 2011;81(1):59–68.

59. Smith BD, Arthur DW, Buchholz TA, et al. Accelerated partial breast irradiation consensus statement from the American Society for Radiation Oncology (ASTRO). Int J Radiat Oncol Biol Phys 2009;74(4):987–1001.

60. Anonymous Statement of the American Society of Human Genetics on genetic testing for breast and ovarian cancer predisposition. Am J Hum Genet 1994; 55:i–iv.

61. Wildiers H, Kunkler I, Biganzoli L, et al. Management of breast cancer in elderly individuals: recommendations of the International Society of Geriatric Oncology. Lancet Oncol 2007;8(12):1101–15.

62. Foulkes WD, Smith IE, Reis JS. Triple-negative breast cancer. N Engl J Med 2010;363(20):1938–48.

63. Chia S. Testing for discordance at metastatic relapse: does it matter? J Clin Oncol 2012;30(6):575–6.

64. Mouridsen H, Chaudri-Ross HA. Efficacy of first-line letrozole versus tamoxifen as a function of age in postmenopausal women with advanced breast cancer. Oncologist 2004;9(5):497–506.

65. Aapro M, Monfardini S, Jirillo A, et al. Management of primary and advanced breast cancer in older unfit patients (medical treatment). Cancer Treat Rev 2009;35(6):503–8.

66. Christman K, Muss HB, Case LD, et al. Chemotherapy of metastatic breast cancer in the elderly. The Piedmont Oncology Association experience. JAMA 1992; 268(1):57–62 [see comment].

67. Miles D, von Minckwitz G, Seidman AD. Combination versus sequential single-agent therapy in metastatic breast cancer. Oncologist 2002;7(Suppl 6):13–9.

68. Slamon DJ, Leyland-Jones B, Shak S, et al. Use of chemotherapy plus a monoclonal antibody against HER2 for metastatic breast cancer that overexpresses HER2. N Engl J Med 2001;344(11):783–92.

69. Gregor M, Zhang N, Niu J, et al. Trastuzumab-related cardiotoxicity among older breast cancer patients. ASCO Meeting Abstract. J Clin Oncol 2012;30(suppl 27): abstract 135.

70. Geyer CE, Forster J, Lindquist D, et al. Lapatinib plus capecitabine for HER2-positive advanced breast cancer. N Engl J Med 2006;355(26):2733–43.

71. Verma S, Miles D, Gianni L, et al. Trastuzumab emtansine for HER2-positive advanced breast cancer. N Engl J Med 2012;367(19):1783–91.

72. Hadji P, Aapro M, Costa L, et al. Antiresorptive treatment options and bone health in cancer patients-safety profiles and clinical considerations. Cancer Treat Rev 2012;38(6):815–24.

73. Stopeck AT, Lipton A, Body JJ, et al. Denosumab compared with zoledronic acid for the treatment of bone metastases in patients with advanced breast cancer: a randomized, double-blind study. J Clin Oncol 2010;28(35):5132–9.

74. Bauman G, Charette M, Reid R, et al. Radiopharmaceuticals for the palliation of painful bone metastasis-a systemic review. Radiother Oncol 2005;75(3):258–70.

75. Temel JS, Greer JA, Muzikansky A, et al. Early palliative care for patients with metastatic non-small-cell lung cancer. N Engl J Med 2010;363(8):733–42.

76. Connor SR, Pyenson B, Fitch K, et al. Comparing hospice and nonhospice patient survival among patients who die within a three-year window. J Pain Symptom Manage 2007;33(3):238–46.

77. Kemeny MM, Peterson BL, Kornblith AB, et al. Barriers to clinical trial participation by older women with breast cancer. J Clin Oncol 2003;21(12):2268–75.

78. Best I. Central role of the research nurse in improving accrual of older persons to cancer treatment trials. J Clin Oncol 2005;23(30):7752–3.

79. Kornblith AB, Kemeny M, Peterson BL, et al. Survey of oncologists' perceptions of barriers to accrual of older patients with breast carcinoma to clinical trials. Cancer 2002;95(5):989–96.

80. Audisio RA, Bozzetti F, Gennari R, et al. The surgical management of elderly cancer patients; recommendations of the SIOG surgical task force. Eur J Cancer 2004;40(7):926–38.

81. Audisio RA, Pope D, Ramesh HS, et al. Shall we operate? Preoperative assessment in elderly cancer patients (PACE) can help. A SIOG surgical task force prospective study. Crit Rev Oncol Hematol 2008;65(2):156–63.

82. Horiot JC. Radiation therapy and the geriatric oncology patient. J Clin Oncol 2007;25(14):1930–5.

83. Lichtman SM, Wildiers H, Chatelut E, et al. International Society of Geriatric Oncology Chemotherapy Taskforce: evaluation of chemotherapy in older patients—an analysis of the medical literature. J Clin Oncol 2007;25(14):1832–43.

84. Lewis JH, Kilgore ML, Goldman DP, et al. Participation of patients 65 years of age or older in cancer clinical trials. J Clin Oncol 2003;21(7):1383–9.

Breast Cancer Survivorship Issues

Daniela Stan, MD[a],*, Charles L. Loprinzi, MD[b],
Kathryn J. Ruddy, MD, MPH[c]

KEYWORDS

- Vasomotor symptoms • Sexual dysfunction • Infertility • Osteoporosis
- Musculoskeletal pain • Cognitive changes • Neuropathy
- Treatment-related cancers

KEY POINTS

- Surveillance after early stage breast cancer should include routine mammograms, physical examinations, and histories, but not blood work or imaging focused on possible distant sites of relapse.
- Vasomotor symptoms, sexual dysfunction, infertility, osteoporosis, musculoskeletal pain, weight gain, cognitive changes, fatigue, neuropathy, congestive heart failure, and treatment-related cancers can all plague survivors of breast cancer.
- Efforts are underway to coordinate follow-up care for survivors of breast cancer and to optimize management of the physical, mental, and emotional sequelae of breast cancer and breast cancer treatment.

SURVEILLANCE OF SURVIVORS OF BREAST CANCER

In the 1980s, it was common to follow early stage survivors of breast cancer with multiple blood tests, chest radiographs, and other imaging (eg, bone scans). This practice was not evidence-based, and arose primarily from clinician biases. When patients are followed on clinical protocols with histories, physical examinations, chest radiographs, blood work, and bone scans, approximately 75% of recurrences are first recognized by history or physical examination.[1] In the other 25% of patients, approximately a third of recurrences are each detected by abnormalities in chest radiographs, bone scans, and liver function tests. Virtually no recurrences are identified

Funding: Dr D. Stan: Internal Mayo Clinic funds; Dr C.L. Loprinzi: This work was supported by United States National Institutes of Health Grant-CA 124477; Dr K.J. Ruddy: Internal Dana Farber Cancer Institute funds.
Conflicts of Interest: Dr D. Stan: None; Dr C.L. Loprinzi: Research funding provided to Mayo Clinic, from Pfizer; Dr K.J. Ruddy: None.
[a] Division of General Internal Medicine, Mayo Clinic, 200 First Street Southwest, Rochester, MN 55905, USA; [b] Medical Oncology, Mayo Clinic, 200 First Street Southwest, Rochester, MN 55905, USA; [c] Medical Oncology, Dana-Farber Cancer Institute, Harvard Medical School, Brookline Avenue, Boston, MA 02215, USA
* Corresponding author.
E-mail address: stan.daniela@mayo.edu

based on complete blood count abnormalities. Although blood work or imaging may identify the first evidence of distant recurrence in a minority of cases, this is only clinically important if detecting these recurrences while a patient is still asymptomatic improves quantity or quality of life (QOL).

In the 1990s, American Society of Clinical Oncology (ASCO) developed practice guidelines regarding follow-up surveillance in patients with a history of breast cancer that had been treated for cure.[2] These guidelines were largely influenced by two Italian studies that prospectively evaluated more intensive surveillance strategies, compared with following a patient by history, physical examination, and mammography.[3,4] These ASCO guidelines were updated, predominantly unchanged, in 2006[5]; they state that the primary surveillance procedures for asymptomatic survivors of breast cancer should include intermittent patient histories and physical examinations every 3 to 6 months during the first 3 years, every 6 to 12 months during years 4 to 5, and annually thereafter; and annual mammography for patients with residual breast tissue, with the first one scheduled at least 6 months after completion of breast radiation therapy. Patients should be educated with regard to symptoms of breast cancer recurrence, and they should be instructed to call a provider if questions or problems arise. Genetic counseling should be offered to those whose personal or family history is suggestive of a genetic cancer syndrome. Regular gynecologic follow-up is recommended for most patients; patients on tamoxifen should be alerted to report abnormal bleeding.

ASCO guidelines specifically recommend against routine blood counts, liver function tests, and tumor markers (eg, carcinoembryonic antigen), and routine radiologic tests other than mammograms (eg, chest radiographs, bone scans, computed tomography scans, positron emission tomography scans, and breast magnetic resonance imaging tests). Newer data, however, do support the use of surveillance breast magnetic resonance imaging in certain patient subsets (eg, those with BRCA mutations and residual breast tissue).[6] ASCO provides patient information material that can be helpful to give to patients who have questions about breast cancer surveillance testing.

BOTHERSOME SYMPTOMS
Vasomotor Symptoms Caused by Chemotherapy-related Amenorrhea and Hormonal Therapies

Vasomotor symptoms occur in 65% to 96% of women treated for breast cancer.[7] In survivors of breast cancer, vasomotor symptoms are often longer lasting and more severe than in the general population. These negatively impact QOL, sleep, and compliance with medications. Breast cancer therapies can cause hot flashes by abruptly interrupting ovarian function (with chemotherapy, ovarian inhibition, and oophorectomy); decreasing estrogen concentrations (aromatase inhibitors [AI]); or decreasing the sensitivity of tissues to estrogen (tamoxifen). Discontinuation of hormone-replacement therapy can also cause problematic symptoms.

Hot flashes are the most common adverse events of adjuvant endocrine therapies, with a prevalence of 50% to 70% in patients treated with tamoxifen.[8] In this setting, the frequency and severity of hot flashes usually increase during the first 3 months of treatment, after which they plateau. Compared with tamoxifen, the AIs are slightly less likely to cause hot flashes.[9] In general, the symptoms that result from chemotherapy-induced menopause are more severe than those associated with natural menopause.

Lifestyle options for hot flash relief (eg, keeping the room cold; avoiding spices, caffeine, and hot fluids; using a fan and cooling pillows; and dressing in layers) are sensible and straightforward. Although extremely effective in alleviating hot flashes in 80% to 90% of patients, hormone-replacement therapy is contraindicated in survivors of breast cancer, especially for those with estrogen receptor–positive tumors, because of an increased risk of recurrence.[10]

A single intramuscular dose of depomedroxyprogesterone acetate was effective in alleviating hot flashes in 75% to 80% of women with breast cancer, and its effect was long-lasting[11,12]; however, the safety of this approach has not been clearly delineated.

Efforts to expand the therapeutic options for vasomotor symptoms have led to trials of the following: (1) newer antidepressants, such as selective serotonin reuptake inhibitors paroxetine, sertraline, fluoxetine, citalopram, and escitalopram, and serotonin-norepinephrine reuptake inhibitors venlafaxine and desvenlafaxine; (2) anticonvulsants, such as gabapentin and pregabalin; and (3) the antihypertensive drug clonidine.

Table 1 provides an overview of treatments for hot flashes. Venlafaxine seems no more effective than gabapentin, but was preferred by the patients in an randomized controlled trial (RCT) with a crossover design.[13] Gabapentin and pregabalin reduce hot flashes in the general population and survivors of breast cancer.[14,15] Clonidine had similar effects in survivors of breast cancer treated with tamoxifen.[16]

Paroxetine, fluoxetine, and sertraline should be used with caution in patients receiving tamoxifen, because they substantially inhibit CYP 2D6, the enzyme converting tamoxifen to its active metabolite, endoxifen. Venlafaxine, desvenlafaxine, citalopram, and escitalopram seem to inhibit CYP 2D6 to a lesser degree and thus may be better choices in patients receiving tamoxifen.[17]

Complementary and alternative methods have been assessed for hot flash treatment, with varying degrees of success. Black cohosh, ginseng, evening primrose oil, wild yam, and phytoestrogens have all been studied prospectively but seem to have minimal, if any, effects.[18] Vitamin E seems to be mildly effective in alleviating hot flashes and can be considered for patients with mild symptoms.[19] Mind-body interventions, such as paced breathing, cognitive behavioral therapy, and yoga, were all suggested to be beneficial in small studies, but systematic reviews revealed methodologic research flaws and, to date, there is no definite proof of benefit.[20] It is possible that acupuncture may be helpful for some patients with hot flashes,[21] but most RCTs of acupuncture versus sham acupuncture have showed no difference between groups.[22] Likewise, a review of RCTs on the benefits of physical exercise for treatment of hot flashes was negative.[23] New data support that hypnosis can be beneficial,[24,25] but additional trials are needed and training is necessary to provide this therapy.

Sexual Dysfunction Caused by Chemotherapy-related Amenorrhea and Hormonal Therapies

Sexuality is an integral part of life and is influenced by physical, psychological, relational, and sociocultural factors.[26] Surgery and radiation for breast cancer may alter sexuality by changing body contour and sensation; in addition, early menopause induced by chemotherapy, and hormonal alterations associated with endocrine therapies, can negatively impact the sexual organs. A recent review of sexual dysfunction in female survivors of breast cancer identified a high prevalence of sexual symptoms (30%–100%), the most commonly reported being decreased libido (23%–64%); decreased arousal or lubrication (20%–48%); dyspareunia (35%–38%); anorgasmy (16%–36%); body image concerns (30%–67%); and poor nipple sensation after nipple-sparing mastectomy (>90%).[26]

Although lumpectomy has been less commonly associated with deterioration in body image compared with mastectomy, sexual functioning seems to be comparable

Table 1
Effectiveness of different interventions for hot flashes

Agent	Dose	% of Patients in Active Arm with ≥50% Decrease in Baseline Hot Flash Score[136,137]	% of Patients in Placebo Arm with ≥50% Decrease in Baseline Hot Flash Score[136,137]	Other Outcomes More Common in Active Arm vs Placebo
MPA[138]	400 mg intramuscularly	72	Comparison with venlafaxine	No placebo data
Megestrol acetate[12]	20 mg BID	63	30	Withdrawal menstrual bleeding
Venlafaxine[139]	37.5 mg/d	54	30	Nausea, appetite loss, dizziness, constipation, dry mouth, sleepiness, improved quality of life
Venlafaxine[139]	75 mg/d	70		
Venlafaxine[139]	150 mg/d	62		
Fluoxetine[140]	20 mg/d	70	52	None
Paroxetine CR[141]	12.5 mg/d	50	49	None
Paroxetine CR[141]	25 mg/d	68		None
Paroxetine[142]	10 mg/d	70	33; 57[a]	No side effects. Improved sleep
Paroxetine[142]	20 mg/d	76		Nausea
Sertraline[143,144]	50 mg/d	40–50	21–38	Nausea, fatigue, diarrhea, anxiety
Sertraline[145]	100 mg/d	56	41	Nausea
Gabapentin[14]	300 mg/d	46	27	Decrease in appetite, decrease in pain
Gabapentin[14,146]	900 mg/d	56–63	27–38	
Gabapentin[147]	2400 mg/d	84	47	Trend toward more headache, dizziness, disorientation, sleep disturbance
Clonidine[16]	0.1 mg/d oral or patch	37	30	Difficulty sleeping, dry mouth, constipation, skin rash from patch, improved quality of life
Vitamin E[148]	800 IU/d	32	30	None
Soy[149]	70–150 mg isoflavones/d	30	?	None
Black cohosh[150]	20 mg/d	20	30	None

All agents were compared with placebo unless otherwise noted.

[a] This study had two placebo arms.

Data from Loprinzi CL, Barton DL, Sloan JA, et al. Mayo Clinic and North Central Cancer Treatment Group hot flash studies: a 20-year experience. Menopause 2008;15(4 Pt 1):655–60; and Loprinzi CL, Sloan J, Stearns V, et al. Newer antidepressants and gabapentin for hot flashes: an individual patient pooled analysis. J Clin Oncol 2009;27(17):2831–7.

after either surgery,[27] regardless of the time since surgery. Women who received chemotherapy are more likely to experience vaginal dryness, dyspareunia, decreased libido, and difficulty achieving orgasm.[28] These symptoms are more prevalent in younger women and it seems that chemotherapy-associated sexual dysfunction usually resolves within 10 years after treatment.[29]

There is strong evidence that treatment with tamoxifen is not associated with sexual dysfunction in most survivors of breast cancer,[30] whereas AIs contribute significantly to dissatisfaction with sexual life. In the Anastrozole, Tamoxifen, Alone and in Combination (ATAC) trial, therapy with anastrazole was associated with more vaginal dryness (16% vs 8%), dyspareunia (18% vs 8%), and decreased libido (16% vs 9%) compared with tamoxifen.[31] Similar findings were shown in a study that examined exemestane versus tamoxifen.[32]

There are several barriers to treatment of sexual dysfunction in survivors of breast cancer. First, many medical providers may be uncomfortable discussing sexuality because of deficiencies in formal training in this field, unfamiliarity with resources for referral, and fear of embarrassing the patient or invading her privacy.[26,33] Patients may be reluctant to be the first to broach this subject. As such, sexual dysfunction may remain unaddressed in a substantial proportion of survivors of breast cancer despite evidence that, given the opportunity, patients would like to discuss this issue.[34]

Second, there is no standard tool for detecting sexual dysfunction in survivors of cancer. Recently, it was proposed that the use of the Female Sexual Function Index[35] or other patient self-reported assessments be implemented for this purpose.[26] A valuable practical approach to assessing cancer-related sexual dysfunction in survivors of cancer, including specific phrases to help opening the discussion, was recently outlined by Bober and Varela.[26]

Treatment of sexual dysfunction necessitates a comprehensive assessment and intervention that addresses the communication between sexual partners and requires sensitivity to cultural and personal values. The quality of one's relationship is the most consistent predictor of sexual satisfaction in survivors of breast cancer.[28]

Vaginal lubricants (Astroglide) and moisturizers (Replens, KY Jelly) are effective in alleviating vaginal dryness and dyspareunia.[36,37] Moisturizers should be used regularly, three to five times a week, to be effective, whereas lubricants are meant to be used as needed (generally before and during sexual activity).

Topical estrogen preparations are more effective than vaginal moisturizers, but their use raises concerns about systemic absorption and possible stimulation of cancer recurrence. Nevertheless, low-dose vaginal estrogens, such as estradiol vaginal ring (Estring), estradiol vaginal tablet (Vagifem), or vaginal conjugated estrogens (Premarin vaginal cream), can be considered for women with significant vaginal symptoms. Systemic absorption of vaginal estrogens is most concerning in women treated with AIs; in these women, vaginal estrogens should be avoided or only used in the short term after thorough counseling regarding potential risks.[38] New data support the use of dehydroepiandrosterone as an agent to help vaginal dryness.[39] Most of the work has been obtained in patients without prior history of breast cancer. Undergoing work is addressing this issue in patients with a prior history of cancer.

Testosterone does not seem to be beneficial for sexual function in survivors of breast cancer.[40] The use of vaginal dilators, vibrators, self-stimulating techniques, and pelvic floor relaxation techniques have been advocated for women with vaginal atrophy and stenosis causing vaginal discomfort and dyspareunia.[41] This treatment is best administered in coordination with a mental health specialist, gynecologist, or counselor with expertise in sexual health. **Box 1** summarizes the sexual dysfunction issues.

Box 1
Sexual dysfunction key points

- The most common sexual symptoms in survivors of breast cancer are (1) decreased libido, arousal, or lubrication; (2) dyspareunia; (3) anorgasmy; (4) body image concerns; and (5) decreased nipple sensation

- Sexual dysfunction does not seem to differ substantially after lumpectomy versus mastectomy

- Chemotherapy and AI therapy, but not tamoxifen, are associated with an increased risk of sexual dysfunction

- It is the responsibility of the provider to open the discussion on sexual dysfunction

- Screening for sexual dysfunction should be performed regularly through objective or self-reported assessment tools

- Hormone-replacement therapy is contraindicated for treatment of sexual dysfunction in survivors of breast cancer

- Testosterone without estrogen does not seem to be helpful in treating sexual dysfunction in female survivors

- Vaginal moisturizers (Replens, KY Jelly) and lubricants (Astroglide) are effective for dyspareunia and vaginal dryness, and should be used as a first-line therapy

- Low-dose vaginal estrogen preparations (Vagifem, Estring, Premarin cream) may be considered for selected women with severe vaginal dryness

- Vaginal dilators, vibrators, self-stimulation, and pelvic relaxation techniques may ameliorate vaginal stenosis and severe dyspareunia

- Referral to mental health specialists, sexual counselors, and gynecologists may be considered for women with severe symptoms

---

Infertility and Delayed Childbearing Caused by Gonadotoxic and Hormonal Therapies

Young survivors of breast cancer may face delayed child-bearing and infertility because of gonadotoxic chemotherapies and time-consuming hormonal therapies. Chemotherapy damages the ovaries and causes earlier menopause and reduced fertility. The most common chemotherapeutics causing premature ovarian failure are the alkylating agents, followed by platinum agents, anthracyclines, and taxanes.[42] Conception of a child is strongly discouraged during any cancer systemic or radiation therapy because of potential teratogenicity. Because a standard endocrine therapy course for a premenopausal woman lasts at least 5 years, natural ovarian aging during this period contributes significantly to infertility in many survivors of breast cancer (even those who did not require chemotherapy).

Infertility and worry about possible future infertility are significant burdens for many survivors. The ability to reproduce has been identified as a major concern in this population,[43] and not all survivors believe that this issue is adequately addressed by their health care providers.[44] For new patients with breast cancer that prioritize the ability to bear children in the future, reproductive options can be maximized by early referral to a reproductive endocrinologist. Before the initiation of systemic treatment, embryo and oocyte cryopreservation, and experimental ovarian tissue cryopreservation, may be considered. If a newly diagnosed premenopausal patient has a male partner with whom she would like to conceive, or if she is willing to use sperm from a donor, she may opt for the most widely available and highly effective fertility preservation technique, embryo cryopreservation (ie, retrieval of eggs followed by fertilization, freezing, and storage). If she prefers to store unfertilized eggs because she does not have access to a desirable sperm source, oocyte cryopreservation (ie, retrieval, freezing, and storage of unfertilized eggs) may be best performed at an experienced center. Embryo and oocyte cryopreservation generally require a 2- to 6-week delay in chemotherapy depending on a woman's menstrual calendar, and may theoretically stimulate the growth of hormonally sensitive cancers because of spikes in estradiol and other hormones during stimulation of ovarian follicle development (which optimizes egg retrieval yields). However, new techniques that use letrozole or tamoxifen during ovarian stimulation prevent high spikes in estradiol levels,[45] and no detrimental impact on prognosis has been associated with this strategy.[46,47] Ovarian tissue cryopreservation (ie, removal, freezing, and storage of a piece of an ovary) is the most invasive and least well tested of these techniques, but it does not require any hormonal stimulation, and it may minimize delays, because it does not require synchronization with the menstrual cycle.[48]

Even if fertility concerns are not addressed until after breast cancer treatment is completed, prompt reproductive endocrinology referral, as soon as possible, is desirable. Options after breast cancer treatment may include in vitro fertilization, use of donor eggs, and early cessation of hormonal therapy when a patient believes that the benefits outweigh the risks. Use of a decision aid at the time of diagnosis may help reduce regrets about fertility-related decisions later.[49] Likewise, online reproductive health and fertility education may improve QOL during the survivorship period.[50]

Osteoporosis Caused by Chemotherapy-related Amenorrhea and Antiestrogen Therapies

Osteoporosis, a metabolic disease of the bone characterized by low bone mineral density (BMD) and changes in bone microarchitecture that increase risk of fractures, is a major health issue in survivors of breast cancer, with a prevalence five times higher than in the general population.[51] Estrogen decreases the activity of bone resorptive cells (osteoclasts) and stimulates bone formation by osteoblasts. Age, natural menopause, chemotherapy-induced amenorrhea, ovarian inhibitors, and AIs are all associated with a low estrogenic state. Tamoxifen seems to have detrimental bone resorptive effects in premenopausal women,[52] but advantageous antiresorptive effects in postmenopausal women.[53]

Chemotherapy-induced premature menopause is associated with rapid bone loss, comparable with that seen with surgical premature menopause.[54] Gonadotropin-releasing hormone (GnRH) agonists (eg, goserelin) cause even more bone loss than chemotherapy.[55] Adjuvant treatment with an AI poses a significantly increased risk of osteoporosis and fractures, although less than that seen with chemotherapy-induced ovarian failure or GnRH agonists.[42] In a bone substudy within the ATAC trial, women treated with anastrozole experienced a decrease in BMD of 6% at the lumbar spine and 7% at the hip after 5 years of therapy (a tamoxifen and a nonrandomized comparator untreated group had a slight BMD increase and slight BMD decrease, respectively).[56] At 10 years, there were more fractures in the anastrozole group than in the tamoxifen group (15% vs 11%), a difference accounted for by fractures during active treatment only, after which there were equal numbers of fractures in the two groups.[57] Similar findings were reported from studies of adjuvant exemestane and letrozole[58,59] versus tamoxifen. Of note, women with a normal BMD, before initiation on AI therapy, did not develop osteoporosis during or after completion of AI therapy.

Risks factors for osteoporosis are classified into modifiable (eg, smoking, caffeine intake, inactivity, muscle weakness, low body weight, low calcium and vitamin D intake, low estrogen levels) and nonmodifiable (eg, family history of fractures, white or Asian race, older age, female gender, height, late menarche, hip geometry). However, most fractures in the general population occur in people with a BMD above the osteoporotic range.[60] The Fracture Assessment Tool (FRAX),[61] which includes modifiable and nonmodifiable risk factors for osteoporosis, may aid assessing an individual's risk of osteoporotic fractures. A 10-year risk of major osteoporotic fractures of greater than or equal to 20% or of hip fracture of greater than or equal to 3%, according to this tool, is considered a clinical indication for bone-strengthening treatment. In women treated with AIs, the FRAX may underestimate the risk of fractures.[62]

In cancer survivors, ASCO guidelines recommend screening for osteoporosis in high-risk women (age ≥65 years; age 60–64 at high risk [family history, previous nontraumatic fracture, weight <70 kg]; those initiating AI therapy; premenopausal women on ovarian suppression), by annual DEXA.[63] Other guidelines (National Comprehensive Cancer Network [NCCN], International Expert Panel), recommend screening only for women initiating an AI therapy with DEXA scans every 1 to 2 years.[62,64] In women with normal BMD at baseline, it is reasonable to repeat testing less frequently. Treatment is recommended for those with a T score less than or equal to −2.5 by the ASCO guidelines, whereas the NCCN recommends treatment for those with a T score less than or equal to −2 or with an FRAX score for which treatment is indicated.

Prevention of bone loss in patients with cancer should start with addressing modifiable risk factors: weight-bearing physical activity; supplemental calcium and vitamin D for a total daily intake (from diet and supplements) of about 1200 mg calcium and 800 IU of vitamin D; smoking cessation; and avoidance of excessive alcohol.[63] Vitamin D deficiency is prevalent in survivors of breast cancer, and measurement of serum 25-hydroxyvitamin D levels (followed by replacement for those with deficiency) may be valuable before starting therapy with bone antiresorptive agents.

Bone antiresorptive therapies recommended for survivors of breast cancer belong to two groups of medications: bisphosphonates (alendronate, residronate, ibandronate, pamidronate, and zoledronate) and a monoclonal antibody to receptor activator nuclear factor kappa-B ligands, of which denosumab is the only one clinically available. Both classes work by inhibiting the activity of osteoclasts. Denosumab is Food and Drug Administration (FDA) approved for use in postmenopausal osteoporosis, women with osteopenia on AI, and women with breast cancer metastatic to the bone. In osteopenic survivors of breast cancer treated with an AI, denosumab (60 mg subcutaneously every 6 months) increased the lumbar spine BMD by 7.6% at 2 years, compared with placebo.[65]

Although starting bisphosphonates at the time of initiation of chemotherapy significantly increases BMD compared with a delayed approach or to a placebo arm,[65,66] this approach lacks long-term follow-up and data proving fewer bone fractures. Recent meta-analyses failed to reveal benefit from up-front versus delayed use of bisphosphonates in women initiating AI therapy, with regard to fractures or survival.[67] Because of concerns about osteonecrosis of the jaw, atypical femoral neck fractures, and esophageal cancer associated with the use of bisphosphonates, the FDA has recommended that the benefits and risks of this therapy be assessed periodically and therapy be discontinued if the risk of fractures has subsided.[68] **Box 2** provides a synopsis of this topic.

Musculoskeletal Complaints Related to AIs

AIs were used in clinical practice for some time before it was widely recognized that they caused arthralgias. One of the earliest clinical trials demonstrating increased risk of musculoskeletal symptoms was the ATAC trial, which reported a 30% incidence of musculoskeletal disorders with anastrozole versus a 24% incidence with

---

Box 2
Osteoporosis key points

- Treatment with AI, GnRH, or chemotherapy poses a significant risk of osteoporosis

- Tamoxifen has a slight bone resorptive effect on BMD in premenopausal women, but has bone protective effects after menopause

- Screening for osteoporosis with DEXA scans every 1 to 2 years is recommended in survivors of breast cancer greater than or equal to 65 years of age, age 60 to 64 at high risk, initiating AI therapy, or premenopausal on ovarian suppression

- Prevention of bone loss can be achieved through weight-bearing physical activity, supplemental calcium and vitamin D, smoking cessation, and avoidance of excessive alcohol intake

- Treatment of osteoporosis is recommended for women with a T score less than or equal to −2.5 or a T score less than or equal to −2 and a high FRAX score ($\geq$20% risk of major osteoporotic fracture or $\geq$3% risk of hip fracture)

- Bisphosphonates (pamidronate, residronate, and zoledronic acid) or denosumab (receptor activator nuclear factor kappa-B ligands inhibitor) can treat or prevent osteoporosis in survivors of breast cancer

- There is no evidence that up-front versus delayed treatment with these medication improves clinically relevant bone outcomes

---

tamoxifen.[69] This statistically significant difference likely underestimated the true incidence of this problem because it required clinician documentation of a clinical problem that had not been identified to possibly be associated with AIs, as opposed to measuring patient-reported symptoms that queried about this toxicity. Because this was not a widely recognized problem at the time, clinicians were likely not attuned to it.

Despite the current paucity of placebo-controlled data regarding patient-reported arthralgias on AIs, these medications seem to cause musculoskeletal symptoms in approximately 50% of patients, with 15% of patients experiencing severe symptoms.[70] Hands and knees are often involved. A few patients develop symptoms within weeks to a month, whereas others first notice symptoms a year or more after drug initiation. The incidence of AI-mediated musculoskeletal symptoms seems to be relatively similar among the three clinically available AIs: (1) anastrozole, (2) letrozole, and (3) exemestane. Joint abnormalities can be seen radiologically in some affected patients.[71]

Although the cause of AI-mediated musculoskeletal symptoms has not been definitively determined, the most likely cause is from estrogen deficiency. In 1925, Cecil and Archer first described "arthritis of the menopause" as the rapid development of hand and knee osteoarthritis after the cessation of menses.

Currently, there are no proved drugs or procedures for patients suffering AI-mediated arthralgias. In clinical practice, nonsteroidal anti-inflammatory medications do seem to help many patients. Phase III clinical trials are planned or ongoing for testosterone, vitamin D, acupuncture, and an omega-3 fatty acid. At this time, the recommended treatment of patients with severe AI arthralgias is to temporarily discontinue the drug. In most cases, symptoms largely resolve within a month or so. At that time, another AI may be tried. Some patients tolerate this better, whereas other patients develop recurrent symptoms. Another option is to switch antiestrogen therapy to tamoxifen. For patients with minimal benefits from antiestrogen therapy (eg, an 80-year-old woman with a 0.5 cm breast cancer) consideration of stopping adjuvant hormonal therapy may be appropriate.

Weight Gain

Weight gain is common in patients with breast cancer treated with chemotherapy (average gain is 2.5–6.2 kg, but is more in premenopausal women and those treated with multiagent regimens),[72] but not usually in patients treated with endocrine therapy alone, compared with placebo.[73] Chemotherapy causes sarcopenic obesity, characterized by loss of lean mass and gain of fat mass. Decreased physical activity caused by fatigue, decreased resting energy expenditure, and, to lesser degree, overeating, have been shown to contribute to obesity after chemotherapy.[74] Weight gain after breast cancer diagnosis is associated with a decreased QOL and an increased risk of cardiovascular disease, diabetes, orthopedic complications, and gallbladder disease. Weight gain might increase breast cancer–specific and overall mortality, although this has not been consistently established.[75]

It remains unclear whether purposeful weight loss after breast cancer treatment impacts breast cancer outcomes. There is strong evidence that implementing a physical exercise program after breast cancer treatment is associated with a decreased risk of cancer recurrence and death, but the mechanism for this is unclear. Large studies of dietary interventions in early survivors of breast cancer have reported a positive effect on disease-free survival only if the intervention was associated with weight loss.[76] Small studies showed success with weight loss through multimodality interventions that included caloric restriction, exercise, and psychologic support.[77] Larger studies are underway to analyze the impact of multimodality approaches on weight loss and survival.

Currently, the American College of Sports Medicine[78] and the American Cancer Society[79] recommend moderate-intensity aerobic activity for greater than or equal to 150 minutes per week; strength training at least 2 days per week; a diet rich in fruits, vegetables, and whole grains; and limiting the ingestion of processed foods, to achieve or maintain a healthy weight.

Cognitive Changes

Cognitive impairment associated with cancer treatments includes problems with attention, concentration, executive function, and working memory. Cross-sectional studies report a high prevalence of cognitive impairment, between 15% and 75%. In some studies that measure pretreatment cognitive functioning, 15% to 25% of patients with breast cancer had worse cognitive function after chemotherapy,[80] whereas other recent studies have been negative.[81] Heterogeneity of the measured outcomes and patient populations, and sometimes a lack of pretreatment cognitive assessment, may account for these conflicting results.

Interestingly, 20% to 30% of patients with breast cancer had a lower than expected cognitive performance before treatment, irrespective of any psychological factors, such as depression, anxiety, fatigue, or anesthesia type. It is postulated that cancer can induce an inflammatory state that induces cognitive dysfunction or that cancer and cognition might have a common risk factor.[82] Cognitive changes after breast cancer treatment were initially attributed wholly to chemotherapy, but evidence is emerging to suggest a role for endocrine therapy. Tamoxifen seems to negatively affect cognitive abilities, whereas AIs do not.[83]

Older patients and those with a lower cognitive reserve are more vulnerable to treatment-induced cognitive deficits.[84] Genetic factors involved in apolipoprotein E and catechol O-methyltransferase metabolism may also contribute to predisposition toward chemotherapy-induced cognitive decline.[85]

Treatment of cognitive dysfunction has been poorly studied. The natural history seems to be one of slow recovery and return to pretreatment levels in about 6 months.

Modafinil and cognitive behavioral training have been studied and found to be promising.[86,87]

Fatigue

Cancer-related fatigue (CRF) is a persistent feeling of emotional, physical, and cognitive exhaustion associated with cancer diagnosis or treatment, out of proportion to recent activity and not relieved by rest.[88] CRF is often identified as the most distressing side effect of cancer diagnosis and treatments. CRF significantly impacts overall QOL and patients consider fatigue to be a major disruptor of daily activities. However, health care providers rarely assess for presence and severity of fatigue, and often attribute less importance to fatigue than do patients.[89] The pathophysiology of fatigue in this population is complex and poorly understood; proposed mechanisms include neurotoxicity of cancer treatments, chronic stress affecting the hypothalamic-pituitary-adrenal axis, systemic inflammatory response, hormonal changes of menopause, anemia, and immune activation.[90]

The prevalence of CRF varies significantly, based on the diagnostic criteria used, and has been reported to be between 15% and 90%.[91] In one study, 21% were found to report persistent fatigue beyond 5 years.[92]

NCCN guidelines recommend fatigue assessments at initial visit, during chemotherapy, and when advanced cancer is diagnosed.[88] The recommended screening tool is a visual analog scale (How would you rate your fatigue from 0–10?) with scores between 1–3, 4–6, and 7–10 representing mild, moderate, and severe fatigue, respectively.

Certain breast cancer treatments are linked to fatigue. Radiation is associated with fatigue that is usually worst late in the course, and persistent fatigue. A psychological mechanism has been proposed, but not proved, for survivors of early stage breast cancer receiving radiation. Receiving both chemotherapy and radiation is known to be associated with a greater risk of CRF than either therapy alone.[92]

Managing fatigue should include, at a minimum, instruction on energy conservation for those with severe symptoms, and treatment of comorbid conditions (eg, insomnia, pain, depression, anemia, cardiomyopathy [CMP], and hypothyroidism).[93] However, improvement in depression or insomnia with pharmacologic interventions has not been found to be associated with decreased fatigue,[94] although bupropion is still under study. Aerobic physical exercise during or after completion of breast cancer treatments was found to reduce fatigue in a recent meta-analysis that included 56 studies (28 of survivors of breast cancer), whereas resistive (eg, strength training) and alternative exercise (eg, yoga and qigong) methods were not found to be helpful.[95] To date, most of the literature does not support that psychostimulants (eg, methylphenidate, modafinil) are very helpful in patients with CRF.

American ginseng did improve the general and physical subscales of fatigue in a double-blind RCT, but not the mental, emotional, and vigor dimensions of fatigue.[96] One small study suggested that guarana, a stimulant from the seeds of an Amazonian plant, improved fatigue, but this needs to be confirmed in larger studies. **Box 3** provides a summary of this topic.

Neuropathy

Although many chemotherapy drugs can cause bothersome neuropathy, taxanes are the most common culprits in patients with breast cancer. This section focuses on paclitaxel-induced neuropathy, because the best natural history information is available with this drug, although docetaxel also causes neuropathy to a slightly lesser

---

Box 3
Fatigue key points

- Fatigue is one of the most distressing cancer-related symptoms and significantly impacts QOL
- Screening for fatigue with a simple visual analog scale is recommended at initial visit, during chemotherapy, and at recurrence
- In patients with fatigue, one must evaluate for anemia, hypothyroidism, and CMP
- Depression and insomnia often coexist with fatigue, and should be treated
- Treatment of fatigue should include energy-conservation measures for those with severe symptoms and aerobic exercise during and after treatment for those able to exercise

---

degree.[97] Despite previous claims, nab-paclitaxel seems to cause as much neuropathy, if not more, than standard paclitaxel.[98]

It was recognized in early clinical trials that paclitaxel caused an acute pain syndrome, which was uncommon with previous chemotherapeutic agents, occurring within days of each dose and largely abating after a few to several days. This pain syndrome became commonly known as "paclitaxel-induced arthralgia/myalgia." In recent years, it has been hypothesized that this pain syndrome is not related to joint or muscle pathology, but is more likely a type of neuropathy.[99,100] In addition to the acute pain syndrome, paclitaxel commonly causes a distal peripheral neuropathy, which commonly presents in a stocking-glove distribution. It is primarily a sensory neuropathy, but some patients have motor or autonomic neuropathy components. This neuropathy, which is the most common dose-limiting toxicity of this drug, commonly occurs over the first several weeks or few months of therapy. Although the symptoms usually lessen after discontinuation of paclitaxel, neuropathy can be persistent and severe for an appreciable subset of patients, and can cause long-term disability. At this time, there is no proved antidote to prevent paclitaxel-induced neuropathy other than dose reduction or discontinuation.

For patients with established paclitaxel-induced neuropathy, there is a dearth of proved effective therapies. Gabapentinoids, such as gabapentin and pregabalin, are commonly used clinically, but a randomized, placebo-controlled, double-blinded clinical trial failed to support this therapy.[101] Duloxetine,[102] Scrambler therapy,[103] a topical preparation of baclofen/amitriptyline/ketamine,[104] and topical menthol have all shown some promise.[105]

Cardiac Toxicity

Radiation therapy, chemotherapy, and endocrine therapy have all been incriminated in cardiotoxicity during treatment of breast cancer. Anthracycline-based chemotherapeutic regimens have been in use since the 1980s, and their cardiotoxicity is well recognized.[106] They can cause a dose-dependent CMP resulting in chronic heart failure. The mechanism by which anthracyclines cause CMP is believed to be a direct toxic effect on the myocytes with generation of free radicals. This syndrome can clinically manifest immediately after administration or after a delay of months or years.[106] Traditionally, it was believed that this heart damage is irreversible (type I cardiac toxicity) and poorly responsive to treatment; however, newer studies have shown that early intervention with angiotensin-converting enzyme inhibitors (ACEI) or β-blockers leads to complete left ventricular ejection fraction recovery.[107]

The incidence of clinical CMP reaches 5% with cumulative doxorubicin and epirubicin doses of 400 mg/m^2 and 920 mg/m^2, respectively.[108] Modern trials, in which the cumulative dose of doxorubicin is much lower (in the range of 240 mg/m^2) have reported a CMP incidence of 0% to 1.6%, and up to 2.1% if taxanes are added.[109] However, the incidence of subclinical heart failure identified through echocardiograms or Multi Gated Acquisition (MUGA) scans is much higher, up to 23% for grade 1 or 2 cardiac toxicity.[110] Factors associated with an increased risk of anthracycline-induced CMP include older age, hypertension, preexisting coronary artery disease, and previous mediastinal radiotherapy.[106]

Data on the natural history of anthracycline-induced CMP are scarce and based mainly on retrospective analyses. One study reported a poor prognosis, compared with other more common causes of CMP, and a 60% 2-year mortality.[111] Newer prospective studies have shown that, if detected early, CMP is treatable and frequently curable with the use of an ACEI or β-blockade.[107] The diagnosis of CMP during chemotherapy may be problematic if it results in a dose decrease, delay, or cessation of further anthracycline treatments, potentially impairing cancer outcomes.

Weekly dosing or prolonged infusion (rather than the standard dosing every 3 weeks) may be considered in patients with the previously mentioned risk factors for possible prevention of anthracycline-induced CMP.[112,113] Pegylated liposomal doxorubicin is less cardiotoxic, but potentially less effective than the parent compound.[114] Dexrazoxane is a cardioprotective medication that was proved to significantly decrease the risk of heart failure and cardiac events during and after treatment with anthracyclines.[115] However, it is FDA approved for use only in patients who require additional doses of anthracyclines after having already received 300 mg/m^2, and consequently it is rarely used. Short-term data on taxanes does not suggest that they increase risk of anthracycline-induced cardiotoxicity.

HER-2 neu-directed therapies are associated with symptomatic cardiac dysfunction in 2% to 4% of patients, whereas 3% to 18% develop asymptomatic CMP, usually reversible with the discontinuation of the drug (type II cardiac dysfunction).[116] Cardiotoxicity is rare in patients who have not received anthracyclines before trastuzumab.[117] Antiangiogenic-based chemotherapy may also cause cardiotoxicity by uncontrolled hypertension.[118]

Radiation therapy, at least by protocols used until the mid-1980s, is associated with an increased risk of dying of cardiac disease and vascular disease; a higher risk has been seen with radiation to the left breast or left chest wall and particularly to the internal mammary chain on either side. The risk increases with the time from radiation and is higher among smokers.[119] Newer radiation techniques deliver a lower dose of cardiac radiation, although parts of the heart and the left anterior descending artery likely continue to receive concerning amounts of radiation.[120] Aggressive treatment of any cardiovascular risk factors is of paramount importance in survivors of breast cancer treated with radiation therapy, especially if left-sided.

Tamoxifen has not been associated with cardiotoxicity, but a recent meta-analysis has demonstrated excess cardiac mortality in women treated with AI for 5 years versus tamoxifen or versus tamoxifen followed by AI for 2 to 3 years.[121]

Early detection of CMP may allow avoidance of irreversible damage[122] but there are no clear guidelines for detection of subclinical CMP. Serial electrocardiograms, echocardiograms, or MUGA scans have been suggested, but these have low sensitivity and specificity in this setting. Troponin I and B-type natriuretic peptide (BNP) are emerging as potential predictive markers for the development of anthracycline-induced CMP and as barometers of response to therapy for this problem.[123] Currently, no cardiac screening is recommended for the average breast cancer survivor. Treatment of asymptomatic or symptomatic CMP should include ACEI or β-blocker, aggressive control of blood pressure, and other cardiovascular risk factors.

TREATMENT-RELATED CANCERS

Patients who receive radiation or chemotherapy for breast cancer may develop therapy-related myelodysplastic syndrome or leukemia. Rates of chronic myelogenous leukemia, acute lymphocytic leukemia, and acute myelogenous leukemia (AML) have all been found to be increased by chemotherapy,[124–126] with alkylating agents, topo-isomerase II inhibitors (associated with 11q23 chromosomal alterations), and platinum compounds all implicated.[127] Out of 16,705 French survivors of breast cancer treated at a single center between 1981 and 1997, at a median follow-up of 10.5 years, 709 patients had developed a second malignancy.[128] Compared with registry data from the general French population, the standardized incidence rate of leukemia was 2.07, and the receipt of chemotherapy was strongly associated with this increased risk. Similarly, in the Danish Cancer Registry, for patients with breast cancer registered between 1977 and 2001, the standardized incidence ratio for acute leukemia was 2.02 compared with the general population.[129] Likewise, an analysis of the National Cancer Institute's Surveillance, Epidemiology, and End Results database showed that AML was diagnosed in the 10 years after the breast cancer diagnosis in 1.8% of women who had received chemotherapy and 1.2% of those who had not.[126] In a later Surveillance, Epidemiology, and End Results analysis of more female survivors of breast cancer, there was an age-dependent elevated risk of later developing AML in women younger than 50 years old (relative risk, 4.14; $P<.001$) and 50 to 64 years old (relative risk, 2.19; $P<.001$), but not in those 65 and older (relative risk, 1.19; $P = .123$) when compared with the expected incidence of AML. Higher stage was associated with an elevated risk of AML (likely caused by a greater likelihood of receiving chemotherapy and radiation with stage III vs stage I disease), and this association was strongest in the youngest women.[130] It is uncertain whether growth factors that support white blood cell counts during chemotherapy contribute to these risks.[126,131]

Alkylating chemotherapy and, more substantially, radiation, can also cause lung cancers, sarcomas, and other solid tumors.[127] In the Danish Cancer Registry, the relative risk of lung cancer in patients who received radiation for breast cancer, compared with those who had not, was 1.33 (95% confidence interval, 1.00–1.77).[129]

Tamoxifen increases the risk of uterine cancer. In the Danish Cancer Registry, patients with breast cancer who received tamoxifen had a standardized incidence ratio for uterine cancer of 1.83, whereas patients with breast cancer who did not receive tamoxifen only had a standardized incidence ratio of 1.04.[129]

Nevertheless, because of low prevalence of secondary malignancies, the NCCN recommends against routine complete blood counts, blood work, or imaging tests to evaluate for new nonbreast malignancies in survivors of breast cancer in general.[132] Patients on tamoxifen are advised to undergo a gynecologic examination annually to monitor for endometrial malignancy. In patients who are known to carry a genetic mutation (eg, p53) that predisposes to a higher risk of a specific malignancy, decisions about screening should be individualized.

ORGANIZING FOLLOW-UP CARE

In recent years, attention to coordinated follow-up for survivors of breast cancer has grown. The Institute of Medicine identified this as a priority for survivors of all cancers.[133] An effort is underway to communicate better to patients and providers about the specifics of the cancer diagnosis and the oncologic care received, such that future care can be better tailored to each survivor's needs. Treatment summaries synopsize an individual's cancer type; stage; methods and doses (where appropriate) of treatment; and toxicities experienced to date. Survivorship care plans lay out a recommended approach to future care, usually including optimal visit frequency and frequency of screening for recurrences, new primaries, and other medical problems.

These treatment summaries and survivorship care plans aim to improve patient understanding and to encourage communication and coordination among primary care providers, oncologists, and other providers (eg, gynecologists, cardiologists, surgeons, and so forth). Ideally, better coordination will help minimize redundant care (ie, repetitive testing and unnecessary visits). Given that health care resources are limited, it is hoped that these efforts streamline follow-up procedures and facilitate efficient and high-quality survivorship care. However, one recent study failed to show a significant benefit to administration of survivorship care plans to patients with breast cancer as part of a 30-minute visit with a nurse practitioner at the completion of curative therapy.[134] Nevertheless, broader implementation of survivorship care coordination for cancer survivors is of great interest to many patients and providers.[135]

SUMMARY

Survivors of breast cancer are confronted with a plethora of cancer treatment-related long-term symptoms, the most common being fatigue, hot flashes, sexual dysfunction, arthralgias, neuropathy, and cognitive dysfunction. Survivors of breast cancer also face cancer treatment-related disease states, such as osteoporosis, cardiac dysfunction, obesity, infertility, and secondary cancers. Evidence-based recommendations for screening, prevention, and early intervention should be implemented to improve QOL and decrease comorbidities in this population.

REFERENCES

1. Pandya KJ, McFadden ET, Kalish LA, et al. A retrospective study of earliest indicators of recurrence in patients on Eastern Cooperative Oncology Group adjuvant chemotherapy trials for breast cancer. A preliminary report. Cancer 1985; 55(1):202–5.
2. Recommended breast cancer surveillance guidelines. American Society of Clinical Oncology. J Clin Oncol 1997;15(5):2149–56.
3. Rosselli Del Turco M, Palli D, Cariddi A, et al. Intensive diagnostic follow-up after treatment of primary breast cancer. A randomized trial. National Research Council Project on Breast Cancer follow-up. JAMA 1994;271(20):1593–7.
4. Impact of follow-up testing on survival and health-related quality of life in breast cancer patients. A multicenter randomized controlled trial. The GIVIO Investigators. JAMA 1994;271(20):1587–92.
5. Khatcheressian JL, Wolff AC, Smith TJ, et al. American Society of Clinical Oncology 2006 update of the breast cancer follow-up and management guidelines in the adjuvant setting. J Clin Oncol 2006;24(31):5091–7.
6. Saslow D, Boetes C, Burke W, et al. American Cancer Society guidelines for breast screening with MRI as an adjunct to mammography. CA Cancer J Clin 2007;57(2):75–89.
7. Gupta P, Sturdee DW, Palin SL, et al. Menopausal symptoms in women treated for breast cancer: the prevalence and severity of symptoms and their perceived effects on quality of life. Climacteric 2006;9(1):49–58.
8. Loprinzi CL, Zahasky KM, Sloan JA, et al. Tamoxifen-induced hot flashes. Clin Breast Cancer 2000;1(1):52–6.
9. Cella D, Fallowfield LJ. Recognition and management of treatment-related side effects for breast cancer patients receiving adjuvant endocrine therapy. Breast Cancer Res Treat 2008;107(2):167–80.

10. North American Menopause Society. Estrogen and progestogen use in post-menopausal women: 2010 position statement of The North American Menopause Society. Menopause 2010;17(2):242–55.

11. Bertelli G, Venturini M, Del Mastro L, et al. Intramuscular depot medroxypro-gesterone versus oral megestrol for the control of postmenopausal hot flashes in breast cancer patients: a randomized study. Ann Oncol 2002; 13(6):883–8.

12. Loprinzi CL, Michalak JC, Quella SK, et al. Megestrol acetate for the prevention of hot flashes. N Engl J Med 1994;331(6):347–52.

13. Bordeleau L, Pritchard KI, Loprinzi CL, et al. Multicenter, randomized, cross-over clinical trial of venlafaxine versus gabapentin for the management of hot flashes in breast cancer survivors. J Clin Oncol 2010;28(35):5147–52.

14. Pandya KJ, Morrow GR, Roscoe JA, et al. Gabapentin for hot flashes in 420 women with breast cancer: a randomised double-blind placebo-controlled trial. Lancet 2005;366(9488):818–24.

15. Loprinzi CL, Qin R, Balcueva EP, et al. Phase III, randomized, double-blind, placebo-controlled evaluation of pregabalin for alleviating hot flashes, N07C1. J Clin Oncol 2010;28(4):641–7.

16. Goldberg RM, Loprinzi CL, O'Fallon JR, et al. Transdermal clonidine for amelio-rating tamoxifen-induced hot flashes. J Clin Oncol 1994;12(1):155–8.

17. Sideras K, Ingle JN, Ames MM, et al. Coprescription of tamoxifen and medica-tions that inhibit CYP2D6. J Clin Oncol 2010;28(16):2768–76.

18. Bordeleau L, Pritchard K, Goodwin P, et al. Therapeutic options for the manage-ment of hot flashes in breast cancer survivors: an evidence-based review. Clin Ther 2007;29(2):230–41.

19. Ziaei S, Kazemnejad A, Zareai M. The effect of vitamin E on hot flashes in meno-pausal women. Gynecol Obstet Invest 2007;64(4):204–7.

20. Tremblay A, Sheeran L, Aranda SK. Psychoeducational interventions to alleviate hot flashes: a systematic review. Menopause 2008;15(1):193–202.

21. Porzio G, Trapasso T, Martelli S, et al. Acupuncture in the treatment of menopause-related symptoms in women taking tamoxifen. Tumori 2002;88(2): 128–30.

22. Vincent A, Barton DL, Mandrekar JN, et al. Acupuncture for hot flashes: a randomized, sham-controlled clinical study. Menopause 2007;14(1):45–52.

23. Daley AJ, Stokes-Lampard HJ, Macarthur C. Exercise to reduce vasomotor and other menopausal symptoms: a review. Maturitas 2009;63(3):176–80.

24. Elkins GR, Fisher WI, Johnson AK, et al. Clinical hypnosis in the treatment of postmenopausal hot flashes: a randomized controlled trial. Menopause 2012. [Epub ahead of print].

25. Elkins G, Marcus J, Stearns V, et al. Randomized trial of a hypnosis intervention for treatment of hot flashes among breast cancer survivors. J Clin Oncol 2008; 26(31):5022–6.

26. Bober SL, Varela VS. Sexuality in adult cancer survivors: challenges and inter-vention. J Clin Oncol 2012;30(30):3712–9.

27. Thors CL, Broeckel JA, Jacobsen PB. Sexual functioning in breast cancer survivors. Cancer Control 2001;8(5):442–8.

28. Ganz PA, Desmond KA, Belin TR, et al. Predictors of sexual health in women after a breast cancer diagnosis. J Clin Oncol 1999;17(8):2371–80.

29. Joly F, Espie M, Marty M, et al. Long-term quality of life in premenopausal women with node-negative localized breast cancer treated with or without adju-vant chemotherapy. Br J Cancer 2000;83(5):577–82.

30. Ganz PA, Rowland JH, Desmond K, et al. Life after breast cancer: understanding women's health-related quality of life and sexual functioning. J Clin Oncol 1998;16(2):501–14.
31. Fallowfield L, Cella D, Cuzick L, et al. Quality of life of postmenopausal women in the Arimidex, Tamoxifen, Alone or in Combination (ATAC) Adjuvant Breast Cancer Trial. J Clin Oncol 2004;22(21):4261–71.
32. Jones SE, Cantrell J, Vukelja S, et al. Comparison of menopausal symptoms during the first year of adjuvant therapy with either exemestane or tamoxifen in early breast cancer: report of a tamoxifen exemestane adjuvant multicenter trial substudy. J Clin Oncol 2007;25(30):4765–71.
33. Katz A. The sounds of silence: sexuality information for cancer patients. J Clin Oncol 2005;23(1):238–41.
34. Reese JB, Keefe FJ, Somers TJ, et al. Coping with sexual concerns after cancer: the use of flexible coping. Support Care Cancer 2010;18(7):785–800.
35. Rosen R, Brown C, Heiman J, et al. The Female Sexual Function Index (FSFI): a multidimensional self-report instrument for the assessment of female sexual function. J Sex Marital Ther 2000;26(2):191–208.
36. Ganz PA, Greendale GA, Petersen L, et al. Managing menopausal symptoms in breast cancer survivors: results of a randomized controlled trial. J Natl Cancer Inst 2000;92(13):1054–64.
37. Loprinzi CL, Abu-Ghazaleh S, Sloan JA, et al. Phase III randomized double-blind study to evaluate the efficacy of a polycarbophil-based vaginal moisturizer in women with breast cancer. J Clin Oncol 1997;15(3):969–73.
38. Kendall A, Dowsett M, Folkerd E, et al. Caution: vaginal estradiol appears to be contraindicated in postmenopausal women on adjuvant aromatase inhibitors. Ann Oncol 2006;17(4):584–7.
39. Labrie F, Archer D, Bouchard C, et al. Intravaginal dehydroepiandrosterone (Prasterone), a physiological and highly efficient treatment of vaginal atrophy. Menopause 2009;16(5):907–22.
40. Barton DL, Wender DB, Sloan JA, et al. Randomized controlled trial to evaluate transdermal testosterone in female cancer survivors with decreased libido; North Central Cancer Treatment Group protocol N02C3. J Natl Cancer Inst 2007;99(9):672–9.
41. Carter J, Goldfrank D, Schover LR. Simple strategies for vaginal health promotion in cancer survivors. J Sex Med 2011;8(2):549–59.
42. Lustberg MB, Reinbolt RE, Shapiro CL. Bone health in adult cancer survivorship. J Clin Oncol 2012;30(30):3665–74.
43. Howard-Anderson J, Ganz PA, Bower JE, et al. Quality of life, fertility concerns, and behavioral health outcomes in younger breast cancer survivors: a systematic review. J Natl Cancer Inst 2012;104(5):386–405.
44. Partridge AH, Gelber S, Peppercorn J, et al. Web-based survey of fertility issues in young women with breast cancer. J Clin Oncol 2004;22(20):4174–83.
45. Oktay K, Hourvitz A, Sahin G, et al. Letrozole reduces estrogen and gonadotropin exposure in women with breast cancer undergoing ovarian stimulation before chemotherapy. J Clin Endocrinol Metab 2006;91(10):3885–90.
46. Oktay K, Buyuk E, Libertella N, et al. Fertility preservation in breast cancer patients: a prospective controlled comparison of ovarian stimulation with tamoxifen and letrozole for embryo cryopreservation. J Clin Oncol 2005;23(19):4347–53.
47. Azim AA, Costantini-Ferrando M, Oktay K. Safety of fertility preservation by ovarian stimulation with letrozole and gonadotropins in patients with breast cancer: a prospective controlled study. J Clin Oncol 2008;26(16):2630–5.

48. Oktay K, Oktem O. Ovarian cryopreservation and transplantation for fertility preservation for medical indications: report of an ongoing experience. Fertil Steril 2010;93(3):762–8.

49. Peate M, Meiser B, Cheah BC, et al. Making hard choices easier: a prospective, multicentre study to assess the efficacy of a fertility-related decision aid in young women with early-stage breast cancer. Br J Cancer 2012;106(6):1053–61.

50. Meneses K, McNees P, Azuero A, et al. Evaluation of the Fertility and Cancer Project (FCP) among young breast cancer survivors. Psychooncology 2010;19(10):1112–5.

51. Kanis JA, McCloskey EV, Powles T, et al. A high incidence of vertebral fracture in women with breast cancer. Br J Cancer 1999;79(7–8):1179–81.

52. Powles TJ, Hickish T, Kanis JA, et al. Effect of tamoxifen on bone mineral density measured by dual-energy x-ray absorptiometry in healthy premenopausal and postmenopausal women. J Clin Oncol 1996;14(1):78–84.

53. Kristensen B, Ejlertsen B, Dalgaard P, et al. Tamoxifen and bone metabolism in postmenopausal low-risk breast cancer patients: a randomized study. J Clin Oncol 1994;12(5):992–7.

54. Shapiro CL, Manola J, Leboff M. Ovarian failure after adjuvant chemotherapy is associated with rapid bone loss in women with early-stage breast cancer. J Clin Oncol 2001;19(14):3306–11.

55. Sverrisdottir A, Fornander T, Jacobsson H, et al. Bone mineral density among premenopausal women with early breast cancer in a randomized trial of adjuvant endocrine therapy. J Clin Oncol 2004;22(18):3694–9.

56. Eastell R, Adams JE, Coleman RE, et al. Effect of anastrozole on bone mineral density: 5-year results from the anastrozole, tamoxifen, alone or in combination trial 18233230. J Clin Oncol 2008;26(7):1051–7.

57. Cuzick J, Sestak I, Baum M, et al. Effect of anastrozole and tamoxifen as adjuvant treatment for early-stage breast cancer: 10-year analysis of the ATAC trial. Lancet Oncol 2010;11(12):1135–41.

58. Coleman RE, Banks LM, Girgis SI, et al. Skeletal effects of exemestane on bone-mineral density, bone biomarkers, and fracture incidence in postmenopausal women with early breast cancer participating in the Intergroup Exemestane Study (IES): a randomised controlled study. Lancet Oncol 2007;8(2):119–27.

59. Perez EA, Josse RG, Pritchard KI, et al. Effect of letrozole versus placebo on bone mineral density in women with primary breast cancer completing 5 or more years of adjuvant tamoxifen: a companion study to NCIC CTG MA.17. J Clin Oncol 2006;24(22):3629–35.

60. Siris ES, Brenneman SK, Barrett-Connor E, et al. The effect of age and bone mineral density on the absolute, excess, and relative risk of fracture in postmenopausal women aged 50-99: results from the National Osteoporosis Risk Assessment (NORA). Osteoporos Int 2006;17(4):565–74.

61. Available at: http://www.shef.ac.uk/FRAX. Accessed February 21, 2013

62. Hadji P, Aapro MS, Body JJ, et al. Management of aromatase inhibitor-associated bone loss in postmenopausal women with breast cancer: practical guidance for prevention and treatment. Ann Oncol 2011;22(12):2546–55.

63. Hillner BE, Ingle JN, Chlebowski RT, et al. American Society of Clinical Oncology 2003 update on the role of bisphosphonates and bone health issues in women with breast cancer. J Clin Oncol 2003;21(21):4042–57.

64. Gralow JR, Biermann JS, Farooki A, et al. NCCN task force report: bone health in cancer care. J Natl Compr Canc Netw 2009;7(Suppl 3):S1–32 [quiz: S33–5].

65. Ellis GK, Bone HG, Chlebowski R, et al. Randomized trial of denosumab in patients receiving adjuvant aromatase inhibitors for nonmetastatic breast cancer. J Clin Oncol 2008;26(30):4875–82.
66. Hershman DL, McMahon DJ, Crew KD, et al. Zoledronic acid prevents bone loss in premenopausal women undergoing adjuvant chemotherapy for early-stage breast cancer. J Clin Oncol 2008;26(29):4739–45.
67. Mauri D, Valachis A, Polyzos NP, et al. Does adjuvant bisphosphonate in early breast cancer modify the natural course of the disease? A meta-analysis of randomized controlled trials. J Natl Compr Canc Netw 2010;8(3):279–86.
68. Whitaker M, Guo J, Kehoe T, et al. Bisphosphonates for osteoporosis: where do we go from here? N Engl J Med 2012;366(22):2048–51.
69. Baum M, Buzdar A, Cuzick J, et al. Anastrozole alone or in combination with tamoxifen versus tamoxifen alone for adjuvant treatment of postmenopausal women with early-stage breast cancer: results of the ATAC (Arimidex, Tamoxifen Alone or in Combination) trial efficacy and safety update analyses. Cancer 2003; 98(9):1802–10.
70. Crew KD, Greenlee H, Capodice J, et al. Prevalence of joint symptoms in postmenopausal women taking aromatase inhibitors for early-stage breast cancer. J Clin Oncol 2007;25(25):3877–83.
71. Morales L, Pans S, Verschueren K, et al. Prospective study to assess short-term intra-articular and tenosynovial changes in the aromatase inhibitor-associated arthralgia syndrome. J Clin Oncol 2008;26(19):3147–52.
72. Goodwin PJ, Ennis M, Pritchard KI, et al. Adjuvant treatment and onset of menopause predict weight gain after breast cancer diagnosis. J Clin Oncol 1999; 17(1):120–9.
73. Sestak I, Harvie M, Howell A, et al. Weight change associated with anastrozole and tamoxifen treatment in postmenopausal women with or at high risk of developing breast cancer. Breast Cancer Res Treat 2012;134(2):727–34.
74. Demark-Wahnefried W, Winer EP, Rimer BK. Why women gain weight with adjuvant chemotherapy for breast cancer. J Clin Oncol 1993;11(7):1418–29.
75. Caan BJ, Emond JA, Natarajan L, et al. Post-diagnosis weight gain and breast cancer recurrence in women with early stage breast cancer. Breast Cancer Res Treat 2006;99(1):47–57.
76. Pierce JP, Natarajan L, Caan BJ, et al. Influence of a diet very high in vegetables, fruit, and fiber and low in fat on prognosis following treatment for breast cancer: the Women's Healthy Eating and Living (WHEL) randomized trial. JAMA 2007;298(3):289–98.
77. Djuric Z, DiLaura NM, Jenkins I, et al. Combining weight-loss counseling with the weight watchers plan for obese breast cancer survivors. Obes Res 2002; 10(7):657–65.
78. Schmitz KH, Courneya KS, Matthews C, et al. American College of Sports Medicine roundtable on exercise guidelines for cancer survivors. Med Sci Sports Exerc 2010;42(7):1409–26.
79. Rock CL, Doyle C, Demark-Wahnefried W, et al. Nutrition and physical activity guidelines for cancer survivors. CA Cancer J Clin 2012;62(4):243–74.
80. Ahles TA, Root JC, Ryan EL. Cancer- and cancer treatment-associated cognitive change: an update on the state of the science. J Clin Oncol 2012;30(30): 3675–86.
81. Hermelink K, Untch M, Lux MP, et al. Cognitive function during neoadjuvant chemotherapy for breast cancer: results of a prospective, multicenter, longitudinal study. Cancer 2007;109(9):1905–13.

82. Ahles TA, Saykin AJ. Candidate mechanisms for chemotherapy-induced cognitive changes. Nat Rev Cancer 2007;7(3):192–201.

83. Schilder CM, Seynaeve C, Beex LV, et al. Effects of tamoxifen and exemestane on cognitive functioning of postmenopausal patients with breast cancer: results from the neuropsychological side study of the tamoxifen and exemestane adjuvant multinational trial. J Clin Oncol 2010;28(8):1294–300.

84. Ahles TA, Saykin AJ, McDonald BC, et al. Longitudinal assessment of cognitive changes associated with adjuvant treatment for breast cancer: impact of age and cognitive reserve. J Clin Oncol 2010;28(29):4434–40.

85. Ahles TA, Saykin AJ, Noll WW, et al. The relationship of APOE genotype to neuropsychological performance in long-term cancer survivors treated with standard dose chemotherapy. Psychooncology 2003;12(6):612–9.

86. Kohli S, Fisher SG, Tra Y, et al. The effect of modafinil on cognitive function in breast cancer survivors. Cancer 2009;115(12):2605–16.

87. Ferguson RJ, McDonald BC, Rocque MA, et al. Development of CBT for chemotherapy-related cognitive change: results of a waitlist control trial. Psychooncology 2012;21(2):176–86.

88. Available at: http://www.nccn.org/professionals/physician_gls/pdf/fatigue.pdf. Accessed February 21, 2013.

89. Vogelzang NJ, Breitbart W, Cella D, et al. Patient, caregiver, and oncologist perceptions of cancer-related fatigue: results of a tripart assessment survey. The Fatigue Coalition. Semin Hematol 1997;34(3 Suppl 2):4–12.

90. Collado-Hidalgo A, Bower JE, Ganz PA, et al. Inflammatory biomarkers for persistent fatigue in breast cancer survivors. Clin Cancer Res 2006;12(9):2759–66.

91. Cella D, Davis K, Breitbart W, et al. Cancer-related fatigue: prevalence of proposed diagnostic criteria in a United States sample of cancer survivors. J Clin Oncol 2001;19(14):3385–91.

92. Bower JE, Ganz PA, Desmond KA, et al. Fatigue in long-term breast carcinoma survivors: a longitudinal investigation. Cancer 2006;106(4):751–8.

93. Available at: http://www.uptodate.com/contents/cancer-related-fatigue-treatment. Accessed February 21, 2013.

94. Zee PC, Ancoli-Israel S, Participants W. Does effective management of sleep disorders reduce cancer-related fatigue? Drugs 2009;69:29–41.

95. Cramp F, Byron-Daniel J. Exercise for the management of cancer-related fatigue in adults. Cochrane Database Syst Rev 2012;(11):CD006145.

96. Barton DL, Soori GS, Bauer BA, et al. Pilot study of Panax quinquefolius (American ginseng) to improve cancer-related fatigue: a randomized, double-blind, dose-finding evaluation: NCCTG trial N03CA. Support Care Cancer 2010;18(2):179–87.

97. Sparano JA, Wang M, Martino S, et al. Weekly paclitaxel in the adjuvant treatment of breast cancer. N Engl J Med 2008;358(16):1663–71.

98. Rugo H, Barry W, Moreno-Aspitia A, et al. Randomized phase III trial of weekly paclitaxel (P) compared to weekly nanoparticle albumin bound nab-paclitaxel (NP) or ixabepilone (Ix) with or without bevacizumab (B) as first-line therapy for locally recurrent or metastatic breast cancer (MBC). J Clin Oncol 2012; 30(Suppl) [abstract CRA1002].

99. Peters CM, Jimenez-Andrade JM, Jonas BM, et al. Intravenous paclitaxel administration in the rat induces a peripheral sensory neuropathy characterized by macrophage infiltration and injury to sensory neurons and their supporting cells. Exp Neurol 2007;203(1):42–54.

100. Loprinzi CL, Reeves BN, Dakhil SR, et al. Natural history of paclitaxel-associated acute pain syndrome: prospective cohort study NCCTG N08C1. J Clin Oncol 2011;29(11):1472–8.
101. Rao R, Michalak J, Sloan J, et al. Efficacy of gabapentin in the management of chemotherapy-induced peripheral neuropathy: a phase 3 randomized, double-blind, placebo-controlled, crossover trial (N00C3). Cancer 2007;110(9): 2110–8.
102. Lavoie Smith EM, Pang H, Cirrincione C, et al. A phase III double blind trial of duloxetine to treat painful chemotherapy-induced peripheral neuropathy (CIPN). J Clin Oncol 2012;30(Suppl) [abstract CRA9013].
103. Smith TJ, Coyne PJ, Parker GL, et al. Pilot trial of a patient-specific cutaneous electrostimulation device (MC5-A Calmare(R)) for chemotherapy-induced peripheral neuropathy. J Pain Symptom Manage 2010;40(6):883–91.
104. Barton DL, Wos EJ, Qin R, et al. A double-blind, placebo-controlled trial of a topical treatment for chemotherapy-induced peripheral neuropathy: NCCTG trial N06CA. Support Care Cancer 2011;19(6):833–41.
105. Storey D, Colvin L, Scott A, et al. Treatment of chemotherapy-induced peripheral neuropathy (CIPN) with topical menthol: a phase I study. J Clin Oncol 2010; 28(15 Suppl):9129.
106. Bird BR, Swain SM. Cardiac toxicity in breast cancer survivors: review of potential cardiac problems. Clin Cancer Res 2008;14(1):14–24.
107. Cardinale D, Colombo A, Lamantia G, et al. Anthracycline-induced cardiomyopathy: clinical relevance and response to pharmacologic therapy. J Am Coll Cardiol 2010;55(3):213–20.
108. Ryberg M, Nielsen D, Skovsgaard T, et al. Epirubicin cardiotoxicity: an analysis of 469 patients with metastatic breast cancer. J Clin Oncol 1998;16(11): 3502–8.
109. Trudeau M, Charbonneau F, Gelmon K, et al. Selection of adjuvant chemotherapy for treatment of node-positive breast cancer. Lancet Oncol 2005; 6(11):886–98.
110. Perez EA, Suman VJ, Davidson NE, et al. Effect of doxorubicin plus cyclophosphamide on left ventricular ejection fraction in patients with breast cancer in the North Central Cancer Treatment Group N9831 Intergroup Adjuvant Trial. J Clin Oncol 2004;22(18):3700–4.
111. Felker GM, Thompson RE, Hare JM, et al. Underlying causes and long-term survival in patients with initially unexplained cardiomyopathy. N Engl J Med 2000; 342(15):1077–84.
112. Torti FM, Bristow MR, Howes AE, et al. Reduced cardiotoxicity of doxorubicin delivered on a weekly schedule. Assessment by endomyocardial biopsy. Ann Intern Med 1983;99(6):745–9.
113. Benjamin RC, Chawla SP, Hortobagyi G. Clinical applications of continuous infusion chemotherapy and concomitant radiation therapy. In: Rosenthal C, Rotman M, editors. Clinical applications of continuous infusion chemotherapy and concomitant radiation therapy. New York: Plenum Press; 1986. p. 19–25.
114. Ewer MS, Von Hoff DD, Benjamin RS. A historical perspective of anthracycline cardiotoxicity. Heart Fail Clin 2011;7(3):363–72.
115. Marty M, Espie M, Llombart A, et al. Multicenter randomized phase III study of the cardioprotective effect of dexrazoxane (Cardioxane) in advanced/metastatic breast cancer patients treated with anthracycline-based chemotherapy. Ann Oncol 2006;17(4):614–22.

116. Piccart-Gebhart MJ, Procter M, Leyland-Jones B, et al. Trastuzumab after adjuvant chemotherapy in HER2-positive breast cancer. N Engl J Med 2005;353(16): 1659–72.

117. Slamon D, Eiermann W, Robert N, et al. Phase III randomized trial comparing doxorubicin and cyclophosphamide followed by docetaxel (AC -> T) with doxorubicin and cyclophosphamide followed by docetaxel and trastuzumab (AC -> TH) with docetaxel, carboplatin and trastuzumab (TCH) in Her2neu positive early breast cancer patients: BCIRG 006 Study. Cancer Res 2009;69(24):500s.

118. Maitland ML, Bakris GL, Black HR, et al. Initial assessment, surveillance, and management of blood pressure in patients receiving vascular endothelial growth factor signaling pathway inhibitors. J Natl Cancer Inst 2010;102(9):596–604.

119. Bouillon K, Haddy N, Delaloge S, et al. Long-term cardiovascular mortality after radiotherapy for breast cancer. J Am Coll Cardiol 2011;57(4):445–52.

120. Taylor CW, Povall JM, McGale P, et al. Cardiac dose from tangential breast cancer radiotherapy in the year 2006. Int J Radiat Oncol Biol Phys 2008; 72(2):501–7.

121. Amir E, Seruga B, Niraula S, et al. Toxicity of adjuvant endocrine therapy in postmenopausal breast cancer patients: a systematic review and meta-analysis. J Natl Cancer Inst 2011;103(17):1299–309.

122. Lenihan DJ, Cardinale DM. Late cardiac effects of cancer treatment. J Clin Oncol 2012;30(30):3657–64.

123. Cardinale D, Sandri MT. Role of biomarkers in chemotherapy-induced cardiotoxicity. Prog Cardiovasc Dis 2010;53(2):121–9.

124. Howard RA, Gilbert ES, Chen BE, et al. Leukemia following breast cancer: an international population-based study of 376,825 women. Breast Cancer Res Treat 2007;105(3):359–68.

125. Arslan C, Ozdemir E, Dogan E, et al. Secondary hematological malignancies after treatment of non-metastatic breast cancer. J BUON 2011;16(4):744–50.

126. Patt DA, Duan Z, Fang S, et al. Acute myeloid leukemia after adjuvant breast cancer therapy in older women: understanding risk. J Clin Oncol 2007;25(25): 3871–6.

127. Wood ME, Vogel V, Ng A, et al. Second malignant neoplasms: assessment and strategies for risk reduction. J Clin Oncol 2012;30(30):3734–45.

128. Kirova YM, De Rycke Y, Gambotti L, et al. Second malignancies after breast cancer: the impact of different treatment modalities. Br J Cancer 2008;98(5):870–4.

129. Andersson M, Jensen MB, Engholm G, et al. Risk of second primary cancer among patients with early operable breast cancer registered or randomised in Danish Breast Cancer Cooperative Group (DBCG) protocols of the 77, 82 and 89 programmes during 1977-2001. Acta Oncol 2008;47(4):755–64.

130. Martin MG, Welch JS, Luo J, et al. Therapy related acute myeloid leukemia in breast cancer survivors, a population-based study. Breast Cancer Res Treat 2009;118(3):593–8.

131. Hershman D, Neugut AI, Jacobson JS, et al. Acute myeloid leukemia or myelodysplastic syndrome following use of granulocyte colony-stimulating factors during breast cancer adjuvant chemotherapy. J Natl Cancer Inst 2007;99(3):196–205.

132. Available at: http://www.nccn.org. 2012. Accessed February 21, 2013.

133. Hewitt MG, Greenfield S, Stovall E. Committee on cancer survivorship: improving care and quality of life National Cancer Policy Board. Delivering cancer survivorship care In: Institute of Medicine and National Research Council of the National Academies, editor. From cancer patient to cancer survivor: lost in transition. Washington, DC: The National Academies Press; 2005. p. 187–321.

134. Grunfeld E, Julian JA, Pond G, et al. Evaluating survivorship care plans: results of a randomized, clinical trial of patients with breast cancer. J Clin Oncol 2011; 29(36):4755–62.

135. Earle CC, Ganz PA. Cancer survivorship care: don't let the perfect be the enemy of the good. J Clin Oncol 2012;30(30):3764–8.

136. Loprinzi CL, Barton DL, Sloan JA, et al. Mayo Clinic and North Central Cancer Treatment Group hot flash studies: a 20-year experience. Menopause 2008; 15(4 Pt 1):655–60.

137. Loprinzi CL, Sloan J, Stearns V, et al. Newer antidepressants and gabapentin for hot flashes: an individual patient pooled analysis. J Clin Oncol 2009;27(17): 2831–7.

138. Loprinzi CL, Levitt R, Barton D, et al. Phase III comparison of depomedroxyprogesterone acetate to venlafaxine for managing hot flashes: North Central Cancer Treatment Group Trial N99C7. J Clin Oncol 2006;24(9):1409–14.

139. Loprinzi CL, Kugler JW, Sloan JA, et al. Venlafaxine in management of hot flashes in survivors of breast cancer: a randomised controlled trial. Lancet 2000;356(9247):2059–63.

140. Loprinzi CL, Sloan JA, Perez EA, et al. Phase III evaluation of fluoxetine for treatment of hot flashes. J Clin Oncol 2002;20(6):1578–83.

141. Stearns V, Beebe KL, Iyengar M, et al. Paroxetine controlled release in the treatment of menopausal hot flashes: a randomized controlled trial. JAMA 2003; 289(21):2827–34.

142. Stearns V, Slack R, Greep N, et al. Paroxetine is an effective treatment for hot flashes: results from a prospective randomized clinical trial. J Clin Oncol 2005;23(28):6919–30.

143. Kimmick GG, Lovato J, McQuellon R, et al. Randomized, double-blind, placebo-controlled, crossover study of sertraline (Zoloft) for the treatment of hot flashes in women with early stage breast cancer taking tamoxifen. Breast J 2006;12(2): 114–22.

144. Gordon PR, Kerwin JP, Boesen KG, et al. Sertraline to treat hot flashes: a randomized controlled, double-blind, crossover trial in a general population. Menopause 2006;13(4):568–75.

145. Grady D, Cohen B, Tice J, et al. Ineffectiveness of sertraline for treatment of menopausal hot flushes: a randomized controlled trial. Obstet Gynecol 2007; 109(4):823–30.

146. Guttuso T Jr, Kurlan R, McDermott MP, et al. Gabapentin's effects on hot flashes in postmenopausal women: a randomized controlled trial. Obstet Gynecol 2003; 101(2):337–45.

147. Reddy SY, Warner H, Guttuso T Jr, et al. Gabapentin, estrogen, and placebo for treating hot flushes: a randomized controlled trial. Obstet Gynecol 2006;108(1): 41–8.

148. Barton DL, Loprinzi CL, Quella SK, et al. Prospective evaluation of vitamin E for hot flashes in breast cancer survivors. J Clin Oncol 1998;16(2):495–500.

149. Quella SK, Loprinzi CL, Barton DL, et al. Evaluation of soy phytoestrogens for the treatment of hot flashes in breast cancer survivors: a North Central Cancer Treatment Group Trial. J Clin Oncol 2000;18(5):1068–74.

150. Pockaj BA, Gallagher JG, Loprinzi CL, et al. Phase III double-blind, randomized, placebo-controlled crossover trial of black cohosh in the management of hot flashes: NCCTG Trial N01CC1. J Clin Oncol 2006;24(18):2836–41.

What Does Breast Cancer Treatment Cost and What Is It Worth?

Michael J. Hassett, MD, MPH[a,b,*], Elena B. Elkin, PhD[c]

KEYWORDS

- Breast cancer • Cost • Value • Cost-effectiveness • Chemotherapy
- Hospitalization

KEY POINTS

- Breast cancer care is costly, and future projections suggest that costs are likely to increase substantially over time.
- Medications and hospitalizations account for a significant proportion of breast cancer costs. Payers are beginning to introduce policies to constrain the growth of costs.
- Some breast cancer treatments may provide better value than others. Cost-effectiveness analysis is the preferred method for assessing the health benefits of medical interventions relative to their costs.
- The pressure for providers and patients to consider costs when making treatment decisions is likely to increase.

INTRODUCTION

Breast cancer is the most commonly diagnosed nondermatologic cancer and the second leading cause of cancer death for women in the United States and, thus, is responsible for substantial morbidity and mortality. Advances in screening and treatment have led to significant improvements in outcomes but have required more and more costly interventions. For these reasons, it should come as no surprise that breast cancer now accounts for the greatest share of cancer-related spending in the United States. Although the costs of breast cancer care are substantial and increasing,

Funding Sources: Dr M.J. Hassett: Susan G. Komen for the Cure, NCI, AHRQ. Dr E.B. Elkin: NCI.
Conflicts of Interest: None.
[a] Department of Medicine, Harvard Medical School, 250 Longwood Avenue, Boston, MA 02115, USA; [b] Department of Medical Oncology, Dana-Farber Cancer Institute, 450 Brookline Avenue, Boston, MA 02215, USA; [c] Department of Epidemiology & Biostatistics, Memorial Sloan-Kettering Cancer Center, 1275 York Avenue, New York, NY 10065, USA
* Corresponding author. Department of Medical Oncology, Dana-Farber Cancer Institute, 450 Brookline Avenue, Boston, MA 02215.
E-mail address: michael_hassett@dfci.harvard.edu

Hematol Oncol Clin N Am 27 (2013) 829–841
http://dx.doi.org/10.1016/j.hoc.2013.05.011
0889-8588/13/$ – see front matter © 2013 Elsevier Inc. All rights reserved.

hemonc.theclinics.com

resources are limited and decisions about which services should and should not be covered are inevitable. In fact, these decisions are already being made; but many people question how these decisions are made and who is making them. In this article, the authors review the magnitude of spending on breast cancer, describe how costs are changing over time, and highlight which treatments and phases of illness have the greatest impact on spending. The authors outline the current efforts to control spending and discuss the role of cost-effectiveness analysis (CEA) as a tool to characterize the value of therapies, facilitate decision making, and set priorities. The authors also explore the roles and responsibilities of providers to determine what breast cancer care is worth.

HOW MUCH WE SPEND AND HOW WE SPEND IT

Annual spending on all cancer care in the United States exceeds $125 billion, and forecasts predict that spending will continue to climb in the years to come.[1] Breast cancer is responsible for the largest share of cancer-related spending, an estimated $16.5 billion or 13% of all cancer-related spending in 2010.[1] Past data demonstrate that the rate of growth in spending for breast cancer has exceeded that observed for lung, colorectal, or prostate cancer.[2] Future projections suggest that breast cancer spending will exceed $20 billion in 2020.[3]

Spending on breast cancer is distributed across the continuum of care, with approximately 23% going to evaluation and management in the year after diagnosis, 41% covering continuing care, and 36% being spent during the last year of life. It is not surprising that continuing care accounts for the largest share of lifetime costs, considering the relatively long survival of patients with breast cancer. The only cancer with a larger proportion of spending going to continuing care is prostate cancer. When compared with other cancers, the total spending for the initial phase of breast cancer care ranks fourth, and it ranks first for the continuing and end-of-life phases of care.

Several investigators have described the per-person costs of breast cancer care. A detailed review by Campbell and Ramsey,[4] which included studies conducted through 2006, found estimates of lifetime direct medical costs ranged from $20,000 to $100,000. Although total costs were greatest during the continuing phase of care, the cost per unit of time was greatest during the initial and terminal phases of care. More contemporary estimates have placed the average annualized net costs for breast cancer care among women younger than 65 years at $27,700 per year during the initial phase, $2200 per year during the continuing phase, and $94,300 per year during the last year of life. For patients aged 65 years and older, costs are lower, especially during the last year of life ($62,900 per year).[1]

An analysis of Medicare data demonstrated that the distribution of costs in the year after diagnosis by type of therapy was 25% for breast cancer surgery, 15% for chemotherapy, 11% for radiation therapy, 18% for other hospitalizations, and 31% for other services.[2] The total costs attributable to breast-conserving therapy and radiation therapy are approximately $15,000 to $26,000, to mastectomy $10,000 to $13,000, and to mastectomy with reconstruction $23,000.[5,6] Newer radiation techniques, such as hyperfractionation and partial-breast irradiation, may be less costly than traditional whole-breast radiation therapy.[7,8] Intensity-modulated radiation therapy, a particularly expensive form of radiation therapy, is not part of routine care for breast cancer.

The 15% of breast cancer costs that have been attributed to chemotherapy for Medicare patients older than 65 years likely represents an underestimate because chemotherapy utilization in women younger than 65 years is significantly higher. When younger patients are included, chemotherapy for curative intent consistently represents one of the most substantial breast cancer costs, ranging from $23,000 to $31,000 per patient.[4,9] Unfortunately, these studies did not include newer, costly chemotherapy agents, so it is hard to know the extent to which these estimates can be generalized to patients receiving care today. One year of trastuzumab, for example, adds approximately $50,000 to $65,000 to the cost of therapy.[10,11] Chemotherapy can also lead to secondary costs from serious adverse effects, such as febrile neutropenia, which amount to between $1000 and $5000 per patient.[9,12,13]

Patients with breast cancer experience significant and burdensome direct and indirect medical costs. For example, out-of-pocket medical costs for patients with breast cancer and their caregivers were estimated at approximately $2700 to $7900, respectively. Out-of-pocket costs may be lower in other countries (eg, $1000 in Canada).[14] Although most patients who work before they are diagnosed with breast cancer continue to work after completing therapy, many lose time at work during or after their treatment. Lost wages from time spent on treatment and disability have been estimated at $4300 and $5900, respectively.[15–18] At a national level, total lost-productivity costs from breast cancer deaths were estimated to be $10.9 billion in 2010; they accounted for 8% of all cancer-related productivity losses, exceeded only by lung and colorectal cancer.[19]

WHAT WE GET FOR WHAT WE SPEND

Although the United States spends substantially more on health care ($8000 per capita or 16.2% of the gross domestic product [GDP]) than any other country (<$5500 per capita or <12% of GDP),[20] its outcomes are not necessarily better and are sometimes worse. For example, an international analysis found years of life lost caused by malignant neoplasm was 895 per 100,000 people in the United States, whereas it was 847 in Canada, 800 in Australia, and 725 in Japan.[21] Interestingly, breast cancer 5-year relative survival rates are higher for the United States (90.5%) than for many other developed countries (eg, 87.1% in Canada, 86.1% in Sweden, or 85.2% in the Netherlands).[22]

Studies have demonstrated clear improvements in the outcomes experienced by patients with breast cancer in the United States over the last 2 decades. In 1990, the age-adjusted mortality rate from invasive breast cancer was 33 per 100,000, whereas in 2009 it had fallen to 22 per 100,000.[23] Since 1990, the annual death rate from breast cancer declined by more than 1.8% per year.[24] Simulation studies suggest that half of this improvement is attributable to screening mammography and half is caused by the use of adjuvant systemic therapy (ie, chemotherapy and hormone therapy).[25]

Improvements in survival that have been attributed to adjuvant systemic therapy are the result of 2 parallel trends. First, there have been significant advances in the efficacy of adjuvant therapies. For example, studies have demonstrated improved outcomes for patients treated with taxanes,[26–28] dose-dense therapy,[29] trastuzumab,[30,31] and aromatase inhibitors.[32] Second, the rate of utilization of adjuvant therapies has increased over time.[33] Despite these gains and widespread efforts to disseminate treatment recommendations via clinical practice guidelines,[34–36] many patients with breast cancer still do not receive proven, recommended therapies.[37–41] The National Cancer Policy Board concluded that "for many Americans with cancer, there is a wide gulf between what could be construed as the ideal and the reality of their experience with cancer care."[42]

There are different theories regarding how quality-improvement efforts could impact costs. Improving quality could reduce spending by cutting hospitalizations, limiting complications, or other mechanisms.[43] Alternatively, improving quality could increase spending by encouraging the use of recommended services that were not previously being delivered.[44,45] A recent systematic review of 61 studies of general medical care found that the association between quality and cost was inconsistent.[46] Few studies have evaluated this relationship for patients with cancer.[47–49] A Surveillance, Epidemiology, and End Results/Medicare–based analysis of chemotherapy for colorectal cancer care found that high-spending regions were more likely to use chemotherapy, regardless of whether it was recommended (stage III), discretionary (stage II), or not recommended (stage I). In an analysis of women with newly diagnosed breast cancer, the authors found that providing recommended therapy was associated with higher cost, whereas avoiding unnecessary therapy was associated with lower cost.[48]

Many of the aforementioned cost estimates focused on treatments provided to patients with local-regional disease. An analysis of women with metastatic disease who were older than 65 years found average spending in the 6 months after diagnosis was approximately $28,000,[47] and the magnitude of spending in the 6 months that preceded death was similar. Although there was significant regional variation in spending, there was not significant regional variation in survival. In the last month of life, the percent of patients who used specific services included the following: more than 1 emergency department visit (40%), more than 1 hospitalization (27%), intensive care unit admission (19%), chemotherapy in the last 14 days of life (17%), and hospice (60%). Inpatient hospitalizations accounted for most of the expenditures and accounted for much of the observed regional variation in spending.

CONTROLLING THE COSTS OF CANCER CARE

Medical therapies are one of the major drivers for the growth of the cost of breast cancer care. Many medications are available to treat breast cancer. A compendium compiled by the National Comprehensive Cancer Network lists 36 medications, including 16 cytotoxic agents, 11 hormonal agents, and 9 biologics/antibodies.[50] Five of these agents were approved for breast cancer in the last 3 years (eribulin, denosumab, everolimus, pertuzumab, and ado-trastuzumab emtansine), and many more agents are the focus of ongoing clinical trials (the Web site clinicaltrials.gov listed >1200 open interventional studies for breast cancer as of April 2013).

A review of spending on cancer drugs by Peter Bach[51] describes how monthly median drug costs are greater for recently approved cancer medications compared with those approved in the more distant past. A group of hematology/oncology specialists[52] reported that 11 of 12 cancer drugs approved by the US Food and Drug Administration in 2012 were priced at more than $100,000 per year. Moreover, the monthly costs of some existing cancer drugs have also increased.[51] These changes, together with an increase in the rate of use of these agents, have contributed significantly to the substantial growth in cancer spending outlined earlier. There are several potential explanations for increases in per-unit drug costs: (1) drug development costs have increased; (2) newer drugs are more targeted than older drugs, so they cannot be used in as many patients; (3) drug approval decisions in the United States are not based on cost; (4) laws and regulatory policies limit payers' ability to negotiate lower drug prices; and (5) there is a general willingness to pay for newer therapies, sometimes without much consideration of the magnitude of clinical benefit they confer.

Several reviewers have outlined the relatively modest incremental benefits associated with new cancer therapies, and some have asserted that costs may be increasing faster than health benefits.[51,53–55] In some cases, providers have elected to forgo the use of payer-approved therapies because they offer marginal benefits and confer substantial costs (eg, a prominent cancer network decided not to use ziv-aflibercept after it was approved in 2012[56,57]). Newer therapies may tend to confer smaller marginal benefits than their predecessors because, as outcomes improve, it becomes harder for newer treatments to yield the same magnitude of benefits conferred by older treatments. Also, newer treatments tend to be more targeted, so their impact on population health is potentially smaller; a nonspecific agent, such as paclitaxel, can be used to treat more patients than a targeted agent, such as pertuzumab.

High drug costs are undesirable because they limit access to potentially beneficial drugs for those with limited means, they preclude spending on other goods and services, and they are unsustainable. Health care payers have recognized the substantial contribution of cancer medicines to the growth in cancer spending and have taken several steps to control expenditures[51]:

1. Coverage for specific treatments has been restricted. A decade ago, epoetin alfa and darbepoetin were the most costly clinic drugs for the Medicare program, accounting for more than $5 billion (or 23%) of all clinic drug expenditures.[54] A change in the coverage policy was made in 2007 that restricted the use of these agents to selected patients. Although the need to make a change was prompted by cost, the new coverage decision was based only on what was medically reasonable and necessary for the Medicare population. As a result of the change, many oncologists had reported a substantial reduction in the use of these agents by 2009.[58] Similar efforts to control costs by limiting overuse have been applied to other targeted cancer medications, such as trastuzumab.
2. Reimbursement rates for specific medications have been reduced. In 2003, the Medicare Modernization Act reduced reimbursement for chemotherapy to 106% of the average national sales price over the previous two-quarters. Jacobson and colleagues[59] demonstrated that this resulted in a significant reduction in the use of the agents most affected by this change (eg, paclitaxel and carboplatin) in the months leading up to its implementation. Private payers use several different mechanisms to change reimbursement rates, most often through the contractual arrangements they form with providers.

Hospitalizations are a second major driver for the growth of cancer care costs. Because this issue has a broad impact that extends well beyond patients with cancer, payers have engaged actively in efforts to limit hospitalization-related expenditures. For decades, payers have used bundled payments to reimburse a standardized payment amount for each admission based on the diagnosis, regardless of the length of stay or specific services provided during the hospitalization. Although this may reduce the cost per admission, it does not affect the overall number of admissions. To that end, payers are trying to identify potentially avoidable hospitalizations (eg, readmissions within 30 days or hospitalizations for ambulatory-care sensitive conditions), and they are introducing financial penalties to reduce the frequency of these events.[60] The impact of these efforts on oncology patients and providers remains unclear. Unfortunately, current measures of avoidable hospitalizations have not been validated among patients with cancer. It may be harder to identify avoidable hospitalizations for patients with cancer because admissions are a frequent component of oncology care: for initial evaluation and management, symptoms and complications of the disease, scheduled treatments, and treatment-related adverse effects.

HOW WE ASSESS THE VALUE OF MEDICAL TREATMENTS

The increasing costs and sometime marginal benefits of new cancer therapies have led to the assertion that some therapies may not always be worth what they cost.

For example, among women with taxane- and anthracycline-resistant metastatic breast cancer, ixabepilone in combination with capecitabine increases progression-free survival by 1.6 months, compared with capecitabine alone.[61,62] But at a price of more than $4000 per cycle, ixabepilone increases the average cost of treatment by more than $20,000. Is one progression-free month worth $12,000? Is this a good value? In the same population of women with previously treated metastatic breast cancer, eribulin adds as much as $25,000 to the cost of treatment, compared with a single-agent regimen, for an extension of 1.5 months of progression-free survival.[63,64] If we are willing to pay $12,000 for an additional progression-free month, should we be willing to pay $16,000? How do we decide if these treatments provide value sufficient to justify their additional cost?

The preferred method for assessing the health benefits of medical interventions relative to their costs is CEA.[65] This approach compares the incremental costs and the incremental health benefits of a new treatment with those associated with an older, standard treatment. The result is the incremental cost-effectiveness ratio (ICER), a comparative, standardized, objective description of the value associated with a new treatment. In a CEA, the effectiveness of an intervention is defined in nonmonetary units, such as cases of disease prevented, lives saved, or life-years saved. Survival outcomes may be adjusted to reflect quality of life, yielding a measure of effectiveness known as quality-adjusted life-years (QALYs). QALYs are a preferred metric for CEAs because they reflect the impact of an intervention on both morbidity and mortality and because they are comparable across treatment modalities and disease areas. These factors are important to consider, particularly when CEA results are used to inform policy decisions.

CEA has been applied to numerous interventions throughout the continuum of breast cancer care, from risk reduction and screening interventions to treatment modalities for early stage disease and supportive care for advanced disease. As demonstrated by the wide range of published ICER estimates, some breast cancer interventions offer substantial value, whereas others offer only a modest benefit at a very high cost. For example, adjusting all published estimates to 2012 US dollars, adjuvant tamoxifen for a 45-year-old woman with node-positive, Estrogen receptor (ER)-positive breast cancer is associated with an ICER of $7000 per QALY when compared with no therapy; adjuvant chemotherapy for a 45-year-old woman with node-negative, hormone receptor–negative breast cancer is associated with an ICER of $8000 per QALY when compared with no therapy.[66] In the metastatic setting, adding bevacizumab to paclitaxel costs $245,000 per QALY compared with paclitaxel alone.[67] For patients who have bony disease, denosumab costs $697,000 per QALY compared with zoledronic acid.[68]

Comparing ICERs shows how the cost-effectiveness of an intervention may be strongly influenced by characteristics of the patient population (such as age and risk of recurrence), the way the intervention is applied (selectively or universally), and the treatment setting. For example, the ICER for contralateral prophylactic mastectomy (vs no prophylactic surgery) is about $5000 per QALY in 45-year-old women, but it is more than $100,000 per QALY in 65-year-old women.[69] Targeted bisphosphonate therapy for fracture prevention in postmenopausal women receiving adjuvant aromatase inhibitor therapy has an ICER of approximately $92,000 per QALY, whereas universal bisphosphonate therapy in the same population costs almost $300,000 per QALY.[70] The addition of trastuzumab to an adjuvant chemotherapy regimen for localized disease is associated with an ICER of $47,000 per QALY,[11] whereas HER2 testing and the addition of trastuzumab to chemotherapy for metastatic disease are associated with an ICER of $185,000 per QALY.[71]

CEAs and other methods can provide useful information about the comparative value of different medical interventions, but they do not inherently tell us how much is too much to spend or how much we should be willing to pay for health benefits. We still must decide where to draw the line. The frequently quoted threshold of $50,000 per QALY dates back at least to the early 1980s.[72] This threshold has often been justified because it approximates the estimated ICER for renal dialysis in patients with end-stage renal disease. Following the Medicare program's decision to cover this service, one could argue that it represents a societal threshold of willingness to pay for gains in population health.[73] However, the persistence of this threshold fails to account for inflation over time. If we were willing to pay $50,000 per QALY in 1982, we should be willing to pay much more 3 decades later.[74] Adjusting for overall inflation, $50,000 in 1982 now has a value that exceeds $115,000; adjusting for inflation based on the cost of medical goods and services specifically, this threshold approaches $200,000 in today's dollars. By several other measures, societal willingness to pay for health gains in the United States is greater than $100,000 per QALY and is likely in the range of $140,000 to $200,000 per QALY.[75,76]

Economic evaluations, such as CEAs, have been criticized as a step toward rationing and, therefore, denying care to patients in need.[77] It is the application of a threshold ratio, rather than the method itself, that is, presumably, the cause of concern. However, using systematic approaches, like CEA, to understand the return on investments in health acknowledges the simple, but often ignored, reality that resources are limited. Every dollar spent on health care is a dollar not spent elsewhere. Recent statements from oncologists protesting the high cost of new cancer drugs and a formulary decision at one prominent hospital against a drug that yielded a similar magnitude of benefit at double the price of a competing drug suggest that these realities are becoming more difficult to ignore.[52–55,78]

WHO MAKES COST DECISIONS AND HOW THEY SHOULD BE MADE

Any effort to distinguish between aspects of breast cancer care that are cost worthwhile and those that are not requires discussing not only how cost decisions are made but also who should make them. In the United States, payers make most cost-related decisions, and the federal government does relatively little to regulate health care spending. The US Food and Drug Administration, for example, only considers safety and effectiveness when making coverage determinations; it does not consider cost-effectiveness. In many other countries, governmental agencies do make coverage and reimbursement decisions that incorporate cost worthiness. A study of coverage decisions for anticancer medications made between 2004 and 2008 found that countries that considered cost-effectiveness had more restrictions and longer time to coverage than the United States.[79]

Historically, insured patients in the United States have not spent much time considering costs when making health care decisions. However, efforts to shift more costs to patients (for example, by increasing copayments and raising deductibles) may change this. And recent payment reform vehicles, such as accountable care organizations and patient-centered medical homes, may further increase the attention patients give to costs. The impact of these new reimbursement mechanisms for oncology care remains unclear. Regardless, out-of-pocket health care costs for patients with cancer are rising, increasing the burden placed on patients. This burden could potentially limit access to expensive treatments, especially for economically disadvantaged populations; and it could cause significant distress. A recent study by Ramsey and colleagues[80] demonstrated higher bankruptcy rates after a cancer diagnosis.

Providers are much more likely to report that they should be responsible for determining whether a drug provides good value than to suggest that patients, the government, or payers should decide.[81] Considering their role as patient advocates, providers may think that they have a duty to offer any treatment that yields a net benefit regardless of its cost. However, as the share of costs borne by patients increases, there may be a greater need for providers to discuss costs with patients. Patients have reported an interest in discussing health care costs with providers.[82] If providers engage in these discussions, they should be prepared to explain the differences in costs and outcomes for the available options. When deciding whether or not treatments offer good value, providers must honestly address their competing interests as taxpayers, business owners, and patient advocates.

Considering that the current rate of growth in health care costs is viewed as unsustainable, cost-related decisions are inevitable. Historically, providers have not considered costs when making most health care decisions, but this is likely to change as new payment mechanisms transfer more economic risk to providers. Providers have a unique and valuable perspective to contribute. There are several ways in which providers could engage in these decisions:

1. Advocate for practical clinical research studies that have the potential to influence health outcomes and costs. At present, the aims of clinical research studies are heavily influenced by pharmaceutical companies who are in the business of developing new drugs and have a fiduciary responsibility to their investors. A large phase III study of a third-in-class drug may have a modest impact on outcomes and could increase costs significantly, whereas a study that describes a new mechanism for improving compliance with an existing generic drug could have a significant impact on outcomes and be cost saving. Currently, resources are much more likely to be directed toward the former study than the latter one.
2. Current medication coverage policies, mostly developed by payers, can vary considerably and often impose significant procedural burdens. Providers should consider taking a more active role in the development of drug reimbursement policies and should encourage the implementation of a consistent, transparent, common-sense approach to drug utilization that prioritizes effectiveness and safety but also considers cost. CEA, even if used without the more politically charged threshold ratio, is the best available tool to inform this process.
3. Providers should work with patients and payers to reduce costly, potentially avoidable, undesirable admissions, especially for patients with metastatic or relapsed disease. Patients consistently report a strong preference to remain at home if possible; but the resources, infrastructure, and wherewithal needed to support this goal are often lacking.
4. Providers should develop the skills and resources needed to ascertain the potential financial impact of treatments on patients and their families and to discuss costs and outcomes of various treatment options with patients.

After decades of discussion about the substantial costs of health care, there now seems to be growing consensus that something needs to be done. Payers are doing more to rein in costs. The efforts of professional societies to identify unnecessary tests, procedures, and treatments are another reflection of this trend.[83] The American Society of Clinical Oncology has participated in this effort and has identified a top-5 list of common, costly procedures in oncology that are not supported by evidence and could represent opportunities to improve value.[84] However, efforts to control costs will probably not end here, and aggressive cost-containment initiatives may pose risks to the health and financial well-being of patients and providers. Active engagement from providers and patients early in the process will be critical to ensuring that the risks do not outweigh the rewards.

REFERENCES

1. Mariotto AB, Yabroff KR, Shao Y, et al. Projections of the cost of cancer care in the United States: 2010-2020. J Natl Cancer Inst 2011;103(2):117–28.
2. Warren JL, Yabroff KR, Meekins A, et al. Evaluation of trends in the cost of initial cancer treatment. J Natl Cancer Inst 2008;100(12):888–97.
3. Yabroff KR, Lund J, Kepka D, et al. Economic burden of cancer in the United States. estimates, projections, and future research. Cancer Epidemiol Biomarkers Prev 2011;20(10):2006–14.
4. Campbell JD, Ramsey SD. The costs of treating breast cancer in the US: a synthesis of published evidence. Pharmacoeconomics 2009;27(3):199–209.
5. Barlow WE, Taplin SH, Yoshida CK, et al. Cost comparison of mastectomy versus breast-conserving therapy for early-stage breast cancer. J Natl Cancer Inst 2001;93(6):447–55.
6. Palit TK, Miltenburg DM, Brunicardi FC. Cost analysis of breast conservation surgery compared with modified radical mastectomy with and without reconstruction. Am J Surg 2000;179(6):441–5.
7. Lanni T, Keisch M, Shah C, et al. A cost comparison analysis of adjuvant radiation therapy techniques after breast-conserving surgery. Breast J 2013;19(2):162–7.
8. Suh WW, Pierce LJ, Vicini FA, et al. A cost comparison analysis of partial versus whole-breast irradiation after breast-conserving surgery for early-stage breast cancer. Int J Radiat Oncol Biol Phys 2005;62(3):790–6.
9. Hassett MJ, O'Malley AJ, Pakes JR, et al. Frequency and cost of chemotherapy-related serious adverse effects in a population sample of women with breast cancer. J Natl Cancer Inst 2006;98(16):1108–17.
10. Hedden L, O'Reilly S, Lohrisch C, et al. Assessing the real-world cost-effectiveness of adjuvant trastuzumab in HER-2/neu positive breast cancer. Oncologist 2012;17(2):164–71.
11. Kurian AW, Thompson RN, Gaw AF, et al. A cost-effectiveness analysis of adjuvant trastuzumab regimens in early HER2/neu-positive breast cancer. J Clin Oncol 2007;25(6):634–41.
12. Bennett CL, Calhoun EA. Evaluating the total costs of chemotherapy-induced febrile neutropenia: results from a pilot study with community oncology cancer patients. Oncologist 2007;12(4):478–83.
13. Gandhi SK, Arguelles L, Boyer JG. Economic impact of neutropenia and febrile neutropenia in breast cancer: estimates from two national databases. Pharmacotherapy 2001;21(6):684–90.
14. Lauzier S, Levesque P, Mondor M, et al. Out-of-pocket costs in the year after early breast cancer among Canadian women and spouses. J Natl Cancer Inst 2013;105(4):280–92.
15. Chirikos TN, Russell-Jacobs A, Cantor AB. Indirect economic effects of long-term breast cancer survival. Cancer Pract 2002;10(5):248–55.
16. Sasser AC, Rousculp MD, Birnbaum HG, et al. Economic burden of osteoporosis, breast cancer, and cardiovascular disease among postmenopausal women in an employed population. Womens Health Issues 2005;15(3):97–108.
17. Given BA, Given CW, Stommel M. Family and out-of-pocket costs for women with breast cancer. Cancer Pract 1994;2(3):187–93.

18. Arozullah AM, Calhoun EA, Wolf M, et al. The financial burden of cancer: estimates from a study of insured women with breast cancer. J Support Oncol 2004;2(3):271–8.

19. Bradley CJ, Yabroff KR, Dahman B, et al. Productivity costs of cancer mortality in the United States: 2000-2020. J Natl Cancer Inst 2008;100(24):1763–70.

20. Development of EC-oa. OECD Health Data 2012. OECD Health Statistics. 2012. Available at: http://www.oecd.org/els/health-systems/oecdhealthdata2012-frequentlyrequesteddata.htm. Accessed May 30, 2013. Downloaded from http://www.oecd.org/els/health-systems/oecdhealthdata2012-frequentlyrequesteddata.htm.

21. Cylus J, Anderson GF. Multinational comparisons of health systems data, 2006, The Commonwealth Fund, May 2007. Available at: http://www.commonwealthfund.org/Publications/Chartbooks/2007/May/Multinational-Comparisons-of-Health-Systems-Data–2006.aspx.

22. Squires D. Multinational comparisons of health systems data, 2011. The Commonwealth Fund, December 2011. Available at: http://www.commonwealthfund.org/Publications/Chartbooks/2011/Dec/Multinational-Comparisons-of-Health-Data-2011.asp.

23. Howlader N, Noone AM, Krapcho M, et al, editors. SEER cancer statistics review, 1975-2009 (vintage 2009 populations). Bethesda (MD): National Cancer Institute; 2012. Available at: http://seer.cancer.gov/csr/1975_2009_pops09/. based on November 2011 SEER data submission, posted to the SEER web site, 2012.

24. Jemal A, Siegel R, Xu J, et al. Cancer statistics, 2010. CA Cancer J Clin 2010; 60(5):277–300.

25. Berry DA, Cronin KA, Plevritis SK, et al. Effect of screening and adjuvant therapy on mortality from breast cancer [see comment]. N Engl J Med 2005;353(17): 1784–92.

26. Henderson IC, Berry DA, Demetri GD, et al. Improved outcomes from adding sequential Paclitaxel but not from escalating Doxorubicin dose in an adjuvant chemotherapy regimen for patients with node-positive primary breast cancer. J Clin Oncol 2003;21(6):976–83.

27. Mamounas EP, Bryant J, Lembersky B, et al. Paclitaxel after doxorubicin plus cyclophosphamide as adjuvant chemotherapy for node-positive breast cancer: results from NSABP B-28. J Clin Oncol 2005;23(16):3686–96.

28. Roche H, Fumoleau P, Spielmann M, et al. Sequential adjuvant epirubicin-based and docetaxel chemotherapy for node-positive breast cancer patients: the FNCLCC PACS 01 Trial. J Clin Oncol 2006;24(36):5664–71.

29. Citron ML, Berry DA, Cirrincione C, et al. Randomized trial of dose-dense versus conventionally scheduled and sequential versus concurrent combination chemotherapy as postoperative adjuvant treatment of node-positive primary breast cancer: first report of Intergroup Trial C9741/Cancer and Leukemia Group B Trial 9741. J Clin Oncol 2003;21(8):1431–9.

30. Romond EH, Perez EA, Bryant J, et al. Trastuzumab plus adjuvant chemotherapy for operable HER2-positive breast cancer. N Engl J Med 2005; 353(16):1673–84.

31. Piccart-Gebhart MJ, Procter M, Leyland-Jones B, et al. Trastuzumab after adjuvant chemotherapy in HER2-positive breast cancer. N Engl J Med 2005;353(16): 1659–72.

32. Dowsett M, Cuzick J, Ingle J, et al. Meta-analysis of breast cancer outcomes in adjuvant trials of aromatase inhibitors versus tamoxifen. J Clin Oncol 2010;28(3): 509–18.

33. Mariotto A, Feuer EJ, Harlan LC, et al. Trends in use of adjuvant multi-agent chemotherapy and tamoxifen for breast cancer in the United States: 1975-1999 [see comment]. J Natl Cancer Inst 2002;94(21):1626–34.
34. Winn RJ, Botnick W, Dozier N. The NCCN guidelines development program. Oncology (Williston Park) 1996;10(Suppl 11):23–8.
35. Senn HJ, Thurlimann B, Goldhirsch A, et al. Comments on the St. Gallen Consensus 2003 on the primary therapy of early breast cancer. Breast 2003; 12(6):569–82.
36. Adjuvant therapy for breast cancer. NIH Consens Statement 2000;17(4):1–35. Available at: http://consensus.nih.gov/2000/2000AdjuvantTherapyBreast Cancer114html.htm.
37. Malin JL, Schuster MA, Kahn KA, et al. Quality of breast cancer care: what do we know? J Clin Oncol 2002;20(21):4381–93.
38. Du XL, Key CR, Osborne C, et al. Discrepancy between consensus recommendations and actual community use of adjuvant chemotherapy in women with breast cancer [see comment]. Ann Intern Med 2003;138(2):90–7 [Erratum appears in Ann Intern Med 2003;139(10):873]. [Summary for patients in Ann Intern Med 2003;138(2):I16; PMID: 12529113].
39. Harlan LC, Abrams J, Warren JL, et al. Adjuvant therapy for breast cancer: practice patterns of community physicians. J Clin Oncol 2002;20(7):1809–17.
40. Palazzi M, De Tomasi D, D'Affronto C, et al. Are international guidelines for the prescription of adjuvant treatment for early breast cancer followed in clinical practice? Results of a population-based study on 1547 patients. Tumori 2002; 88(6):503–6.
41. Hassett MJ, Hughes ME, Niland JC, et al. Selecting high priority quality measures for breast cancer quality improvement. Med Care 2008;46(8): 762–70.
42. Hewitt ME, Simone JV, National Cancer Policy Board (U.S.). Ensuring quality cancer care [paper, electronic resource]. Washington, DC: National Academy Press; 1999.
43. Huerta TR, Ford EW, Peterson LT, et al. Testing the hospital value proposition: an empirical analysis of efficiency and quality. Health Care Manage Rev 2008; 33(4):341–9.
44. Anderson GF, Chalkidou K. Spending on medical care: more is better? JAMA 2008;299(20):2444–5.
45. Fisher E, Skinner J. Comment on Silber et al.: aggressive treatment styles and surgical outcomes. Health Serv Res 2010;45(6 Pt 2):1893–902 [discussion: 1908–11].
46. Hussey PS, Wertheimer S, Mehrotra A. The association between health care quality and cost. Ann Intern Med 2013;158(1):27–34.
47. Brooks GA, Li L, Sharma DB, et al. Regional variation in spending and survival for older adults with advanced cancer. J Natl Cancer Inst 2013;105(9): 634–42.
48. Hassett MJ, Neville BA, Weeks JC. The relationship between cost, quality and outcomes among women with breast cancer in SEER/Medicare. J Clin Oncol 2011;29. abstract 6001.
49. Landrum MB, Meara ER, Chandra A, et al. Is spending more always wasteful? The appropriateness of care and outcomes among colorectal cancer patients. Health Aff (Millwood) 2008;27(1):159–68.
50. Network TNCC. NCCN drugs & biologics compendium. Fort Washington, PA: The National Comprehensive Cancer Network, Inc; 2013.

51. Bach PB. Limits on Medicare's ability to control rising spending on cancer drugs. N Engl J Med 2009;360(6):626–33.

52. Experts in chronic myeloid leukemia. The price of drugs for chronic myeloid leukemia (CML); a reflection of the unsustainable prices of cancer drugs: from the perspective of a large group of CML experts. Blood 2013. [Epub ahead of print].

53. Schrag D. The price tag on progress–chemotherapy for colorectal cancer [see comment]. N Engl J Med 2004;351(4):317–9.

54. Meropol NJ, Schulman KA. Cost of cancer care: issues and implications. J Clin Oncol 2007;25(2):180–6.

55. Fojo T, Grady C. How much is life worth: cetuximab, non-small cell lung cancer, and the $440 billion question. J Natl Cancer Inst 2009;101(15):1044–8.

56. Bach PB, Saltz L, Wittes RE, editors. Cancer care, cost matters. New York: The New York Times; 2012. Op-Ed.

57. Goldberg P. MSKCC bars zaltrap from formulary, triggering debate over drug pricing. Cancer Lett 2012;38(41):1–2.

58. Hinkel J. Clinicians report on changes in the use of ESA's, outpatient blood transfusions, and supplemental iron as interventions for anemia. eBulletin. 2009. Available at: http://www.nccn.org/about/news/ebulletin/2009-10-12/esa.asp. Accessed April 10, 2013.

59. Jacobson M, Earle CC, Price M, et al. How Medicare's payment cuts for cancer chemotherapy drugs changed patterns of treatment. Health Aff (Millwood) 2010;29(7):1391–9.

60. Jha AK, Orav EJ, Epstein AM. Public reporting of discharge planning and rates of readmissions. N Engl J Med 2009;361(27):2637–45.

61. Reed SD, Li Y, Anstrom KJ, et al. Cost effectiveness of ixabepilone plus capecitabine for metastatic breast cancer progressing after anthracycline and taxane treatment. J Clin Oncol 2009;27(13):2185–91.

62. Fornier M. Ixabepilone plus capecitabine for breast cancer patients with an early metastatic relapse after adjuvant chemotherapy: two clinical trials. Clin Breast Cancer 2010;10(5):352–8.

63. Lopes G, Gluck S, Avancha K, et al. A cost effectiveness study of eribulin versus standard single-agent cytotoxic chemotherapy for women with previously treated metastatic breast cancer. Breast Cancer Res Treat 2013;137(1):187–93.

64. Cortes J, O'Shaughnessy J, Loesch D, et al. Eribulin monotherapy versus treatment of physician's choice in patients with metastatic breast cancer (EMBRACE): a phase 3 open-label randomised study. Lancet 2011;377(9769):914–23.

65. Russell LB, Gold MR, Siegel JE, et al. The role of cost-effectiveness analysis in health and medicine. Panel on Cost-Effectiveness in Health and Medicine. JAMA 1996;276(14):1172–7.

66. Smith TJ, Hillner BE. The efficacy and cost-effectiveness of adjuvant therapy of early breast cancer in premenopausal women. J Clin Oncol 1993;11(4):771–6.

67. Refaat T, Choi M, Gaber G, et al. Markov model and cost-effectiveness analysis of bevacizumab in HER2-negative metastatic breast cancer. Am J Clin Oncol 2013. [Epub ahead of print].

68. Snedecor SJ, Carter JA, Kaura S, et al. Cost-effectiveness of denosumab versus zoledronic acid in the management of skeletal metastases secondary to breast cancer. Clin Ther 2012;34(6):1334–49.

69. Zendejas B, Moriarty JP, O'Byrne J, et al. Cost-effectiveness of contralateral prophylactic mastectomy versus routine surveillance in patients with unilateral breast cancer. J Clin Oncol 2011;29(22):2993–3000.

70. Ito K, Blinder VS, Elkin EB. Cost effectiveness of fracture prevention in postmenopausal women who receive aromatase inhibitors for early breast cancer. J Clin Oncol 2012;30(13):1468–75.
71. Elkin EB, Weinstein MC, Winer EP, et al. HER-2 testing and trastuzumab therapy for metastatic breast cancer: a cost-effectiveness analysis. J Clin Oncol 2004; 22(5):854–63.
72. Hirth RA, Chernew ME, Miller E, et al. Willingness to pay for a quality-adjusted life year: in search of a standard. Med Decis Making 2000;20(3):332–42.
73. Bobinac A, van Exel NJ, Rutten FF, et al. Valuing QALY gains by applying a societal perspective. Health Econ 2012. [Epub ahead of print].
74. Ubol PA, Hirth RA, Chernew ME, et al. What is the price of life and why doesn't It increase at the rate of inflation? Arch Intern Med 2003;163:1637–41.
75. Hillner BE, Smith TJ. Efficacy does not necessarily translate to cost effectiveness: a case study in the challenges associated with 21st-century cancer drug pricing. J Clin Oncol 2009;27(13):2111–3.
76. Smith TJ, Hillner BE. Bending the cost curve in cancer care. N Engl J Med 2011; 364(21):2060–5.
77. Weinstein MC, Skinner JA. Comparative effectiveness and health care spending–implications for reform. N Engl J Med 2010;362(5):460–5.
78. Schnipper LE, Meropol NJ, Brock DW. Value and cancer care: toward an equitable future. Clin Cancer Res 2010;16(24):6004–8.
79. Mason A, Drummond M, Ramsey S, et al. Comparison of anticancer drug coverage decisions in the United States and United Kingdom: does the evidence support the rhetoric? J Clin Oncol 2010;28(20):3234–8.
80. Ramsey S, Fedorenko CR, Snell K, et al. Cancer diagnosis as a risk factor for personal bankruptcy. J Clin Oncol 2011;29(Suppl). abstract 6007.
81. Neumann PJ, Palmer JA, Nadler E, et al. Cancer therapy costs influence treatment: a national survey of oncologists. Health Aff (Millwood) 2010;29(1): 196–202.
82. Howe R, Hassett MJ, Wheelock A, et al. Cost of cancer care: the impact of disclosure on willingness to pay and treatment preferences. J Clin Oncol 2012;30(suppl 34; abstr 15). Paper presented at: ASCO Quality Care Symposium. San Diego, 2012.
83. Foundation A. Choosing Wisely. 2012. Available at: http://choosingwisely.org/. Accessed December 11, 2012.
84. Schnipper LE, Smith TJ, Raghavan D, et al. American Society of Clinical Oncology identifies five key opportunities to improve care and reduce costs: the top five list for oncology. J Clin Oncol 2012;30(14):1715–24.

How to Develop and Deliver Pathway-Based Care

Adam Brufsky, MD, PhD[a],*, Kathleen Lokay, BBA[b]

KEYWORDS

- Pathway-based care • Via Pathways • Cancer • UPMC

KEY POINTS

- Experience at UPMC CancerCenter and other institutions suggest that adoption of clinical pathways programs can improve quality, reduce unwarranted variability and reduce the growth rate of cancer costs.
- A robust pathways program can serve as a vehicle for demonstrating the value of an institution's cancer care to key stakeholders such as payers, referring physicians and patients.
- An effective program must engage the practicing oncologists in the development and implementation of the clinical pathways.

OVERVIEW

Cancer care in the United States faces several key challenges today that are causing payers, referring physicians, and patients alike to question the value of the care, both in terms of outcomes and costs. New technologies in the form of pharmaceuticals and biologics, prognostic tests, and new radiation therapy tools and techniques offer the promise of improved outcomes but their cost-effectiveness is often unclear. Oncologists themselves are caught in the middle because they are prescribers of such technologies and often the entity billing for such services but with limited ability to impact the pricing models for these services. Finally, as the complexity of oncology care continues to increase because of the advances in the understanding of the pathogenesis of the many subtypes of cancer, the community-based oncologist who cares for patients with all cancer subtypes is confronted with maintaining an up-to-date knowledge base that is expanding rapidly. Although no single solution exists for solving these issues in cancer today, the experience at the University of Pittsburgh Medical Center (UPMC) has demonstrated that a clinical pathways program imbedded in a point-of-care, patient-specific, Web-based decision support tool can reduce unwarranted variability, drive adherence to evidence-based medicine, and, in the process, reduce the growth rate in the total cost of cancer care. By prioritizing the right care for the right

[a] University of Pittsburgh, Magee-Women's Hospital, 300 Halket Street, Suite 4628, Pittsburgh, PA 15213, USA; [b] D3 Oncology Solutions, an affiliate of UPMC, 5750 Centre Avenue, Suite 500, Pittsburgh, PA 15206, USA
* Corresponding author.
E-mail address: brufskyam@upmc.edu

Hematol Oncol Clin N Am 27 (2013) 843–850
http://dx.doi.org/10.1016/j.hoc.2013.05.010
0889-8588/13/$ – see front matter © 2013 Elsevier Inc. All rights reserved.

patient presentation and reducing the use of therapies without demonstrable incremental value, oncologists using a clinical pathways program can provide a better solution to the rising costs of cancer than more blunt approaches such as rate reductions or prior authorization programs. Recent articles in the ASCO Post[1] and JNCCN[2] point, respectively, to the growing acceptance and adoption of clinical pathways as a tool for managing the costs of cancer care. These articles also highlight the challenges including the need for transparency and diligence to ensure quality is not inadvertently compromised for the sake of cost reductions. Numerous other articles and surveys published over the last few years similarly cite the pathways trend in oncology and its promise for improving the value of cancer care.[3–5]

HISTORICAL AND CURRENT FACTORS DRIVING UPMC TO DEVELOP AND USE CLINICAL PATHWAYS

By 2004, UPMC CancerCenter (UPMC-CC) had expanded to approximately 40 sites of service in a 100-mile radius in Western Pennsylvania. Concerns over the consistency and quality of care across such a diverse network were validated through the results of internal surveys (internal UPMC unpublished data, 2004) that demonstrated wide variability in approaches to cancer care. Pressures and concerns from the large payers in the region were also driving an imperative to collaborate around a solution to containing the rising costs. Additionally, with the University of Pittsburgh Cancer Institute as its National Cancer Institute–designated cancer center, UPMC-CC needed tools for increasing awareness of, and accrual to, clinical trials. The solution for all of these needs was the development and implementation of the Via Pathways to improve quality, ensure consistency of care, reduce hospital admissions, and reduce the total cost of care. The program has served UPMC-CC well for more than 8 years to date and is now a key foundation for UPMC's overall accountable care strategy.

DIFFERENCES BETWEEN VIA PATHWAYS AND GUIDELINES

Although excellent sources of oncology guidelines exist today, adherence to these guidelines is more difficult to assess, especially in community-based oncology practice, where more than 80% of cancer care is delivered. A recent analysis by IntrinsiQ of their dataset of more than 17 000 patients per month suggests that, for non–small cell lung cancer, adherence to guidelines is 100% for first-line therapy but only 60% for second- and third-line therapy (personal e-mail correspondence with IntrinsiQ [Ed Kissell], September 2009). Even within guidelines, case studies routinely collected through physician surveys by reputable third parties suggest that a significant amount of unexplained variability exists, in large part because of the inclusive nature of multiple options as standards of care. Case study surveys conducted in 2005 within the UPMC-CC revealed a significant amount of variability within guidelines that could not be easily explained. No one will dispute that cancer is a very complex disease, and the nature of decision making depends highly on physician judgment for each unique patient. However, experiences in other fields of business suggest that oncology care will benefit from a certain level of standardization for most clinical presentations (eg, pathways).

DEVELOPMENT AND MAINTENANCE OF THE VIA PATHWAYS

Starting in 2005, UPMC-CC developed and maintained algorithms (Via Pathways) for oncology clinical decision making that UPMC-CC physicians use to inform their decision making for any given state and stage of cancer. This development and maintenance has been time intensive and has involved the mutual cooperation of most of the academic and clinical experts at UPMC-CC as well as numerous physicians from other academic- and community-based practices.

A physician committee exists for each major disease category (eg, colorectal; see full list later) and is led by 2 chairpersons: an academically based oncologist specializing in that disease and a community-based oncologist with a background and patient concentration in that disease. The committees convene quarterly to review new clinical literature, pathway results, and the appropriateness of the granularity of the algorithms (eg, defining the states and stages of disease and unique patient scenarios at which decisions should be made). Through their collaborative work, a single best treatment of most of the clinical scenarios in oncology care is defined. These best treatments are based on reviewing the literature in a consistent decision hierarchy. First, the committees look for the most effective treatment based on the existing literature. In cases when there is a single best (most effective) treatment, that becomes the Via Pathway for that case. However, if there is more than one treatment with comparable efficacy, then the committee looks for the least toxic therapy with the goal of maximizing patient quality of life and outcomes and minimizing unnecessary costs of toxicity management, such as hospitalizations. Finally, if there is more than one treatment with comparable efficacy and toxicity, the committees look for the least costly alternative to reduce unnecessary health care expenditures without compromising clinical benefits.

In addition to a single best therapy as the primary pathway, the committees will include options for common scenarios, such as neuropathy, poor performance status, drug shortages, and so forth. However, such options are only presented and counted as *on pathway* when the physician notes the specific scenarios. For those less frequently occurring patient scenarios not addressed by the pathway, it is anticipated and expected that physicians will choose a treatment *off pathway*. There is no penalty for such decisions; in fact, adherence rates approaching 100% would be concerning. The expectation of Via Pathways' disease committees is adherence rates in the 70% to 80% range overall.

The following table delineates the current diseases and specialties covered by the Via Pathways, with each having a separate physician disease committee.

Via Oncology Pathways Disease Coverage

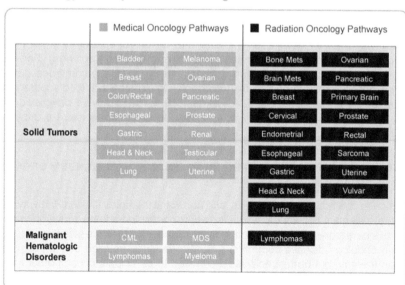

	Medical Oncology Pathways		Radiation Oncology Pathways	
Solid Tumors	Bladder	Melanoma	Bone Mets	Ovarian
	Breast	Ovarian	Brain Mets	Pancreatic
	Colon/Rectal	Pancreatic	Breast	Primary Brain
	Esophageal	Prostate	Cervical	Prostate
	Gastric	Renal	Endometrial	Rectal
	Head & Neck	Testicular	Esophageal	Sarcoma
	Lung	Uterine	Gastric	Uterine
			Head & Neck	Vulvar
			Lung	
Malignant Hematologic Disorders	CML	MDS	Lymphomas	
	Lymphomas	Myeloma		

A key part of the continuous quality improvement of the Via Pathways is the detailed reporting that is provided to the disease committees. These reports provide information for every branch of the disease pathway, including the on-pathway rate, which therapies were selected off pathway, and the reasons for choosing off-pathway alternatives. This information provides insight into areas where the Via Pathways may need further analysis or additional presentations and options added.

KEY CHALLENGES FOR THE VIA PATHWAYS DISEASE COMMITTEES

Among the challenges that face each disease committee are differences in established practice patterns in various practices and regions of the country. With most patient presentations lacking head-to-head comparisons, the committees must evaluate multiple studies with various patient populations and end points. Although levels of evidence clearly impact the decision process, the disease committees must also have the flexibility to give more weight to phase II studies with improvements in efficacy or toxicities than older phase III studies with poorer results. Additionally, the disease committees struggle with decisions over very expensive therapies whereby very little improvement in outcomes has been shown. Finally, when there is little or no data but physicians still need to make decisions (eg, surveillance), the committees think that a well-documented consensus-based recommendation is still preferred in an effort to drive standardization of care.

IMBEDDING DATA-DRIVEN PERSONALIZED MEDICINE WITHIN THE VIA PATHWAYS

As part of the quarterly disease committee process for the Via Pathways, the committees review not only data regarding alternative treatments but also biomarkers and other prognostic testing to encourage use of personalized medicine where the data are appropriate. The same level of rigor is applied to all, with the additional criteria for inclusion on biomarkers and prognostic tests of whether the results actually drive care decisions. If the data are robust and show a positive impact on care decisions, the pathways are updated to include these tests as recommendations in the pathways (examples include anaplastic lymphoma kinase translocation positive, which triggers recommendation of crizotinib; epidermal growth factor receptor mutation triggers recommendation of erlotinib; and so forth). For those tests without adequate data or firm clinical relevance, the committees develop literature-based explanations to be included in the pathways to discourage the ordering of these high-cost tests. As a result, the Via Pathways drive evidence-based personalized medicine only when it has been shown to make a difference in patient care.

EXPANDING PATHWAYS BEYOND DRUG TREATMENT TO THE CONTINUUM OF CANCER CARE

In addition to chemotherapy, biologics, and hormonal therapies, the Via Pathways also incorporate elements of workup (including appropriate biomarkers), radiation therapy, supportive care, surveillance recommendations, and advance care planning. Separate radiation oncology disease committees exist to develop detailed content for use in radiation therapy, but both specialties are invited to participate in each other's committees to ensure that the multidisciplinary recommendations are in concordance with the medical and radiation oncology pathways.

PHYSICIAN ENGAGEMENT STRATEGIES

Several strategies have been successful in engaging oncologists both at UPMC and other markets in the adoption of and adherence to the Via Pathways. Key to their support is an understanding of the realities of the rising costs of cancer care and the likely changes that will be imposed by payers if no alternative solutions are proposed. Beyond this compelling reason, other factors that drive physician acceptance include (1) creating an open and transparent disease committee process that allows participation by all physicians, (2) allowing patients' unique scenarios to be addressed in the pathways, (3) supporting accrual to clinical trials, and (4) emphasizing that treating off pathway is not a negative outcome but an expected one because of the nature of the unique patient scenarios encountered daily.

DECISION SUPPORT TOOLS ARE CRITICAL FOR THE USE AND MEASUREMENT OF CLINICAL PATHWAYS

The development and maintenance of the clinical content of the Via Pathways is certainly the most critical component of reducing unwarranted variability and adhering to evidence-based medicine. However, without tools to deliver such content to the oncologists and measure their adherence to the pathways, the clinical content alone is no more valuable than other online resources or reference textbooks. Within UPMC, the need for such a tool became evident quickly after the development of the clinical pathways and implementation of a cumbersome paper-based process. Significant investment was made by UPMC into the development of a Web-based software application for the delivery of the Via Pathways via a decision support tool to the physicians. The delivery format is patient specific and provided on a real-time basis. The Via Pathways are navigated through a question-and-answer–type format whereby the critical questions that drive that disease-specific pathway are presented and the physician is navigated to the appropriate branch of the decision tree based on his or her response. Finally, at the end of each node of the decision tree, local clinical trial options are presented, followed by the pathway treatment option, including the full details of the order (drugs, doses, schedule, other medications, and so forth). An easy-to-use process is also available for selecting an off-pathway treatment. Physicians are never prevented from going off pathway but, rather, asked to describe the reason for going off pathway (from a predefined list).

MAKING ACCRUAL TO CLINICAL TRIALS A PRIORITY WITHIN PATHWAYS

The Via Pathways also support UPMC-CC's mission of clinical research excellence by presenting clinical trials at the appropriate patient presentation for consideration by the treating physician. The UPMC-CC physician lead for each trial designates the placement of the trial within the existing algorithms for that disease, and the Via Pathways staff uses a proprietary content authoring tool to place that trial within the Via Pathways portal. UPMC-CC staff then use functionality within the software to denote a trial as open or closed to accrual on a specific date, which triggers when trials appear in the Via Pathways. These clinical trials appear in the pathways portal at the appropriate branch when navigating for a specific patient and are placed first before any Via Pathways' standard-of-care options. Selection of the clinical trial sends an internal e-mail message to the designated research coordinator for that disease, indicating the physician's desire to have the patient screened for the trial. If the patient does accrue, the selection of the trial is counted as *on pathway*. If the patient does not accrue to the trial, the physician must select a reason for nonaccrual from a list of structured text options. This information is reported back to the research group on a periodic basis. Additionally, the Via Pathways are also able to provide critical reports to the research leaders regarding patient totals for prior periods for the various states/stages of disease for new trial evaluation.

Table 1
Metastatic, Her2Neu negative/unknown

	Treatment	Selected (%)
First Line (n = 35)	*Paclitaxel 80 mg/m² D1, D8, D15 every 28 d (n = 13)*	37
	For patients with prior taxane or oral therapy desired *Capecitabine 2000 mg/m² daily in 2 divided doses 14 d on 7 d off every 21 d (n = 10)*	29
	For patients with prior hypersensitivity or steroid contraindicated *Paclitaxel (protein bound) 100 mg/m² D1, D8, D15 every 28 d (n = 5)*	14
	For patients with prior hypersensitivity or steroid contraindicated when weekly therapy is not possible *Paclitaxel (protein bound) 260 mg/m² every 21 d (n = 1)*	3
	Clinical trial (n = 2)	6
	Other: off pathway (n = 4)	11
Second Line (n = 26)	No prior taxane *Paclitaxel 80 mg/m² D1, D8, D15 every 28 d (n = 2)*	8
	If prior taxane OR oral therapy desired *Capecitabine 2000 mg/m² daily in 2 divided doses 14 d on 7 d off every 21 d (n = 9)*	35
	If not a candidate for capecitabine *Doxorubicin 20 mg/m² weekly (n = 2)*	8
	If prior anthracycline *Vinorelbine 25 mg/m² D1, D8, D15 every 28 d (n = 2)*	8
	Clinical trial (n = 1)	4
	Other: off pathway (n = 10)	38
Third Line (n = 18)	If no prior anthracycline *Doxorubicin 20 mg/m² weekly (n = 6)*	33
	If prior anthracycline *Eribulin mesylate every 21 d (n = 5)*	28
	Other: off pathway (n = 7)	39
Fourth Line and Beyond (n = 22)	*Eribulin mesylate every 21 d (n = 9)*	41
	Gemcitabine 1000 mg/m² D1, D8, D15 every 28 d (n = 1)	5
	Liposomal doxorubicin 50 mg/m² every 28 d (n = 3)	14
	Vinorelbine 25 mg/m² D1, D8, D15 every 28 d (n = 2)	9
	Clinical trial (n = 1)	5
	Other: off pathway (n = 6)	27

Abbreviation: D, day.
n = 101; on-pathway rate: 73.3%.

RESULTS OF VIA PATHWAYS USE

Currently at UPMC, approximately 90 medical and gynecologic oncologists and 30 radiation oncologists use the Via Pathways in their daily patient care. These oncologists practice in 40 sites of service, including a flagship academic center in the heart of Pittsburgh and community-based sites over a 100-mile radius throughout Western Pennsylvania. For the 12 months ending December 31, 2012, the UPMC medical oncologists confirmed a pathways status for 97% (unpublished internal UPMC and Via Pathways data, 2013) of their patient visits (186 000 visits) and achieved an on-pathway rate of 78% (unpublished internal UPMC and Via Pathways data) for their treatment decisions (13 800 treatment decisions). The original premise of Via Pathways was to find the minimum number of therapies to meet the needs of most of the patient scenarios. This result seems to reflect that the goals of reducing unwarranted variability, adhering to evidence-based medicine, and ensuring that each patient's care is personalized, have been achieved. Other practices using the Via Pathways have generated comparable results.

BREAST CANCER TREATMENT PATTERNS AT UPMC-CC

An analysis of the patterns of care for breast cancer within UPMC-CC for the most recent quarter (ending March 31, 2013) was performed to describe utilization patterns and concordance with the Via Pathways. The analysis included new chemotherapy treatment decisions for all lines of metastatic breast cancer for patients seen and documented by the UPMC-CC oncologists in the Via Pathways portal.

Table 2
Metastatic, Her2Neu positive

	Treatment	Selected (%)
First Line (n = 15)	Docetaxel + trastuzumab + pertuzumab q21 d until progression or toxicity (n = 12)	80
	Other: off pathway (n = 3)	20
Second Line (n = 5)	Capecitabine daily in 2 divided doses 14 d on 7 d off every 21 d with concurrent lapatinib daily (n = 5)	100
Third Line (n = 5)	If prior taxane Vinorelbine D1, D8, D15 every 28 d with concurrent trastuzumab q week (n = 1)	20
	If prior taxane AND prior vinorelbine tartrate (Navelbine) Gemcitabine D1, D8 every 21 d with concurrent trastuzumab q week (n = 1)	20
	Other: off pathway (n = 3)	60
Fourth Line and Beyond (n = 9)	Capecitabine daily in 2 divided doses 14 d on 7 d off every 21 d with concurrent trastuzumab q week (n = 1)	11
	Lapatinib 1000 mg daily + trastuzumab 2 mg/kg weekly (n = 1)	11
	Other: off pathway (n = 7)	78

n = 34; on-pathway rate, 61.8%.

For this time period and this population of decisions, the on-pathway rate (treatment decisions per the Via Pathways recommendation divided by all treatment decisions) was 70% (N = 135). **Tables 1** and **2** describe the frequency and description of treatment decisions according to the Via Pathways as well as accrual to clinical trials. All off-pathways decisions are aggregated and described as *other*. These data are reported as is based on physician answers to questions within the Via Pathways portal (decision support software application) and have not been validated against original medical records.

SUMMARY

The results from the UPMC experience with Via Pathways as well as those reported by other pathways programs[6] suggest that these are effective models for improving quality, reducing unwarranted variability in care, and reducing the rate of growth in the cost of cancer care. A robust pathways program that reduces unwarranted variability can serve as the vehicle to improve the value of cancer care to patients, payers, and providers through increasing quality and decreasing costs. Finally, oncologists must take an active role in defining and implementing cost-effective care for patients, payers, and referring physicians or suffer the alternatives that potentially compromise quality, access to care, and practice viability. If appropriately implemented, clinical pathways are one possible solution to improving the quality and cost-effectiveness of cancer care that also serves to preserve physician decision making; ensure access to evidence-based personalized medicine; and eliminate non–value-added administrative hurdles, such as prior authorizations.

REFERENCE

1. McGiveney WT. The future of clinical guidelines in Oncology. ASCO Post 2013; 4(6):78.
2. DeMartino JK, Larsen JK. Equity in cancer care: pathways, protocols and guidelines. J Natl Compr Canc Netw 2012;10:S1–9.
3. Butcher L. How oncologists are bending the cancer cost curve. Oncology Times 2012;35(1):5–6.
4. Phillips C. Clinical pathways in cancer care catching on. NCI Cancer Bulletin 2012;9(17).
5. Decision Resources. Impact of Payer Imposed Strategies on Market Access in Oncology: Clinical Pathways, Accountable Care Organization Contracting, Specialty Pharmacy, and the Evolution of the Buy and Bill Model. Press Release dated December 10, 2012.
6. Neubauer MA, Hoverman JR, Kolodziej M, et al. Cost effectiveness of evidence-based treatment guidelines for the treatment of non-small-cell lung cancer in the community setting. J Oncol Pract 2010;6(1):12–8.

Ibrutinib (PCI-32765) in Chronic Lymphocytic Leukemia

Nitin Jain, MD, Susan O'Brien, MD*

KEYWORDS

- B-cell receptor inhibitor • Bruton tyrosine kinase inhibitor • Ibrutinib • PCI-32765
- Chronic lymphocytic leukemia

KEY POINTS

- B-cell receptor (BCR) signaling plays a crucial role in pathogenesis of chronic lymphocytic leukemia (CLL).
- Many kinases in the BCR signaling pathway are being explored as therapeutic targets such as Src family kinases, spleen tyrosine kinase, phosphoinositide 3 kinase, and Bruton tyrosine kinase (BTK).
- Ibrutinib (PCI-32765) is a selective, irreversible, and oral inhibitor of BTK.
- Preclinical data suggest that ibrutinib affects both CLL cell survival/proliferation as well as CLL cell migration/homing.
- Preliminary clinical data in patients with CLL is encouraging, with a 67% response rate in the 420-mg dose cohort in the relapsed/refractory CLL setting.
- Combination of ibrutinib with monoclonal antibodies and chemoimmunotherapy has also shown favorable early results.
- BCR inhibitors will likely become an important component of CLL therapeutics in the near future.

INTRODUCTION

Chronic lymphocytic leukemia (CLL) is the most common leukemia in adults in the Western world, with approximately 16,060 men and women expected to be diagnosed with CLL in year 2012 in the United States.[1] Most patients with CLL do not need treatment at diagnosis; however, most patients need CLL-directed therapy in their life time. Chemoimmunotherapy is the current standard of care for patients with CLL needing treatment.[2] One of the commonly used regimens is FCR (fludarabine, cyclophosphamide, rituximab). Tam and colleagues[3] reported long-term follow-up of the FCR regimen for frontline treatment of CLL with a complete remission (CR) rate of 72%

Department of Leukemia, MD Anderson Cancer Center, 1515 Holcombe Boulevard, Houston, TX 77030, USA
* Corresponding author. Department of Leukemia, MD Anderson Cancer Center, 1515 Holcombe Boulevard, Unit 428, Houston, TX 77030.
E-mail address: sobrien@mdanderson.org

Hematol Oncol Clin N Am 27 (2013) 851–860
http://dx.doi.org/10.1016/j.hoc.2013.01.006
0889-8588/13/$ – see front matter © 2013 Elsevier Inc. All rights reserved.

and median progression-free survival (PFS) of 80 months. Despite these impressive results, certain subgroups of patients treated with chemoimmunotherapy have less than optimal outcomes. These patients include older adults (>65 years old), those with poor-risk cytogenetics (del[17p], del[11q]), and patients with relapsed/refractory disease.[2–4] Many approaches have been undertaken to improve the outcome of patients with CLL, including incorporation of drugs such as lenalidomide, ofatumumab, alemtuzumab, and bendamustine.[5–11] These treatment strategies offer options after relapse after chemoimmunotherapy, but outcomes are still less than satisfactory, with approximately 4500 patients expected to die from CLL in the United States in the year 2012.[2] This situation underscores the need to develop better therapeutics for patients with CLL.

B-cell receptor (BCR) activation signaling plays a crucial role in the pathogenesis in CLL.[12–15] The BCR signaling pathway consists of immunoglobulin bound to the cell membrane, which attaches to a heterodimer consisting of CD79a and CD79b.[15–17] Binding of a ligand to the membrane immunoglobulin leads to recruitment and phosphorylation of spleen tyrosine kinase (SYK) and Src family kinases (LYN), which in turn recruit and phosphorylate many kinases and adapter proteins, including Bruton tyrosine kinase (BTK). BTK is a nonreceptor tyrosine kinase of the Tec kinase family and plays a crucial role in BCR signaling.[18,19] BTK is expressed in non–T-cell hematopoietic cell lineages.[20,21] The BTK gene is located on chromosome Xq21.33-q22, and mutations in this gene result in X-linked agammaglobulinemia, a condition characterized by marked reduction in mature B cells, severe hypogammaglobulinemia, and increased susceptibility to infections.[22] BTK activates downstream molecules such as nuclear factor κB (NF-κB) and mitogen-activated protein kinase (MAPK) kinase (MEK)/extracellular signal regulated kinase (ERK), which are involved in many cellular processes, including proliferation, survival, differentiation, apoptosis, and metabolism. Gene expression profiling has shown that BCR signaling is the most expressed signaling pathway in patients with CLL.[14] BCR signaling is enhanced in patients with poor prognostic markers such as ZAP-70 overexpression and those with unmutated immunoglobulin heavy chain gene (*IGHV*) rearrangement.[23,24] Activated BCR signaling has also been shown to be required for cell survival in the activated B-cell subtype of diffuse large B-cell lymphoma (DLBCL).[25] Thus, multiple lines of data point to the crucial role of BCR signaling in CLL and other B-cell lymphoid malignancies. Many kinases in the BCR signaling pathway are being pursued as therapeutic targets in CLL, including LYN,[26] SYK,[27–29] phosphoinositide 3 kinase (PI3K),[30–32] and BTK.[16,17]

Ibrutinib (formerly PCI-32765, Pharmacyclics, Sunnyvale, CA) (**Fig. 1**) is an oral, selective, and irreversible inhibitor of BTK and is the focus of this article. Ibrutinib was initially developed by Celera Genomics (now Quest Diagnostics, Madison, NJ) and acquired by Pharmacyclics in 2006. Ibrutinib forms a specific bond with the cysteine-481 of BTK.[33] It leads to highly potent BTK inhibition with an IC_{50} (half maximal inhibitory concentration) of 0.5 nM (**Table 1**).[34] Ibrutinib is orally administered with daily dosing and has no cytotoxic effect on T cells.[35]

PRECLINICAL STUDIES

Honigberg and colleagues[34] showed that in a B-cell lymphoma cell line (DOHH2), ibrutinib irreversibly inhibited autophosphorylation of BTK (IC_{50} 11 nM) and phosphorylation of downstream kinases such as ERK. Phosphorylation of upstream kinases such as SYK was not affected. These investigators also showed that ibrutinib blocked the transcriptional upregulation of B-cell activation genes in primary cultures of human peripheral B cells.[34] In a mouse model for lupus nephritis, ibrutinib reduced

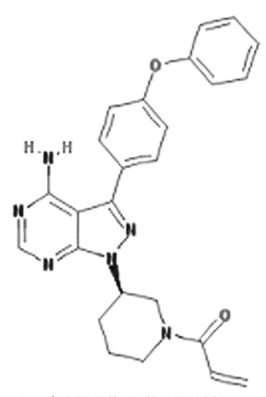

Fig. 1. Chemical structure of PCI-32765 (ibrutinib), a BTK inhibitor.

proteinuria, lowered anti-dsDNA antibody levels, and improved glomerular function, indicating the potential role for ibrutinib in autoimmune diseases.[34] Clinical activity of ibrutinib with once daily oral dosing was also seen in naturally occurring B-cell lymphoma in dogs.[34]

Herman and colleagues[35] reported that BTK mRNA expression was significantly higher in CLL (CD19+) cells compared with normal B cells. These investigators also noted that baseline BTK protein expression was highly variable in the CLL cells and protein expression did not correlate with known prognostic markers such as age, cytogenetics, *IGHV* status, and ZAP-70 expression. Treatment of CLL cells with ibrutinib induced apoptosis in a dose-dependent and time-dependent manner, which was independent of baseline cytogenetics, *IGHV* mutational status, or baseline BTK protein expression but dependent on caspase-pathway activation.[35] Ibrutinib also induced apoptosis in normal B cells, but this was significantly less than that seen in CLL cells, indicating that CLL cells are more sensitive to ibrutinib than normal B cells. Ibrutinib treatment of CLL cells inhibited downstream signaling pathways, including ERK1/2 phosphorylation, CD40L-induced AKT phosphorylation, and CD40L-induced NF-kB DNA binding.[35]

Ponader and colleagues[36] evaluated the role of the tissue microenvironment of CLL cells and its effect on treatment with ibrutinib. They reported that ibrutinib treatment significantly inhibited CLL cell migration and survival in a nurselike cell coculture assay. In this model, ibrutinib treatment significantly decreased the levels of CCL3 and CCL4 and inhibited chemotaxis toward CXCL12 and CXCL13. In an adoptive transfer TCL1 mouse model, ibrutinib treatment was reported to delay CLL disease

Table 1
Inhibition of selected kinases by ibrutinib

Kinase	IC$_{50}$ (nM)	Fold Selectivity for BTK Inhibition
BTK	0.5	—
BLK	0.5	1
BMX	0.8	1.6
CSK	2.3	4.6
FGR	2.3	4.6
EGFR	5.6	11.2
ErbB2	9.4	18.8
ITK	10.7	21.4
JAK3	16.1	32.2
RET	36.5	73
FLT3	73	146
TEC	78	156
ABL	86	172
c-SRC	171	342
LYN	200	400
PDGFRα	718	1436
JAK1	>10,000	>10,000
JAK2	>10,000	>10,000
PI3K	>10,000	>10,000
PLK1	>10,000	>10,000
SYK	>10,000	>10,000

Abbreviations: ABL, Abelson tyrosine-protein kinase; BLK, B lymphoid tyrosine kinase; BMX, Bone marrow kinase on chromosome X; BTK, Bruton Tyrosine Kinase; c-SRC, Src oncogene; CSK, c-Src tyrosine kinase; EGFR, Epidermal growth factor receptor; ErbB2, v-erb-b2 erythroblastic leukemia viral oncogene homolog 2; FGR, Gardner-Rasheed feline sarcoma viral (v-fgr) oncogene homolog; FLT3, fms-related tyrosine kinase 3; ITK, IL2-inducible T-cell kinase; JAK1, Janus kinase 1; JAK2, Janus kinase 2; JAK3, Janus kinase 3; LYN, v-yes-1 Yamaguchi sarcoma viral related oncogene homolog; PDGFRα, platelet-derived growth factor receptor alpha; PLK1, Polo-like kinase 1; PI3K, phosphatidylinositol 3-kinase; RET, Rearranged during Transfection; SYK, spleen tyrosine kinase; TEC, transient erythroblastopenia of childhood.

Data from Honigberg LA, Smith AM, Sirisawad M, et al. The Bruton tyrosine kinase inhibitor PCI-32765 blocks B-cell activation and is efficacious in models of autoimmune disease and B-cell malignancy. Proc Natl Acad Sci U S A 2010;107(29):13075–80.

progression.[36] Overall, the preclinical data suggest that ibrutinib is a selective, irreversible BTK inhibitor with effect on both CLL cell survival/proliferation and CLL cell migration/homing.[15]

CLINICAL STUDIES

Clinical studies with ibrutinib have been published only in abstract form. Ibrutinib was evaluated in a phase 1 study in patients with CLL and lymphoma (small lymphocytic lymphoma (SLL), follicular lymphoma, mantle cell lymphoma [MCL], DLBCL, marginal zone lymphoma, Waldenstrom macroglobulinemia) with a 28-day-on/7-day-off schedule in 5 dose-cohorts (1.25–12.5 mg/kg orally daily) and once daily continuous dose in 2 dose cohorts (8.3 mg/kg and 560 mg fixed dose).[37] Fifty-six patients with relapsed/refractory disease (median 3 previous regimens [range 1–10]) were enrolled.

No dose-limiting toxicity was observed. Maximum tolerated dose was not reached. Of the 50 evaluable patients, 30 (60%) patients achieved an objective response rate (ORR) (23% CR, 77% partial response [PR]). Responses were seen in all non-Hodgkin lymphoma (NHL) subtypes and irrespective of the dose levels. A unique pattern of response was noted, with a transient lymphocytosis lasting a few months. Transient lymphocytosis was also noted by Ponader and colleagues[36] in an adoptive transfer TCL1 mouse model after treatment with ibrutinib. Transient lymphocytosis is postulated to be caused by an initial compartment shift of CLL cells from lymphatic tissues into the peripheral blood.

In a phase 1B/2 study (PCYC-1102), patients with relapsed/refractory CLL and older adults (≥65 years) with untreated CLL were treated with 2 fixed doses of ibrutinib (420 mg daily and 840 mg daily).[38] Ibrutinib was given orally once daily for 28-day cycles until disease progression. Patient enrollment occurred from May 2010 to July 2011. Sixty-one patients were enrolled in the relapsed/refractory cohort (420-mg cohort, n = 27; 840-mg cohort, n = 34). The median age was 64 years (range, 40–81 years). The median number of previous therapies for the 420-mg cohort was 3 (2–10), and for the 840-mg cohort, it was 5 (1–12). High-risk molecular features were present in most of the patients (unmutated *IGHV*: 79%; del[17p]: 36%; del [11q]: 39%). The median follow-up for the 420-mg cohort was 12.6 months, and for the 840-mg cohort, it was 9.3 months. Seventy-five percent of the patients were still on the study at the time of last follow-up. Treatment was well tolerated, with most adverse events being grade 1/2 (diarrhea, fatigue, and nausea). Six patients needed dose reduction (2 in the 420-mg cohort, 4 in the 840-mg cohort). Grade 3/4 hematologic toxicity (neutropenia, anemia, thrombocytopenia), irrespective of attribution, was seen in 8%, 7%, 7% (420-mg cohort) and 21%, 12%, 9% (840-mg cohort), respectively. ORR was noted to be 67% (63% PR, 4% CR) in the 420-mg cohort and 68% (all PR) in the 840-mg cohort. An additional 22% (420-mg cohort) and 24% (840-mg cohort) of patients achieved nodal PR (>50% reduction in aggregate lymph node size) with residual lymphocytosis. Maximum change in tumor burden is shown in **Fig. 2**. Clinical responses were independent of the high-risk molecular

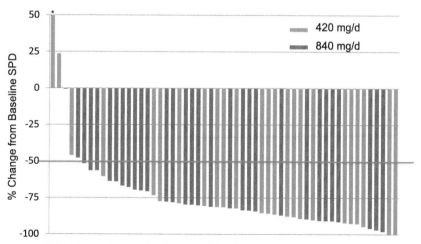

*Patient developed progressive disease, but did not have tumor measurements available
Limited to patients with measurable disease at baseline (n=55)

Fig. 2. Maximum change in tumor burden in patients with relapsed/refractory CLL treated with single-agent ibrutinib (PCYC-1102 trial).

features. Seventy-four percent of the patients with unmutated *IGHV*, 65% with del(17p), and 73% with del(11q) responded. Most clinical responses were nodal responses in the first 4 to 5 months of therapy, which then improved to PR/CR with continued treatment over the next few months. Estimated 18-month PFS was 87.7% in the 420-mg cohort.[39] A transient lymphocytosis typically peaking within the first 2 months of treatment, followed by gradual resolution over the next 6 to 8 months, was noted (**Fig. 3**).

In the update of the data presented at the European Hematology Association meeting in June 2012, O'Brien and colleagues[39] reported the outcomes of 31 treatment-naive older patients (420 mg, n = 26; 840 mg, n = 5). Enrollment in the 840-mg cohort was terminated after similar results were noted between the 420-mg and 840-mg cohort in the relapsed/refractory cohort. Median age was 71 years (range, 65–84 years), with 75% of patients being older than 70 years. Forty-three percent of patients had unmutated *IGHV* and 6% had del(17p). Most of the adverse events (AE) were mild (grade 1–2) and included diarrhea, nausea, and fatigue. Grade 3 nonhematologic AE potentially related to the drug were seen in 6 (19%) patients (diarrhea, 4 patients; hyponatremia, 2 patients; hemorrhagic enterocolitis, 1 patient). No grade 4 nonhematologic toxicity was seen. Hematologic toxicity of grade 3 or higher was seen in 4 (12%) patients and included 2 patients each with anemia and thrombocytopenia. Neutropenia was not observed. In the 420-mg cohort, only 4 of the 26 patients have discontinued therapy, and only 1 patient for disease progression. With a median follow-up of 14.4 months on the 420-mg cohort, 81% achieved a response (69% PR, 12% complete response) by the International Workshop on Chronic Lymphocytic Leukemia criteria. An additional 12% of patients achieved a nodal response. Fifty percent of patients with baseline thrombocytopenia or anemia noted sustained improvement in blood counts. The responses were independent of high-risk features. Ninety-two percent of patients with unmutated *IGHV* responded. There were 2 patients with del(17p), and both responded. The estimated 15-month median PFS for the 420-mg cohort was 96%.

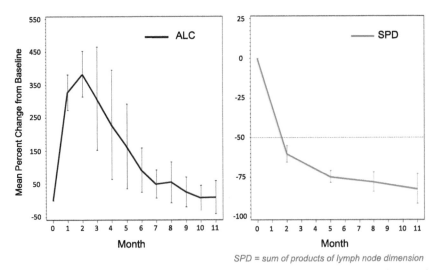

SPD = sum of products of lymph node dimension

Fig. 3. Characteristic response pattern with transient lymphocytosis typically peaking within the first 2 months of treatment, followed by gradual resolution over the next 6 to 8 months. Decrease in lymphadenopathy was consistent from the beginning. Data derived from patients with relapsed/refractory CLL treated with single -agent ibrutinib (PCYC-1102 trial).

Given the impressive single-agent activity of ibrutinib in patients with CLL, trials exploring combinations of ibrutinib with either monoclonal antibodies (rituximab or ofatumumab) or with chemotherapy (bendamustine or FCR) have been initiated. Some of these trials have been reported in abstract form. Preliminary data have been reported for ibrutinib in combination with ofatumumab (PCYC-1109-CA trial).[40] Patients with relapsed/refractory CLL following 2 or more previous therapies, including a purine-nucleoside analogue, were treated with ibrutinib 420 mg daily with addition of ofatumumab from cycle 2 onwards. Twenty-four patients with CLL/prolymphocytic leukemia (PLL) and 3 with Richter transformation were treated. The median age was 66 (range 51–85). High-risk cytogenetics were seen in most patients (10 patients with del[17p] and 9 patients with del[11q]). Most AE were grade 1 to 2. All patients with CLL/PLL and 2 of the 3 patients with Richter transformation achieved PR.

Brown and colleagues[41] reported preliminary data on the combination of ibrutinib with bendamustine/rituximab (PCYC-1108-CA) in relapsed/refractory patients with CLL. Thirty patients were enrolled, with a median age of 62 years (range 41–82 years). The median number of previous therapies was 2 (range 1–4). Twenty-three percent had deletion 17p, and 43% had deletion 11q. No added toxicity was observed with the addition of ibrutinib. With a median follow-up of 8.1 months, 23 of the 30 patients were still on study, with only 2 patients coming off protocol for disease progression. The ORR was 93% (13% CR, 80% PR), which is higher than the 59% seen with bendamustine-rituximab in historical controls. As with single-agent ibrutinib, responses were independent of high-risk genetic and molecular features.

Ibrutinib has also been evaluated in other lymphoid malignancies, including MCL, DLBCL, Waldenstrom macroglobulinemia, and multiple myeloma. In the preliminary results of a phase 2 study (PCYC-1104), Wang and colleagues[42] reported outcomes of 48 relapsed/refractory patients with MCL (29 bortezomib-naive; 19 bortezomib-exposed) who were treated with single-agent ibrutinib. Ibrutinib was administered orally at 560 mg daily until disease progression. The median age was 67 years (range, 62–72 years). Therapy was well tolerated, with most frequently reported AE being grade 1 or 2 diarrhea, fatigue, and nausea (similar to the CLL study). The ORR was 67% (16 of the 24 evaluable patients). Responses were seen in both bortezomib-naive and bortezomib-exposed cohorts.

Many ongoing/planned trials are exploring the role of ibrutinib in hematologic malignancies. Some examples include ibrutinib as a single agent in Waldenstrom macroglobulinemia and multiple myeloma, ibrutinib with rituximab in CLL, ibrutinib with bendamustine/rituximab in relapsed DLBCL/MCL, ibrutinib with R-CHOP chemotherapy in newly diagnosed DLBCL. A phase 3 randomized, open-label registration trial of ibrutinib versus ofatumumab in patients with relapsed or refractory CLL (RESONATE trial) has been initiated.[43] The primary end point of this trial is PFS, with key secondary end points being overall response rate, overall survival, and quality of life measures. Another planned phase 3 study includes a randomized study of bendamustine/rituximab plus ibrutinib versus bendamustine/rituximab plus placebo in relapsed or refractory patients with CLL/SLL.

SUMMARY

It is clear from the preclinical and preliminary clinical data (as stated earlier) that BTK inhibitors (along with other BCR signaling pathway inhibitors) are going to revolutionize the treatment of patients with CLL. Besides ibrutinib, there are other BTK inhibitors in clinical development, such as AVL-292 (Avila Therapeutics, now part of Celgene Corporation, Summit, NJ) and ONO-WG-307 (Ono Pharmaceutical, Osaka, Japan).

In the coming few years, there will be a barrage of preclinical and clinical data with these drugs. Thus far, the clinical responses with ibrutinib have been impressive, with manageable toxicities. It is likely that ibrutinib and other drugs targeting the BCR pathway will become an integral component of CLL and NHL therapy.

REFERENCES

1. Howlader N, Noone AM, Krapcho M, et al. SEER cancer statistics review, 1975-2009 (Vintage 2009 Populations). Bethesda (MD): National Cancer Institute; 2012. Available at: http://seer.cancer.gov/csr/1975_2009_pops09/. based on November 2011 SEER data submission, posted to the SEER web site. Accessed October 5, 2012.
2. Gribben JG, O'Brien S. Update on therapy of chronic lymphocytic leukemia. J Clin Oncol 2011;29(5):544–50.
3. Tam CS, O'Brien S, Wierda W, et al. Long-term results of the fludarabine, cyclophosphamide, and rituximab regimen as initial therapy of chronic lymphocytic leukemia. Blood 2008;112(4):975–80.
4. Dohner H, Stilgenbauer S, Benner A, et al. Genomic aberrations and survival in chronic lymphocytic leukemia. N Engl J Med 2000;343(26):1910–6.
5. Badoux XC, Keating MJ, Wen S, et al. Lenalidomide as initial therapy of elderly patients with chronic lymphocytic leukemia. Blood 2011;118(13):3489–98.
6. Ferrajoli A, Lee BN, Schlette EJ, et al. Lenalidomide induces complete and partial remissions in patients with relapsed and refractory chronic lymphocytic leukemia. Blood 2008;111(11):5291–7.
7. Wierda WG, Kipps TJ, Durig J, et al. Chemoimmunotherapy with O-FC in previously untreated patients with chronic lymphocytic leukemia. Blood 2011;117(24):6450–8.
8. O'Brien SM, Kantarjian HM, Thomas DA, et al. Alemtuzumab as treatment for residual disease after chemotherapy in patients with chronic lymphocytic leukemia. Cancer 2003;98(12):2657–63.
9. Elter T, Gercheva-Kyuchukova L, Pylylpenko H, et al. Fludarabine plus alemtuzumab versus fludarabine alone in patients with previously treated chronic lymphocytic leukaemia: a randomised phase 3 trial. Lancet Oncol 2011;12(13):1204–13.
10. Fischer K, Cramer P, Busch R, et al. Bendamustine combined with rituximab in patients with relapsed and/or refractory chronic lymphocytic leukemia: a multicenter phase II trial of the German Chronic Lymphocytic Leukemia Study Group. J Clin Oncol 2011;29(26):3559–66.
11. Fischer K, Cramer P, Busch R, et al. Bendamustine in combination with rituximab for previously untreated patients with chronic lymphocytic leukemia: a multicenter phase II trial of the German Chronic Lymphocytic Leukemia Study Group. J Clin Oncol 2012;30(26):3209–16.
12. Chiorazzi N, Ferrarini M. B cell chronic lymphocytic leukemia: lessons learned from studies of the B cell antigen receptor. Annu Rev Immunol 2003;21:841–94.
13. Stevenson FK, Caligaris-Cappio F. Chronic lymphocytic leukemia: revelations from the B-cell receptor. Blood 2004;103(12):4389–95.
14. Herishanu Y, Perez-Galan P, Liu D, et al. The lymph node microenvironment promotes B-cell receptor signaling, NF-kappaB activation, and tumor proliferation in chronic lymphocytic leukemia. Blood 2011;117(2):563–74.
15. Burger JA. Nurture versus nature: the microenvironment in chronic lymphocytic leukemia. Hematology Am Soc Hematol Educ Program 2011;2011:96–103.
16. Woyach JA, Johnson AJ, Byrd JC. The B-cell receptor signaling pathway as a therapeutic target in CLL. Blood 2012;120(6):1175–84.

17. Wiestner A. Emerging role of kinase targeted strategies in chronic lymphocytic leukemia. Blood 2012;120(24):4684–91.
18. Khan WN. Regulation of B lymphocyte development and activation by Bruton's tyrosine kinase. Immunol Res 2001;23(2–3):147–56.
19. Satterthwaite AB, Witte ON. The role of Bruton's tyrosine kinase in B-cell development and function: a genetic perspective. Immunol Rev 2000;175:120–7.
20. Smith CI, Baskin B, Humire-Greiff P, et al. Expression of Bruton's agammaglobulinemia tyrosine kinase gene, BTK, is selectively down-regulated in T lymphocytes and plasma cells. J Immunol 1994;152(2):557–65.
21. Genevier HC, Hinshelwood S, Gaspar HB, et al. Expression of Bruton's tyrosine kinase protein within the B cell lineage. Eur J Immunol 1994;24(12):3100–5.
22. Conley ME, Dobbs AK, Farmer DM, et al. Primary B cell immunodeficiencies: comparisons and contrasts. Annu Rev Immunol 2009;27:199–227.
23. Chen L, Widhopf G, Huynh L, et al. Expression of ZAP-70 is associated with increased B-cell receptor signaling in chronic lymphocytic leukemia. Blood 2002;100(13):4609–14.
24. Rosenwald A, Alizadeh AA, Widhopf G, et al. Relation of gene expression phenotype to immunoglobulin mutation genotype in B cell chronic lymphocytic leukemia. J Exp Med 2001;194(11):1639–47.
25. Davis RE, Ngo VN, Lenz G, et al. Chronic active B-cell-receptor signalling in diffuse large B-cell lymphoma. Nature 2010;463(7277):88–92.
26. Contri A, Brunati AM, Trentin L, et al. Chronic lymphocytic leukemia B cells contain anomalous Lyn tyrosine kinase, a putative contribution to defective apoptosis. J Clin Invest 2005;115(2):369–78.
27. Hoellenriegel J, Coffey GP, Sinha U, et al. Selective, novel spleen tyrosine kinase (Syk) inhibitors suppress chronic lymphocytic leukemia B-cell activation and migration. Leukemia 2012;26(7):1576–83.
28. Friedberg JW, Sharman J, Sweetenham J, et al. Inhibition of Syk with fostamatinib disodium has significant clinical activity in non-Hodgkin lymphoma and chronic lymphocytic leukemia. Blood 2010;115(13):2578–85.
29. Buchner M, Baer C, Prinz G, et al. Spleen tyrosine kinase inhibition prevents chemokine- and integrin-mediated stromal protective effects in chronic lymphocytic leukemia. Blood 2010;115(22):4497–506.
30. Herman SE, Gordon AL, Wagner AJ, et al. Phosphatidylinositol 3-kinase-delta inhibitor CAL-101 shows promising preclinical activity in chronic lymphocytic leukemia by antagonizing intrinsic and extrinsic cellular survival signals. Blood 2010;116(12):2078–88.
31. Hoellenriegel J, Meadows SA, Sivina M, et al. The phosphoinositide 3'-kinase delta inhibitor, CAL-101, inhibits B-cell receptor signaling and chemokine networks in chronic lymphocytic leukemia. Blood 2011;118(13):3603–12.
32. Lannutti BJ, Meadows SA, Herman SE, et al. CAL-101, a p110delta selective phosphatidylinositol-3-kinase inhibitor for the treatment of B-cell malignancies, inhibits PI3K signaling and cellular viability. Blood 2011;117(2):591–4.
33. Pan Z, Scheerens H, Li SJ, et al. Discovery of selective irreversible inhibitors for Bruton's tyrosine kinase. ChemMedChem 2007;2(1):58–61.
34. Honigberg LA, Smith AM, Sirisawad M, et al. The Bruton tyrosine kinase inhibitor PCI-32765 blocks B-cell activation and is efficacious in models of autoimmune disease and B-cell malignancy. Proc Natl Acad Sci U S A 2010;107(29):13075–80.
35. Herman SE, Gordon AL, Hertlein E, et al. Bruton tyrosine kinase represents a promising therapeutic target for treatment of chronic lymphocytic leukemia and is effectively targeted by PCI-32765. Blood 2011;117(23):6287–96.

36. Ponader S, Chen SS, Buggy JJ, et al. The Bruton tyrosine kinase inhibitor PCI-32765 thwarts chronic lymphocytic leukemia cell survival and tissue homing in vitro and in vivo. Blood 2012;119(5):1182–9.

37. Advani RH, Sharman JP, Smith SM, et al. The Btk Inhibitor PCI-32765 is highly active and well tolerated in patients with relapsed/refractory B cell malignancies: final results from a phase I study. 11th International Conference on Malignant Lymphoma Meeting Abstract. Lugano, Switzerland. June 15, 2011. p. 153a.

38. O'Brien S, Burger JA, Blum KA, et al. The Bruton's tyrosine kinase (BTK) inhibitor PCI-32765 induces durable responses in relapsed or refractory (R/R) chronic lymphocytic leukemia/small lymphocytic lymphoma (CLL/SLL): follow-up of a phase Ib/II study. American Society of Hematology Annual Meeting Abstracts. San Diego, USA. December 13, 2011. p. 983a.

39. O'Brien S, Furman R, Coutre S, et al. The Bruton's Tyrosine kinase inhibitor ibrutinib is highly active and tolerable in relapsed or refractory and treatment naive CLL patients, updated results of a phase IB/II study. European Hematology Meeting Annual Abstracts. Amsterdam, The Netherlands. June 16, 2012. p. 542a.

40. Jaglowski SM, Jones JA, Flynn JM, et al. A phase Ib/II study evaluating activity and tolerability of BTK inhibitor PCI-32765 and ofatumumab in patients with chronic lymphocytic leukemia/small lymphocytic lymphoma (CLL/SLL) and related diseases. American Society of Clinical Oncology Annual Meeting Abstracts. Chicago, USA. June 4, 2012. p. 6508a.

41. Brown J, Barrientos J, Flinn I, et al. The Bruton's tyrosine kinase (Btk) inhibitor ibrutinib combined with bendamustine and rituximab is active and tolerable in patients with relapsed/refractory CLL, interim results of a phase Ib/II study. European Hematology Meeting Annual Abstracts. Amsterdam, The Netherlands. June 16, 2012. p. 543a.

42. Wang L, Martin P, Blum KA, et al. The Bruton's tyrosine kinase inhibitor PCI-32765 is highly active as single-agent therapy in previously-treated mantle cell lymphoma (MCL): preliminary results of a phase II trial. American Society of Hematology Annual Meeting Abstracts. San Diego, USA. December 13, 2011. p. 442a.

43. Available at: http://clinicaltrials.gov/ct2/show/NCT01578707?term=ibrutinib&rank=6. Accessed August 25, 2012.

Index

Note: Page numbers of article titles are in **boldface** type.

Hematol Oncol Clin N Am 27 (2013) 861–869
http://dx.doi.org/10.1016/S0889-8588(13)00092-0
0889-8588/13/$ – see front matter © 2013 Elsevier Inc. All rights reserved.

hemonc.theclinics.com

Moving?

Make sure your subscription moves with you!

To notify us of your new address, find your **Clinics Account Number** (located on your mailing label above your name), and contact customer service at:

Email: journalscustomerservice-usa@elsevier.com

800-654-2452 (subscribers in the U.S. & Canada)
314-447-8871 (subscribers outside of the U.S. & Canada)

Fax number: 314-447-8029

Elsevier Health Sciences Division
Subscription Customer Service
3251 Riverport Lane
Maryland Heights, MO 63043

*To ensure uninterrupted delivery of your subscription, please notify us at least 4 weeks in advance of move.

Printed and bound by CPI Group (UK) Ltd, Croydon, CR0 4YY

03/10/2024

01040494-0002